INSIGHTS INTO VARIOUS ASPECTS OF ORAL HEALTH

Edited by **Jane Francis Manakil**

Insights into Various Aspects of Oral Health
http://dx.doi.org/10.5772/65997
Edited by Jane Francis Manakil

Contributors

Metin Çalışır, Ana Lourdes Zamora Perez, Zùñiga Guillermo, Belinda Gómez-Meda, Yveth Ortiz-García, Gabriela Morales-Velazquez, Blanca Lazalde-Ramos, Celia Guerrero Velazques, María Guadalupe Sánchez-Parada, Hiroyasu Endo, Terry Rees, Hideo Niwa, Kayo Kuyama, Morio Iijima, Ryuuichi Imamura, Takao Kato, Kenji Doi, Hirotsugu Yamamoto, Takanori Ito, Vikram Niranjan, Vikas Kathuria, Venkatraman J, Arpana Salve, Maen Hussni Zreaqat, Rozita Hassan, Abdulfattah Hanoun, Liliana Porojan, Florin Topala, Sorin Porojan, Jorge Gamonal, Paulo Beltrão, Ahmed A. Madfa, Elham M Senan, Kostas Spiropoulos

Published by InTech
Janeza Trdine 9, 51000 Rijeka, Croatia

Publishing Process Manager Edi Lipovic
Technical Editor SPi Global
Cover InTech Design team

First published September, 2017
Printed in Croatia
Legal deposit, Croatia: National and University Library in Zagreb

Additional hard copies can be obtained from orders@intechopen.com

Insights into Various Aspects of Oral Health, Edited by Jane Francis Manakil
p. cm.
Print ISBN 978-953-51-3531-9
Online ISBN 978-953-51-3532-6

For EU product safety concerns:
IN TECH d.o.o., Prolaz Marije Krucifikse Kozulić 3, 51000 Rijeka, Croatia,
info@intechopen.com or visit our website at intechopen.com.

Meet the editor

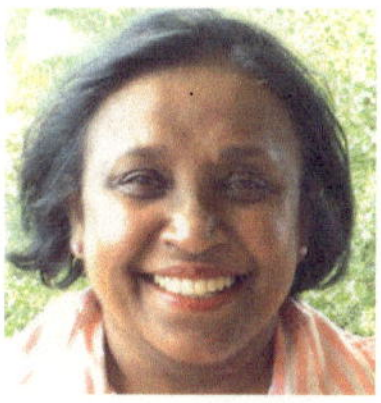

Jane Francis Manakil is an academic and a clinician in the School of Dentistry at Griffith University, Australia. She holds a PhD degree and a Graduate Certificate in Clinical Dentistry from the University of Queensland, Australia, and she is a member of the Royal Australasian College of Dental Surgeons. She completed her speciality in the field of periodontology (1989) and BDS in 1985. She has three decades of clinical experience, with skills covering all aspects of general dentistry, primarily in the speciality of periodontology. She has clinical and research interests include learning and teaching, relationship between periodontitis and systemic health and practice in the field of periodontics. She has edited a book, reviewed articles and has publications in peer-reviewed journals with multiple citations.

Contents

Preface

Evidence-based dentistry is a concept held in high regard in the field of clinical dentistry for decades. The concept is based on the systematic approach of amalgamating established scientific and clinical evidence and relevant clinical application in everyday practice. An unbiased analytical approach of all relevant data should be undertaken in order to deliver the best care for the patient. This analysis involves the integration of the evidence into various aspects of clinical management and the oral status, as it relates to oral health and systemic risk factors.

In *Insights into Various Aspects of Oral Health,* a comprehensive web-based resource, the aim is to combine the scientific literature with the clinical evidence. Here, there is evidenced literature with clinical applications on systemic health, risk factors and periodontal disease, functional rehabilitation and innovative restorative material science. This web resource is a collaboration of numerous specialists and researchers from around the world showcasing varied topics from aspects of oral health status to clinical management. Due to the extensive nature of the areas presented in this resource, limitations are inevitable. An incorporation of review, research studies and clinical management of the following topics are covered:

- Relationship Between the Periodontal Diseases and the Systemic Health
- Functional Rehabilitation of the Dental Status
- Innovations in Dental Restorations
- Research Guidelines on Oral Health Promotion

The subject matter has relevance to a broad oral healthcommunity, including educators and dental students with interests in different subject areas of dentistry. The judicious integration of various topics is designed to give readers an insight into evidenced studies and review different aspects of the oral health status. This book has an international perspective, covering contemporary research on periodontal disease, functional occlusal rehabilitation, research on the biomimetic restorative materials and guidelines on oral health promotion strategies.

Information presented on periodontal status ranges from the diagnostics of specific disease or disorder causing desquamative gingivitis (DG) to the increase of oxidative stress seen in chronic inflammatory conditions and genetic risk factors associated with periodontitis. An investigative review is undertaken on the similarities in pathophysiology of both chronic obstructive pulmonary disease and chronic periodontitis, due to high levels of the pro-inflammatory cytokines, such as CRP and TNF-α and proteases, associated with these chronic inflammatory conditions. Microbial interference therapy using different modalities in the treatment of advanced to aggressive periodontitis has been an ongoing treatment for years, but increasingly the side effects and transient nature of this approach have compromised the goal of the outcome. In this book, a review is presented on an alternative treatment involving non-surgical treatment and probiotic intake. This can lead to host modulation and microbial regulation and contribute to successful periodontal treatment outcomes.

Further, another aspect of oral health is the clinical management of cleft lip and palate (CLP) —the most common congenital deformity of the orofacial region. This chapter highlights the concepts and direction for treatment associated with clefts, with the aim of restoring aesthetics and functional impairments through various modalities. Also addressed is MEAW therapy in restoring aesthetics and occlusal function in the correction of class II deep bite malocclusion together with a hypo-divergent skeletal pattern. This is a difficult situation to treat due to insufficient vertical dimension, combined with steepness of the occlusal plane and strong muscle patterns present in these types of patients. The evidence-based patient cases presented here support MEAW therapy as an effective method of restoring this malocclusion.

In addition, an insight into bioinspired innovative restorative material, which has the ability to combine diverse material properties into a single structure of functionally graded material (FGM), is presented here. The advantage of this system is the integration of dissimilar materials with minimal internal stress and reduced stress concentration at the interface resulting in a free surface intersection. The potential for delamination between layers is eliminated in the graded structure, unlike in traditional core-veneer fabrication, and has applications in implant dentistry, direct-filling tooth restoratives, crowns, dental prosthetics, dental posts, etc.

An analytical input of a digital simulation for providing a biomechanical explanation of the clinical behaviour of ceramic bilayer crowns is also presented here. Finite element analysis (FEA) is a powerful and flexible computational tool that models dental structures and devices, simulates occlusal loading conditions and predicts stress and strain distribution. This can provide design guidelines for the development of complex structures and has the capability to predict clinical survival of all-ceramic restorative prostheses, based on functional loading in the posterior region, hence predicting better crown outcomes.

Oral health promotion involves strategic planning, integrative activities, evidence-based concepts, evaluation, policy making and effective and sustainable intervention. In this endeavour, along with the consideration of the above factors, contributing and limiting elements such as fiscal limitations, regional factors and the comprehension of the population to create healthy living conditions are addressed here. The action programme is influenced by community empowerment, creating a sustainable supporting environment originating from local experiences and strengths. Oral health promotion has a wide scientific scope, with evidences and strategies varying in each region, so a platform to share an amalgamated global strategy is a challenging exercise and is the objective of this chapter.

Jane Francis Manakil, BDS, MDS, PhD, GCHE, MRACDS (Periodontology)
Senior Lecturer, School of Dentistry and Oral Health,
Griffith University, Queensland,
Australia

Section 1

Relationship Between the Periodontal Diseases and the Systemic Health

Chapter 1

Desquamative Gingivitis

Hiroyasu Endo, Terry D. Rees, Hideo Niwa,
Kayo Kuyama, Morio Iijima, Ryuuichi Imamura,
Takao Kato, Kenji Doi, Hirotsugu Yamamoto and
Takanori Ito

Additional information is available at the end of the chapter

http://dx.doi.org/10.5772/intechopen.69268

Abstract

Desquamative gingivitis (DG) is characterized by erythematous, epithelial desquamation, erosion of the gingival epithelium, and blister formation on the gingiva. DG is a clinical feature of a variety of diseases or disorders. Most cases of DG are associated with mucocutaneous diseases, the most common ones being lichen planus, mucous membrane pemphigoid, and pemphigus vulgaris. Proper diagnosis of the underlying cause is important because the prognosis varies, depending on the disease. This chapter presents the underlying etiology that is most commonly associated with DG. The current literature on the diagnostic and management modalities of patients with DG is reviewed.

Keywords: gingival diseases/pemphigus/pemphigoid, benign mucous membrane/lichen planus, oral/hypersensitivity/autoimmune diseases

1. Introduction

Manifestations of desquamative gingivitis (DG) include erythematous gingiva, epithelial desquamation, and erosion of the gingival epithelium, as well as blister formation on the gingiva [1, 2] (**Figure 1**). The DG lesions may be localized or generalized and may extend into the alveolar mucosa. Similar lesions are often found on the buccal mucosa, tongue, and palate in the oral cavity. The signs of DG are clearly different from those of dental plaque-induced gingivitis. Patients having DG may be asymptomatic or symptomatic [3]. Most symptomatic patients complain of mild or moderate oral discomfort, gingival soreness, or a burning sensation [4, 5]. DG occurs more often in females than males; approximately 80% of the patients are female [4–8]. Most patients with DG are middle-aged and older, although rare cases have

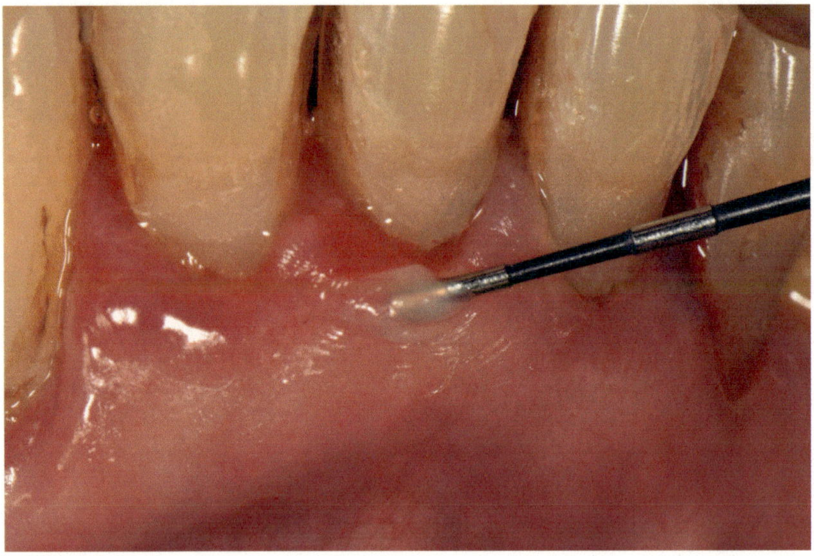

Figure 1. Desquamative lesions on the attached gingiva. Gentle palpation with the periodontal probe elicited some desquamation of the gingival surface (positive Nikolsky's sign).

been observed in children [4, 6, 8, 9]. Early investigators believed that there was a single etiology for DG. However, it is apparent that the condition is a nonspecific manifestation of several diseases or disorders and therefore has multiple etiologies [1, 2]. Most cases of DG are associated with mucocutaneous diseases, the most common ones being lichen planus (LP), mucous membrane pemphigoid (MMP), and pemphigus vulgaris (PV) [1, 2, 4–8, 10, 11]. A variety of other potential causes, such as lupus erythematosus [12], mixed connective tissue disease [5, 10], graft versus host disease [13], erythema multiforme [14], epidermolysis bullosa [15, 16], epidermolysis bullosa acquisita [17], Kindler syndrome [18], chronic ulcerative stomatitis [10, 19, 20], lichen planus pemphigoides [21, 22], plasmacytosis [23], plasma cell gingivitis [24], orofacial granulomatosis [25, 26], foreign body granulomas [27], candidal infection [28], and linear IgA disease [29, 30], may cause DG lesions. Factitious injury of the gingiva may also present with clinical features consistent with DG [31–34], which was suggestive of mucocutaneous diseases including MMP [32, 33] or PV [34]. Contact stomatitis due to dental hygiene products, dental materials, or food flavorings and preservatives may mimic DG [1, 11, 25, 35–39], while several systemic disorders, including Crohn's disease [40], psoriasis [41–43], sarcoidosis [44], and adverse drug reactions [38, 45], may possess some but usually not all of the clinical features of DG.

2. Diagnosis

It is very important to accurately diagnose diseases or disorders causing DG because the prognosis varies widely, depending on the cause. Although PV rarely occurs, it is a potentially life-threatening disease, so it is important to diagnose and treat it in its early stages. Airway obstruction due to laryngeal scarring and blindness due to conjunctival scarring would certainly deteriorate the quality of life for MMP patients. Early recognition and treatment of the lesions can prevent serious complications. Histopathological examination and direct immunofluorescence (DIF) testing of biopsied tissues are often required to determine the underlying etiology of DG [6–8, 10]. For histopathological study, the biopsy site should be selected from an area of intact epithelium and include perilesional tissue. This may require two separate biopsies, one lesional and one non-lesional. The perilesional tissue or non-lesional biopsy site should show a nonspecific inflammatory response in suspected non-autoimmune disorders such as LP, erythema multiforme, foreign body gingivitis, factitious disorder, and contact stomatitis [1, 7, 10]. In contrast, the DIF test should be performed on normal-appearing tissue rather than perilesional sites in suspected autoimmune diseases such as MMP, PV, and chronic ulcerative stomatitis [1, 7, 10, 46, 47]. Since immune deposits in autoimmune bullous disease are present in all oral tissue, a positive result from DIF tests may be obtained from biopsies taken from distant normal mucosa [46]. The DIF test is considered to be the best diagnostic evidence for MMP, PV, chronic ulcerative stomatitis, and other autoimmune disorders; therefore, DIF testing is often essential in obtaining a final diagnosis since clinical features may be so similar [6–8, 10, 47, 48]. On the other hand, DIF findings are supportive but not diagnostic for LP, psoriasis, lupus erythematosus, and mixed connective tissue disease because the DIF features of these diseases can also be found in other conditions [6, 10, 48]. A negative result from DIF tests should be anticipated in biopsies of contact stomatitis [1].

Biopsy sites appearing to have an intact epithelial surface should be selected. If lesions are present at several mucosal sites, including the gingiva, it is usually best not to use the gingiva for the biopsy [1, 49, 50]. However, in approximately half of DG cases, the gingiva was the only site of involvement [50, 51]. In these cases, the gingiva should be selected for the biopsy. Rees and Burkhart [1] described the six steps to be considered when a gingival biopsy is required in DG patients. They highlight the importance of careful site selection for gingival biopsies in order to obtain diagnostic tissue samples. An inadequate surgical site selection may easily lead to the loss of the gingival epithelium, since the biopsied gingival tissue is thin and tends to be fragile. The stab-and-roll biopsy technique is a procedure specially designed to prevent the epithelium from being removed from the biopsy specimen [1, 46, 52]. This biopsy technique prevents the occurrence of lateral shear forces. The operator applies gentle pressure on the gingiva with the tip of a #15 blade until the bone surface is reached and then the blade is rolled from the tip along the entire cutting edge. If a larger specimen is needed, the tip of the blade can be repositioned and the rolling stroke extended. The gingival epithelium was well maintained, and the relationship with the underlying connective tissue was diagnostic from the gingiva of DG patients using the stab-and-roll biopsy technique [1, 46, 52].

3. Oral mucosal diseases or disorders that are associated with DG

3.1. Lichen planus (LP)

LP is a relatively common, T-cell-mediated chronic inflammatory disease of unknown etiology. LP commonly occurs in middle-aged and older people, and women are affected more frequently than men [53, 54]. The lesions are found in multiple regions including the skin, genitalia, or oral mucosa, although they are confined to the gingiva alone in some cases [53–56] (**Figures 2** and **3**). In many instances, atrophic, ulcerative, and bullous forms are combined as erosive LP. The reticular, popular, and plaque-like forms of LP are often asymptomatic, whereas erosive forms may be quite painful when a patient is eating spicy foods or performing oral hygiene procedures [53–55, 57] (**Figures 4–6**). For these reasons, erosive LP usually requires treatment. Histopathologically, specimens may demonstrate hyperortho- or hyperparakeratosis, degenerative changes to the basal cells, and band-like subepithelial infiltrate composed of lymphocytes [11] (**Figure 7**). When available, DIF testing is also valuable in establishing the diagnosis, although DIF findings are only suggestive, rather than diagnostic, of LP [6, 10, 48, 58]. Characteristic DIF findings in oral LP include a linear pattern of anti-fibrin or anti-fibrinogen in the basement membrane zone and, to a lesser degree, the presence of IgM or IgG deposits in cytoid bodies [6, 10, 48, 58] (**Figure 8**).

3.2. Mucous membrane pemphigoid (MMP)

MMP is an autoimmune, subepithelial blistering disease that affects mucous membranes. Most patients with MMP are between 60 and 80 years of age [59–61]. However, on relatively rare occasions, MMP has been reported in children [9]. Women are affected nearly two times more frequently than men [59–61]. MMP can involve any oral mucosal site, although the gingiva is affected far more often than other oral tissues [52, 59–62] (**Figures 9–13**). In more than half of early developing cases, the gingiva is the only site of lesions [61, 63]. Extraoral areas including the conjunctiva, skin, pharynx, nose, larynx, genitalia, anus, and esophagus may also be affected [52, 62, 64, 65]. Scarring of the mucous membranes is often considered the clinical hallmark of MMP, although scarring is rarely a feature of oral MMP [52, 64, 65].

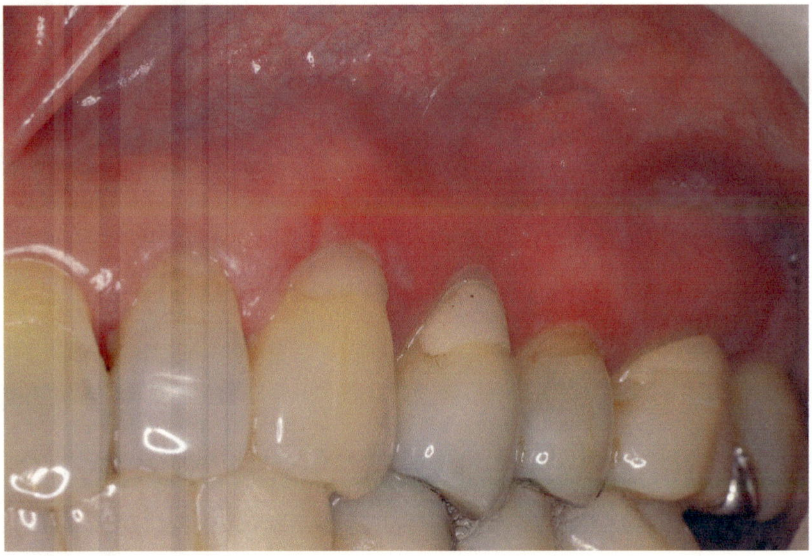

Figure 2. Desquamative gingivitis associated with oral lichen planus. Erythematous lesions on the attached gingiva.

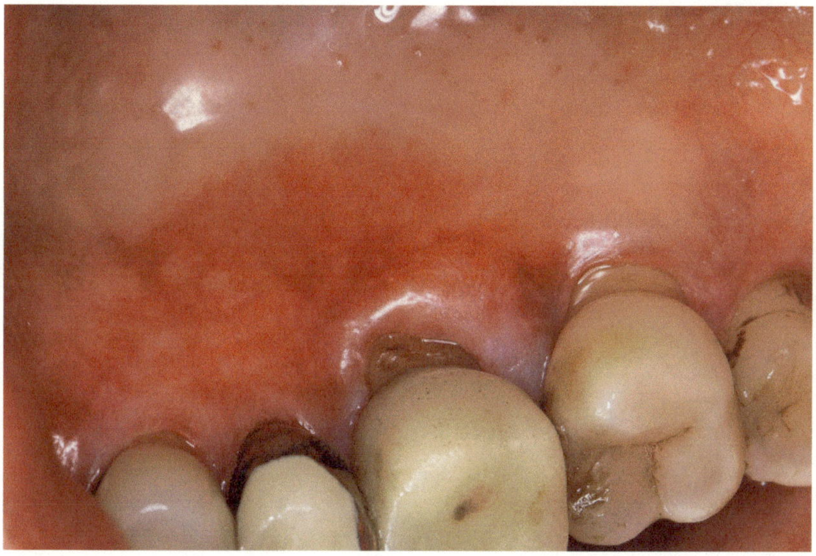

Figure 3. Desquamative gingivitis associated with oral lichen planus. Patchy erythematous lesion was found on the palatal mucosa.

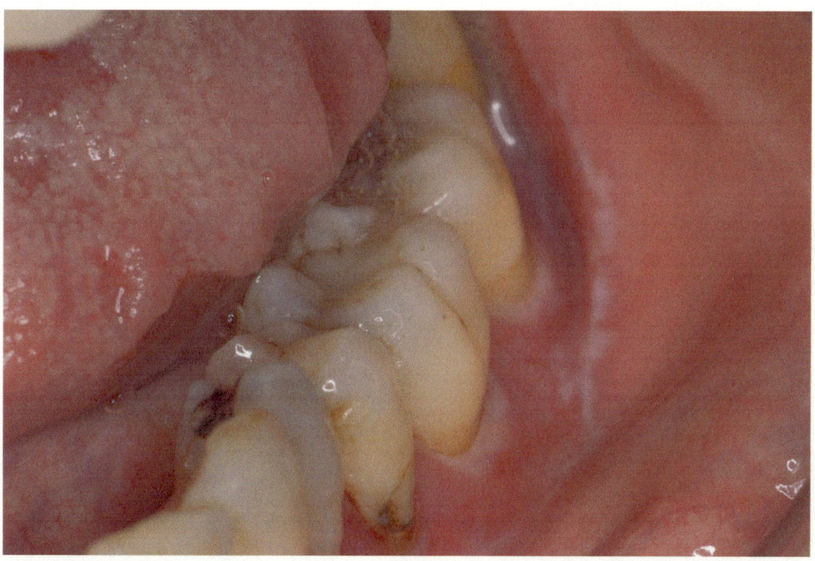

Figure 4. Desquamative gingivitis associated with oral lichen planus. Reticular lesions of buccal mucosa in addition to gingiva.

Multiple target antigens of MMP were identified in cell-to-basement membrane adhesion components by the presence of circulating autoantibodies in the patients' serum. These antigens include bullous pemphigoid antigens (BP180 and BP230), $\alpha 6$ $\beta 4$ integrin, type VII collagen, and laminin 332 [62, 63, 66, 67]. The loss of cell-to-basement membrane adhesion

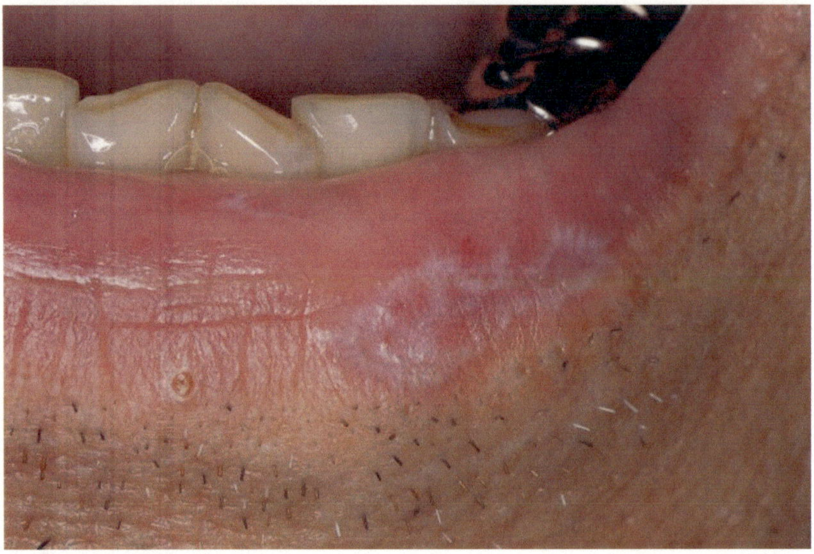

Figure 5. Extraoral lesion associated with oral lichen planus. The reticular lesion was observed on the lip.

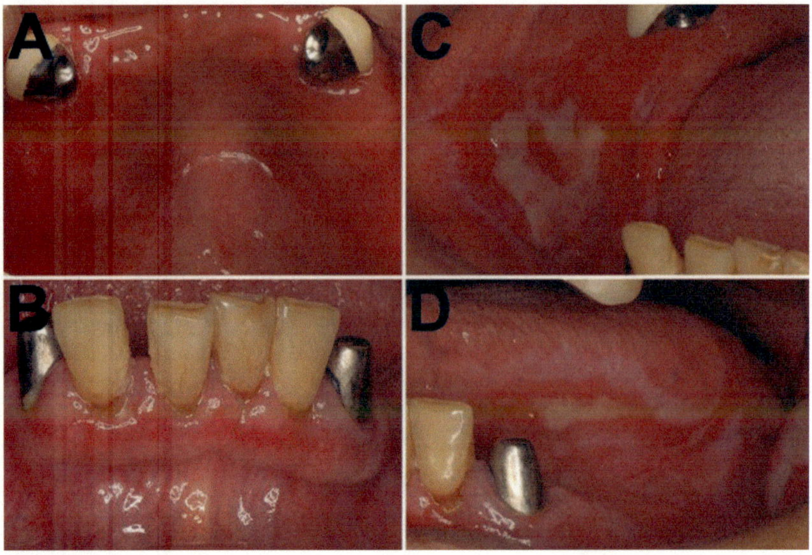

Figure 6. Oral lichen planus patient. The examination revealed diffuse erythematous lesions on the gingiva (A and B). Lesions were also found on the buccal mucosa (C) and tongue (D).

caused by these antibodies may result in subepithelial blistering. Histopathologically, MMP is characterized by subepithelial bulla formation [11] (**Figure 14**). During DIF testing, the linear deposition of complement component C3, IgG, or other immunoglobulin is observed in a linear pattern along the basement membrane zone [48, 62] (**Figure 15**).

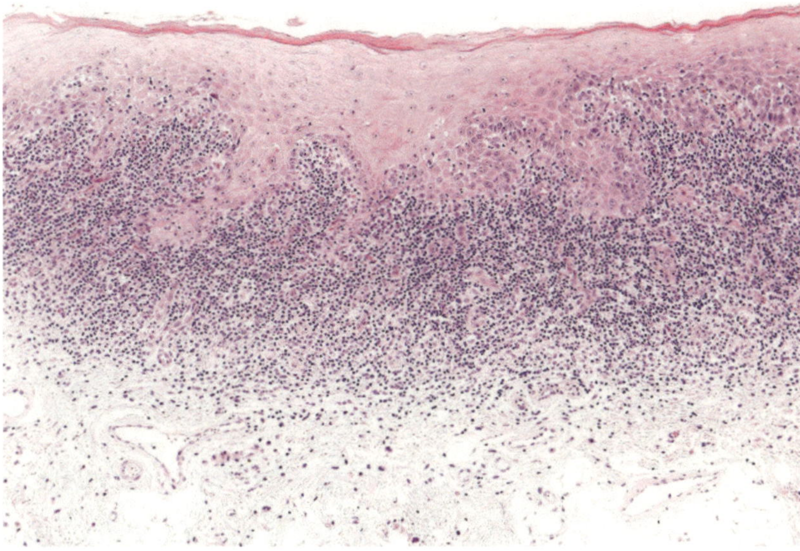

Figure 7. Hematoxylin-eosin-stained section of oral lichen planus. The basal layer liquefaction and shortened rete ridges were found. A band-like infiltration of lymphocytes in the lamina propria was also observed.

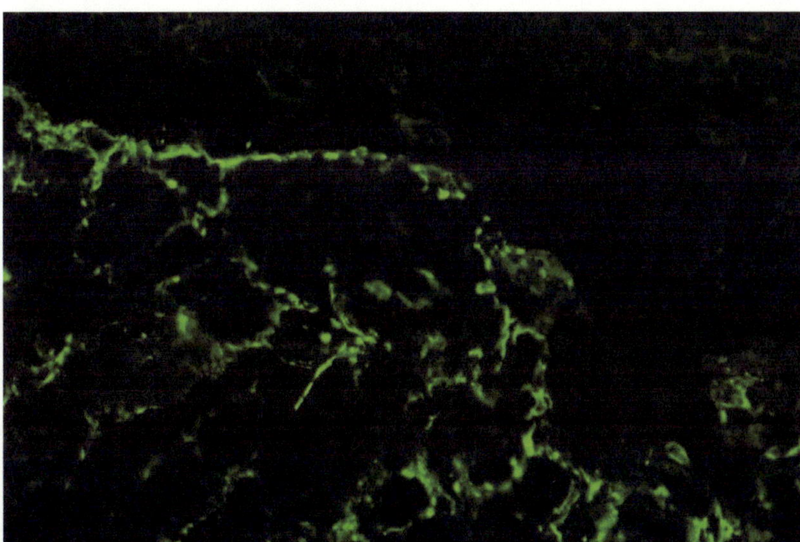

Figure 8. Direct immunofluorescence of oral lichen planus. A linear deposition of fibrinogen at the basement membrane zone was found.

3.3. Pemphigus vulgaris (PV)

PV is an autoimmune blistering disease characterized by acantholysis in the epithelium. Most patients with PV are middle-aged and elderly [68–71]. The disease is equally common in men and women [71], and it is a potentially life-threatening disease [72]. Characteristics

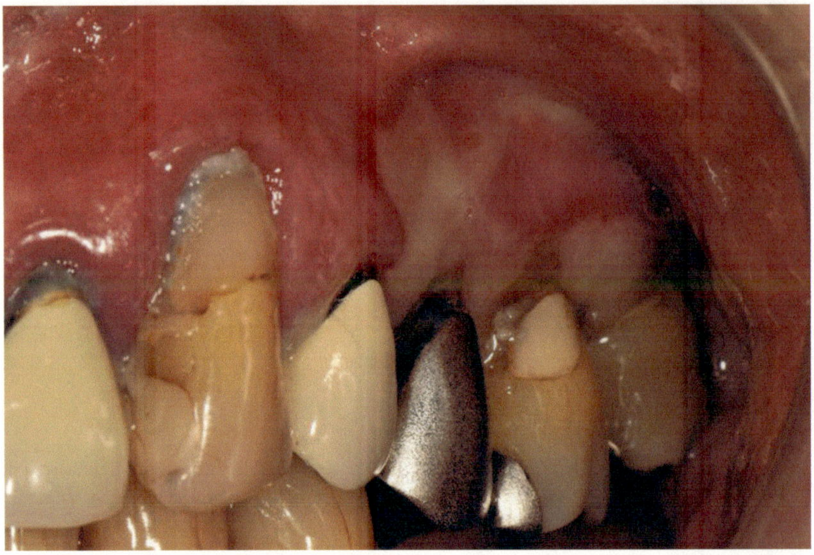

Figure 9. Desquamative gingivitis associated with mucous membrane pemphigoid. Ulcerated gingival surface was observed.

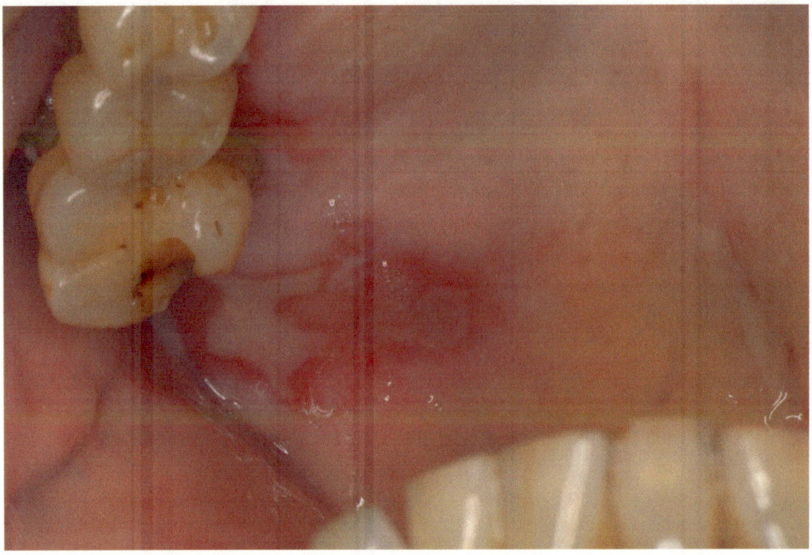

Figure 10. Desquamative gingivitis associated with mucous membrane pemphigoid. Ulceration of the palatal mucosa.

of the PV lesions are flaccid bulla formation, erosion, and ulceration in the skin or mucosa [1, 68] (**Figures 16–19**). PV frequently begins with oral lesions and later progresses to involve the skin [73, 74] (**Figure 20**). Oral lesions are the most common evidence and develop in almost all patients having PV [68, 71]. Lesions may affect the gingiva, and occasionally, the gingiva is the only site of involvement in early lesions [69, 73–75]. Circulating PV autoantibodies

http://dx.doi.org/10.5772/intechopen.69268

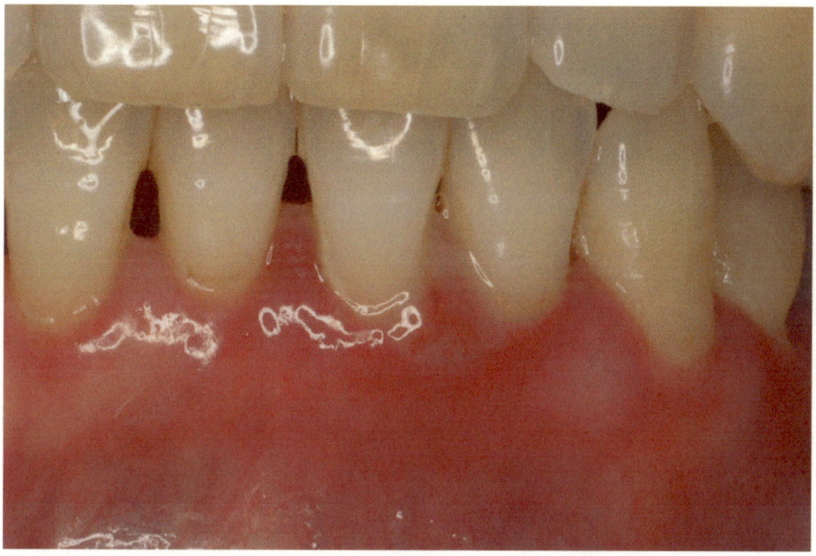

Figure 11. Desquamative lesions featuring gingival erythema associated with mucous membrane pemphigoid.

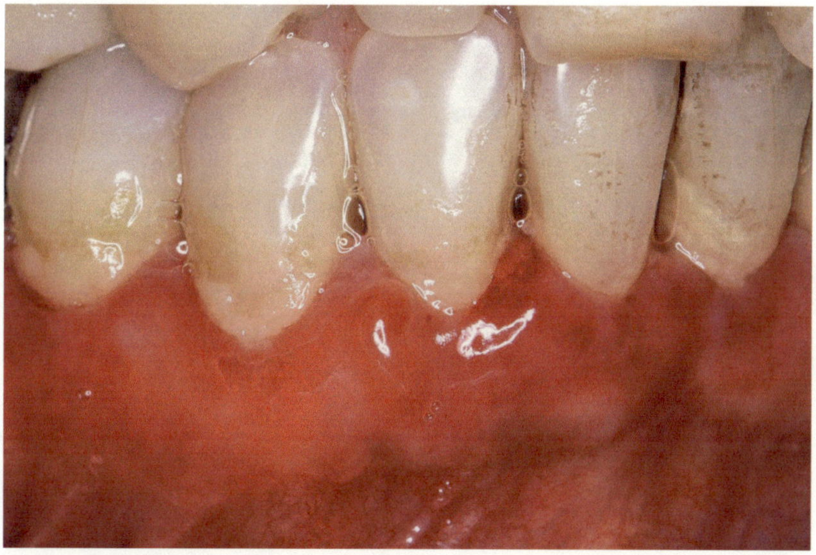

Figure 12. Localized blister formation on the gingiva associated with mucous membrane pemphigoid.

in the serum are pathogenic, and they can cause acantholysis in the epithelium [76]. More than 50 proteins have been reported to specifically react with pemphigus IgG autoantibodies [77], but it has been determined that the principal autoantigens in pemphigus patients are desmogleins, which are the components of desmosomes in the epidermis and mucous membranes [78, 79]. Almost all patients with PV lesions restricted to the oral mucosa have only anti-desmoglein 3 antibody in the serum, whereas patients with advanced cases involving

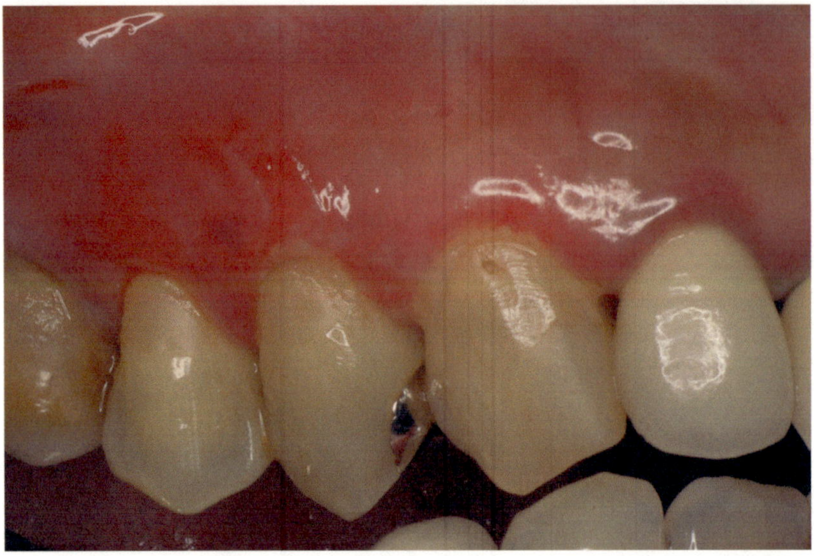

Figure 13. Desquamative lesions on the attached gingiva associated with mucous membrane pemphigoid.

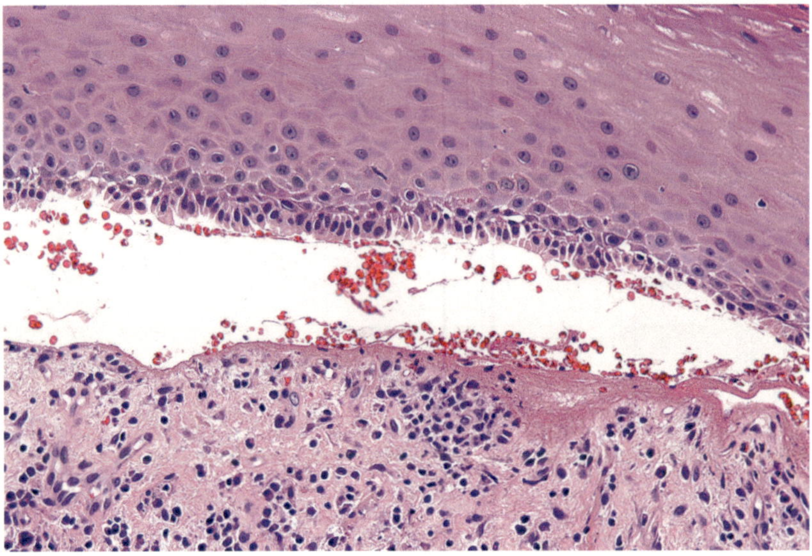

Figure 14. Hematoxylin-eosin-stained section of mucous membrane pemphigoid. A subepithelial blister formation was found.

the oral mucosa and skin may have both anti-desmoglein 3 and anti-desmoglein 1 antibodies [73, 74]. Histopathologically, PV is characterized by acantholysis and a suprabasilar split in the epithelium [11] (**Figure 21**). Tzanck cells are often found in intraepithelial clefts [80]. In the DIF examination of PV patients, the deposition of IgG and/or C3 is found in the intercellular spaces of the epithelium [48] (**Figure 22**).

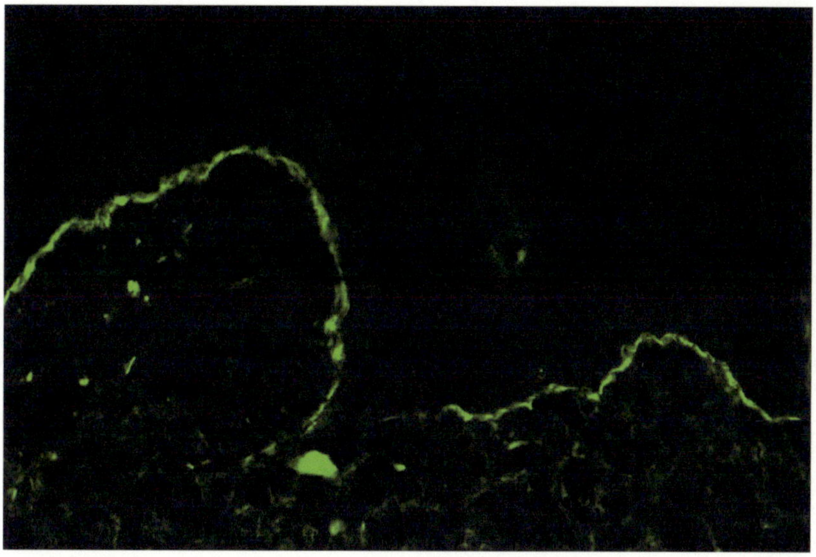

Figure 15. Direct immunofluorescence of the mucous membrane pemphigoid. A linear deposition of IgG at the basement membrane zone was found.

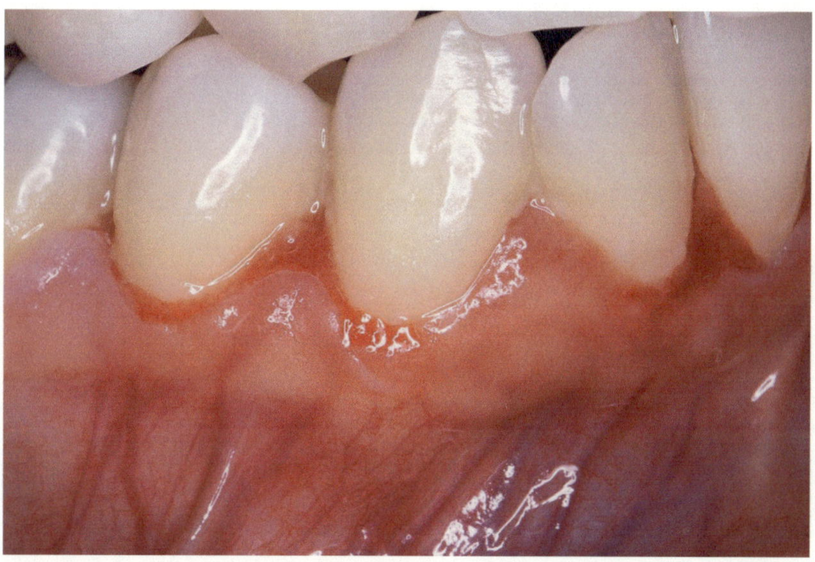

Figure 16. Desquamative gingivitis associated with pemphigus vulgaris. Eroded gingival surface with ragged edges was observed.

3.4. Contact hypersensitivity reactions as cause of DG

Localized or generalized DG is sometimes elicited by contact hypersensitivity reactions to various foodstuffs, preservatives, oral hygiene products, and dental restorative materials [11, 25, 35–39, 81]. Toothpaste hypersensitivity reactions may occur in various oral or perioral

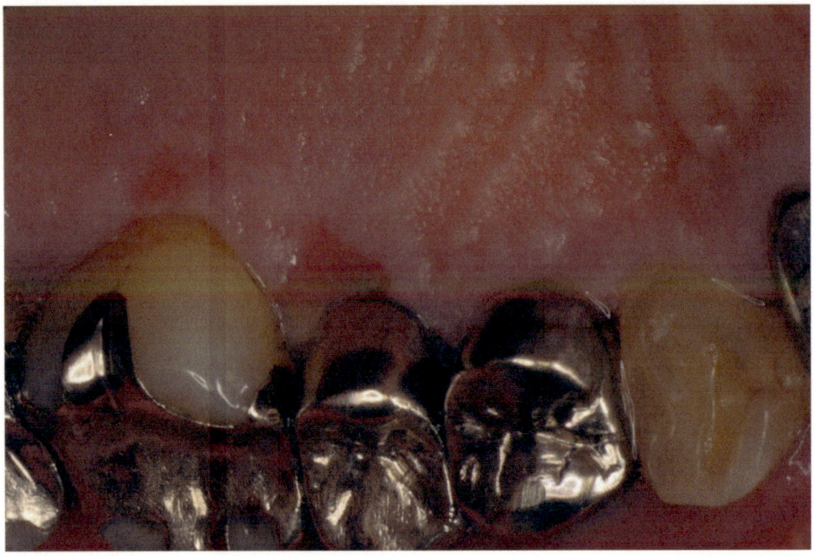

Figure 17. Desquamative gingivitis associated with pemphigus vulgaris. Localized erosions of the palatal mucosa.

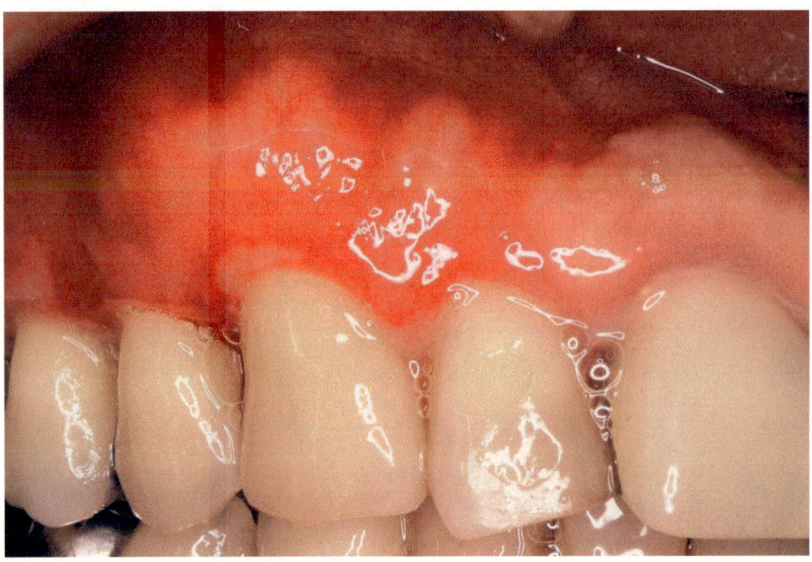

Figure 18. Mild erythema and ulceration of gingiva associated with pemphigus vulgaris.

sites, but the gingiva was the most common site of onset [24, 35, 36, 39, 81] (**Figure 23**). Erythema has been expressed as a "velvet-like appearance of the gingiva" or "fiery red gingiva" [35]. Epithelial sloughing is the most common irritant effect associated with toothpastes and mouthwashes [1, 2, 35, 82] (**Figure 24**). Allergy to dental restorative materials usually causes localized DG in gingival or other mucosal tissues directly contacting the allergen [1, 11]. Gingival contact hypersensitivity lesions are usually not biopsied. However, if a biopsy

http://dx.doi.org/10.5772/intechopen.69268

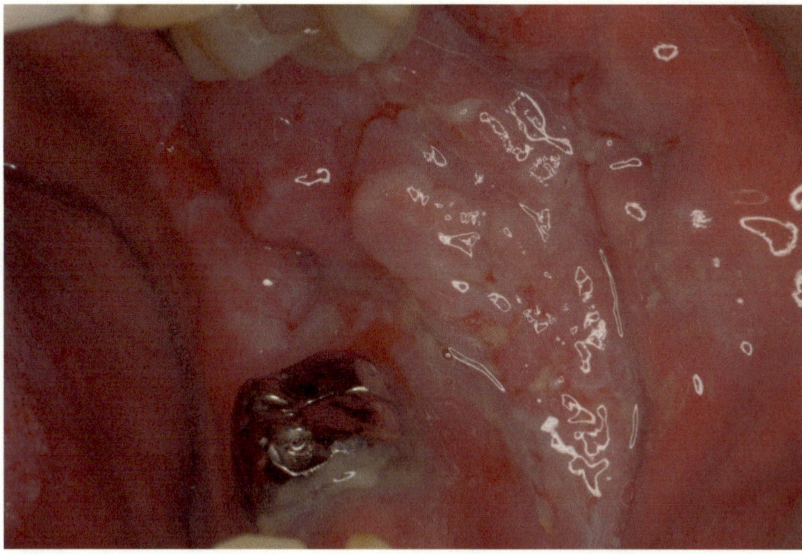

Figure 19. Pseudomembrane-covered erosion of buccal mucosa associated with pemphigus vulgaris.

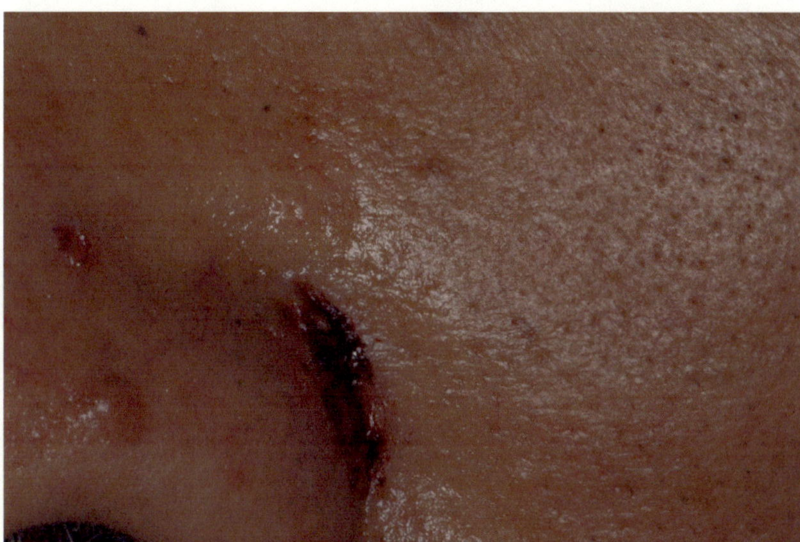

Figure 20. Skin involvement in a desquamative gingivitis associated with pemphigus vulgaris.

is performed, these lesions present with non-specific histopathologic findings with submucosal perivascular inflammatory cell infiltration [11, 35, 36]. The existence of focal granulomatous inflammation and/or multinucleated giant cells in the deep layer of the lamina propria was also described in some cases studying contact hypersensitivity stomatitis [25, 81]. DIF is not indicated because it is routinely negative [11]. To treat contact hypersensitivity reactions, the allergen should be identified and removed. To do so, patients should be questioned

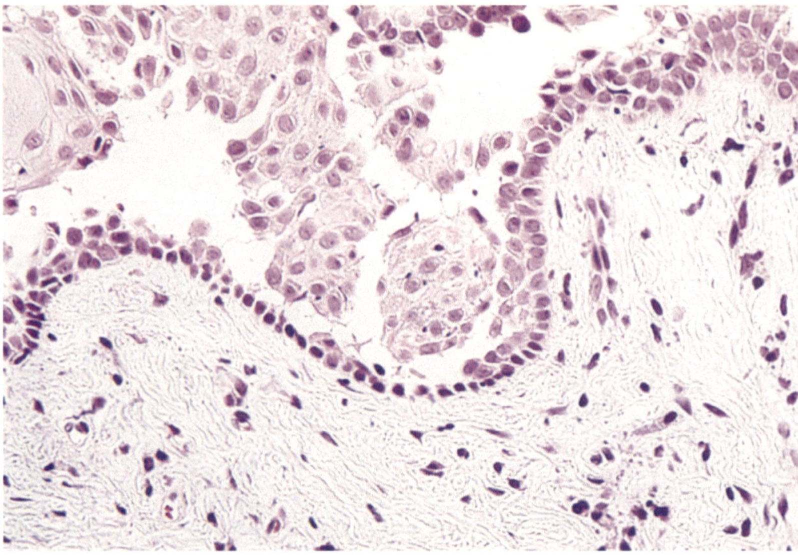

Figure 21. Hematoxylin-eosin-stained section of pemphigus vulgaris. Acantholys was recognized.

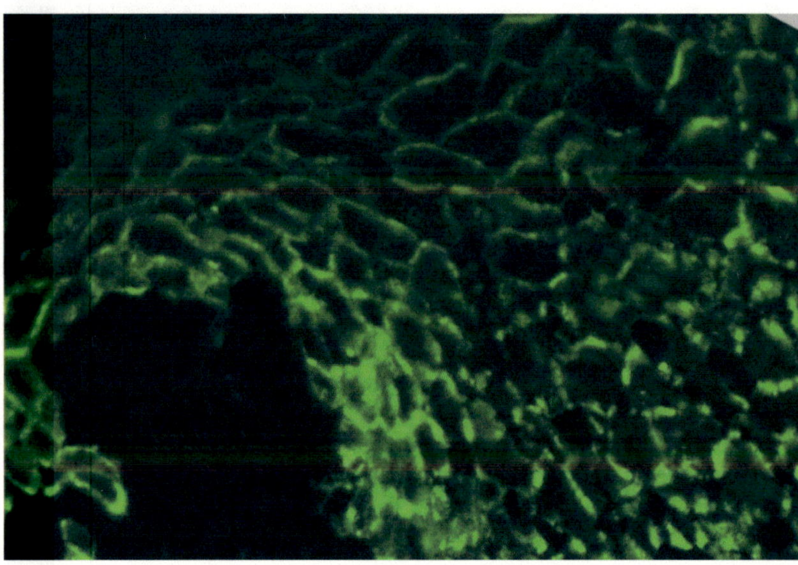

Figure 22. Direct immunofluorescence of pemphigus vulgaris. An intercellular deposition of IgG was seen.

regarding the type(s) of oral hygiene products they use, and a 1–2-week food diary may help identify causative agents [35]. Patch testing may be required to identify the allergen or to confirm a specific allergen in a dental hygiene product or in a dental restoration. Patients are considered to have allergic reactions to a relevant allergen if their patch test results are

http://dx.doi.org/10.5772/intechopen.69268

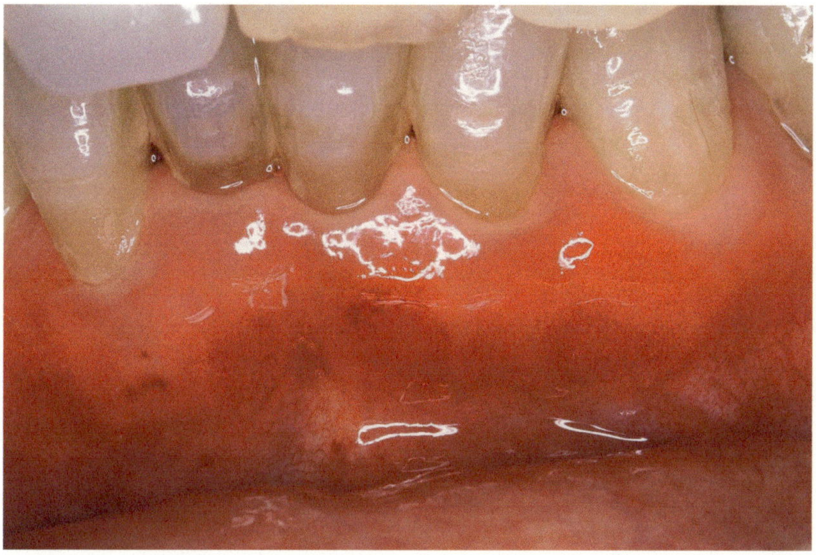

Figure 23. Contact hypersensitivity reactions caused by toothpaste. Localized erythematous and edematous lesions were found on the gingiva.

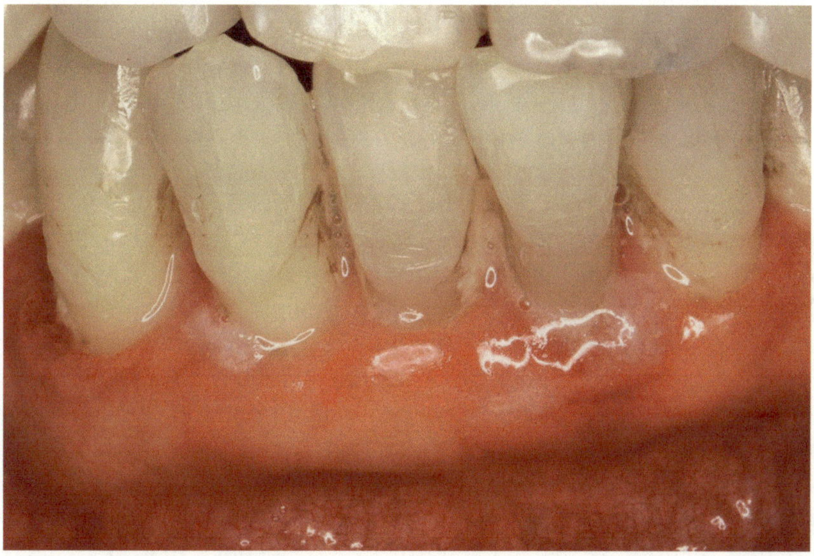

Figure 24. Contact hypersensitivity reactions caused by mouth rinse. Epithelial sloughing was noted.

positive [35, 81]. However, diagnosis of contact hypersensitivity reactions may be confirmed simply by the discontinuation of the causative agent(s) resulting in the remission of clinical signs and symptoms [35, 36, 81].

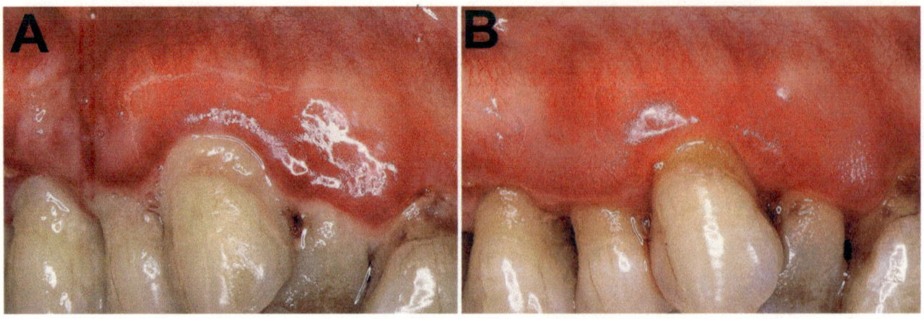

Figure 25. Desquamative gingivitis associated with mucous membrane pemphigoid. The initial examination revealed moderate erythema and swelling of the gingiva with plaque and calculus deposits (A). Treatment response. The condition of the gingiva improved due to a topical corticosteroid therapy combined with effective plaque control (B).

4. Managing DG patients

The specific disease or disorder causing DG, the severity of the gingival lesions, the presence or absence of extraoral involvements, and the medical history of the patient are the key factors in determining the selection of a topical or systemic immunosuppressive therapy [1, 2, 69, 83]. The patients diagnosed as having an autoimmune disease should be closely followed because they may require immediate referral to other health care experts especially if they develop extraoral lesions. After MMP is diagnosed from DG or concomitant lesions, patients should undergo examination by medical specialists including an ophthalmologist and an otolaryngologist, and the presence or absence of extraoral lesions should be determined. PV patients with exclusively oral lesions should be followed closely and referred to other experts immediately if they develop lesions elsewhere on the body. Management of the specific disease or disorder causing DG may best be provided by a specialist in oral medicine, oral pathology, periodontics, or oral surgery, but the dentist may still be responsible for maintaining the dental and periodontal health of the patient. This is important because periodontal and dental considerations are often observed in DG patients, but the literature contains minimal information regarding the periodontal and dental management of these individuals. Plaque-induced gingivitis is almost universal in patients with symptomatic DG, and an effective therapeutic protocol should include non-surgical periodontal therapy consisting of oral hygiene instruction, scaling, and root planting [2, 84–89] (**Figure 25**). We believe that excessively vigorous scaling and root planting can be unnecessarily damaging to DG-affected lesions, and we prefer a sequential gingival management approach that features gentle supragingival and slight subgingival debridement which can be repeated at two-week intervals resulting in gradual improvement in periodontal status until an acceptable level of periodontal health has been achieved. The relationship between the existence of DG lesions and the progression of periodontal diseases is inconclusive, although some but not all studies

http://dx.doi.org/10.5772/intechopen.69268

demonstrated a correlation between compromised periodontal status and autoimmune bullous diseases affecting the mouth [90–96]. There are several reports on periodontal surgery or dental implant therapy performed on patients having DG [15–17, 73, 97–100]. Tissue sloughing and a lack of tissue elasticity caused by active autoimmune bullous disease can disturb the manipulation of the mucosal flap. Strict mucosal disease control prior to surgery may reduce the surgical complications [101]. Implant therapy is likely to enhance the quality of life in patients with systemic diseases and may help them maintain long-term masticatory function. Patients with DG are often unable to wear tissue-borne prostheses because of discomfort. This tissue irritation and oral pain can be increased if the appliances are ill fitting or damaged. A dental implant-supported prosthesis improves the stabilization of the prosthesis, resulting in a higher degree of comfort. Published case reports indicated that DG patients can be successfully managed with dental implants. These reports suggest that the degree of disease control may be more important than the nature of the disease itself in regard to the effects on osseointegration. Penarrocha et al. [98] reported that implants can be successfully placed and used to support dental prostheses in patients with recessive dystrophic epidermolysis bullosa. A total of 38 implants were placed in six totally edentulous patients. Only one implant failed to achieve osseointegration. The average follow-up from implant placement was 5.5 years. The implant-supported prostheses were associated with improvements in the patients' comfort and function, esthetics and appearance, taste, speech, and self-esteem. Altin et al. [99] presented a case of PV rehabilitation using a successful implant-supported prosthesis with a 32-month follow-up. They concluded that the implant treatment may be considered as a good alternative to a tissue-borne prosthesis in PV patients. Esposito et al. [100] reported implant retained overdentures for two patients with severe oral LP. The patients were often unable to wear tissue-borne prostheses because of the discomfort. There was good integration of the implants with no clinical or radiographic evidence of bone loss, and the soft-tissue/implant response was excellent. Lesions occasionally flared-up but were successfully treated with topical steroids. There was no evidence of potential implant failure as a result of these flare-ups. Although these descriptions of successful management using dental implants for patients with DG are promising, further studies are needed since these were individual case reports.

5. Conclusion

DG is a clinical manifestation that is common to several diseases or disorders. It is important to diagnose the diseases causing DG because the prognosis varies, depending on the disease. Histopathological examination and DIF testing are often required to establish the final diagnosis. The patients diagnosed with autoimmune diseases such as MMP or PV should be closely followed because they must be immediately referred to other experts when they develop lesions on parts of their body other than the oral cavity.

Abbreviations

DG	Desquamative gingivitis
LP	Lichen planus
MMP	Mucous membrane pemphigoid
PV	Pemphigus vulgaris
DIF	Direct immunofluorescence

Author details

Hiroyasu Endo[1*], Terry D. Rees[2], Hideo Niwa[3], Kayo Kuyama[4], Morio Iijima[5], Ryuuichi Imamura[6], Takao Kato[7], Kenji Doi[1], Hirotsugu Yamamoto[4] and Takanori Ito[1]

*Address all correspondence to: endo.hiroyasu@nihon-u.ac.jp

1 Department of Oral Diagnosis, School of Dentistry at Matsudo, Nihon University, Matsudo, Japan

2 Department of Periodontics, Texas A&M College of Dentistry, Dallas, Texas, USA

3 Department of Head and Neck Surgery, School of Dentistry at Matsudo, Nihon University, Matsudo, Japan

4 Department of Oral Pathology, School of Dentistry at Matsudo, Nihon University, Matsudo, Japan

5 Department of Removable Prosthodontics, School of Dentistry at Matsudo, Nihon University, Matsudo, Japan

6 Department of Maxillofacial Orthodontics, School of Dentistry at Matsudo, Nihon University, Matsudo, Japan

7 Department of Oral Implantology, School of Dentistry at Matsudo, Nihon University, Matsudo, Japan

References

[1] Rees TD, Burkhart N. Desquamative Gingivitis [Internet]. 2016. Available from: https://www.dentalcare.com/en-us/professional-education/ce-courses/ce481 [Accessed: February 9, 2017]

[2] Endo H, Rees TD. Diagnosis and management of desquamative gingivitis. In: Panagakos FS, Davies RM, editors. Gingival Diseases – Their Aetiology, Prevention and Treatment. Rijeka, Croatia: InTech; 2011. pp. 171-188. Available from: http://www.intechopen.

com/articles/show/title/diagnosis-and-management-of-desquamative-gingivitis [Accessed: February 9, 2017]

[3] Nisengard RJ, Levine RA. Diagnosis and management of desquamative gingivitis. Periodontal Insights. 1995;**2**:4-10

[4] Lo Russo L, Fierro G, Guiglia R, et al. Epidemiology of desquamative gingivitis: Evaluation of 125 patients and review of the literature. International Journal of Dermatology. 2009;**48**:1049-1052

[5] Leao JC, Ingafou M, Khan A, Scully C, Porter S. Desquamative gingivitis: Retrospective analysis of disease associations of a large cohort. Oral Diseases. 2008;**14**:556-560

[6] Nisengard RJ, Neiders M. Desquamative lesions of the gingiva. Journal of Periodontology. 1981;**52**:500-510

[7] Nisengard RJ, Rogers 3rd RS. The treatment of desquamative gingival lesions. Journal of Periodontology. 1987;**58**:167-172

[8] Rinaggio J, Crossland DM, Zeid MY. A determination of the range of oral conditions submitted for microscopic and direct immunofluorescence analysis. Journal of Periodontology. 2007;**78**:1904-1910

[9] Cheng YS, Rees TD, Wright JM, Plemons JM. Childhood oral pemphigoid: A case report and review of the literature. Journal of Oral Pathology & Medicine. 2001;**30**:372-377

[10] Suresh L, Neiders ME. Definitive and differential diagnosis of desquamative gingivitis through direct immunofluorescence studies. Journal of Periodontology. 2012;**83**:1270-1278. DOI: 10.1902/jop.2012.110627

[11] Rees TD. Desquamative gingivitis/mucocutaneous diseases commonly affecting the gingiva. In: Harpenau LA, Kao RT, Lundergan WP, Sanz M, editors. Hall's Critical Decisions in Periodontology and Dental Implantology. 5th ed. Connecticut, USA: People's Medical Publishing House; 2013. pp. 68-73

[12] Kranti K, Seshan H, Juliet J. Discoid lupus erythematosus involving gingiva. Journal of Indian Society of Periodontology. 2012;**16**:126-128. DOI: 10.4103/0972-124X.94621

[13] Bassim CW, Fassil H, Mays JW, et al. Oral disease profiles in chronic graft versus host disease. Journal of Dental Research. 2015;**94**:547-554. DOI: 10.1177/0022034515570942

[14] Ayangco L, Rogers 3rd RS. Oral manifestations of erythema multiforme. Dermatologic Clinics. 2003;**21**:195-205

[15] Brain JH, Paul BF, Assad DA. Periodontal plastic surgery in a dystrophic epidermolysis bullosa patient: Review and case report. Journal of Periodontology. 1999;**70**:1392-1396

[16] Buduneli E, Ilgenli T, Buduneli N, Ozdemir F. Acellular dermal matrix allograft used to gain attached gingiva in a case of epidermolysis bullosa. Journal of Clinical Periodontology. 2003;**30**:1011-1015

[17] Hakki SS, Celenligil-Nazliel H, Karaduman A, et al. Epidermolysis bullosa acquisita: Clinical manifestations, microscopic findings, and surgical periodontal therapy. A case report. Journal of Periodontology. 2001;**72**:550-558

[18] Ricketts DN, Morgan CL, McGregor JM, Morgan PR. Kindler syndrome: A rare cause of desquamative lesions of the gingiva. Oral Surgery, Oral Medicine, Oral Pathology, Oral Radiology, and Endodontics. 1997;**84**:488-491

[19] Lorenzana ER, Rees TD, Glass M, Detweiler JG. Chronic ulcerative stomatitis: A case report. Journal of Periodontology. 2000;**71**:104-111

[20] Qari H, Villasante C, Richert J, Rees TD, Kessler H. The diagnostic challenges of separating chronic ulcerative stomatitis from oral lichen planus. Oral Surgery, Oral Medicine, Oral Pathology and Oral Radiology. 2015;**120**:622-627. DOI: 10.1016/j.oooo.2015.07.018

[21] Sultan A, Stojanov IJ, Lerman MA, et al. Oral lichen planus pemphigoides: A series of four cases. Oral Surgery, Oral Medicine, Oral Pathology and Oral Radiology. 2015;**120**:58-68. DOI: 10.1016/j.oooo.2015.03.012

[22] Mignogna MD, Fortuna G, Leuci S, Stasio L, Mezza E, Ruoppo E. Lichen planus pemphigoides, a possible example of epitope spreading. Oral Surgery, Oral Medicine, Oral Pathology, Oral Radiology, and Endodontics. 2010;**109**:837-843. DOI: 10.1016/j.tripleo.2009.12.044

[23] Gupta SR, Gupta R, Saran RK, Krishnan S. Plasma cell mucositis with gingival enlargement and severe periodontitis. Journal of Indian Society of Periodontology. 2014;**18**:379-384. DOI: 10.4103/0972-124X.134583

[24] Mishra MB, Sharma S, Sharma A. Plasma cell gingivitis: An occasional case report. The New York State Dental Journal. 2015;**81**:57-60

[25] Rees TD. Orofacial granulomatosis and related conditions. Periodontology 2000. 1999; **21**:145-157

[26] Mignogna MD, Fedele S, Lo Russo L, Lo Muzio L. Orofacial granulomatosis with gingival onset. Journal of Clinical Periodontology. 2001;**28**:692-696

[27] Gravitis K, Daley TD, Lochhead MA. Management of patients with foreign body gingivitis: Report of 2 cases with histologic findings. Journal of the Canadian Dental Association. 2005;**71**:105-109

[28] Yalamanchili PS, Potluri S, Surapaneni H, Basha MH, Davanapelly P. Candidal infection of the gingiva mimicking desquamative gingivitis: A case report. Journal of Clinical and Diagnostic Research. 2016;**10**:ZD04-ZD05. DOI: 10.7860/JCDR/2016/17413.7367

[29] Porter SR, Bain SE, Scully CM. Linear IgA disease manifesting as recalcitrant desquamative gingivitis. Oral Surgery, Oral Medicine, Oral Pathology. 1992;**74**:179-182

[30] O'Regan E, Bane A, Flint S, Timon C, Toner M. Linear IgA disease presenting as desquamative gingivitis: A pattern poorly recognized in medicine. Archives of Otolaryngology – Head and Neck Surgery. 2004;**130**:469-472

[31] McGrath KG, Pick R, Leboff-Ries E, Patterson R. Factitious desquamative gingivitis simulating a possible immunologic disease. The Journal of Allergy and Clinical Immunology. 1985;**75**:44-46

[32] Heasman PA, MacLeod I, Smith DG. Factitious gingival ulceration: As presenting sign of Munchausen's syndrome? Journal of Periodontology. 1994;**65**:442-447

[33] Kotansky K, Goldberg M, Tenenbaum HC, Mock D. Factitious injury of the oral mucosa: A case series. Journal of Periodontology. 1995;**66**:241-245

[34] Zonuz AT, Treister N, Mehdipour F, Farahani RM, Tubbs RS, Shoja MM. Factitial pemphigus-like lesions. Medicina Oral Patologia Oral y Cirugia Bucal. 2007;**12**:E205-E208

[35] Endo H, Rees TD. Clinical features of cinnamon-induced contact stomatitis. Compendium of Continuing Education in Dentistry. 2006;**27**:403-409; quiz 410, 421

[36] Endo H, Rees TD, Sisilia F, et al. Atypical gingival manifestations that mimic mucocutaneous diseases in a patient with contact stomatitis caused by toothpaste. Journal of Implant and Advanced Clinical Dentistry. 2010;**2**:101-106

[37] Lamey PJ, Lewis MA, Rees TD, Fowler C, Binnie WH, Forsyth A. Sensitivity reaction to the cinnamonaldehyde component of toothpaste. British Dental Journal. 1990;**168**:115-118

[38] Rees TD. Drugs and oral disorders. Periodontology 2000. 1998;**18**:21-36

[39] Singh B, Sharma A, Garg A. Herbal oral gel induced contact stomatitis along with desquamative gingivitis due to a coloring agent. Journal of Indian Society of Periodontology. 2015;**19**:569-572. DOI: 10.4103/0972-124X.167165

[40] Ayangco L, Rogers 3rd RS, Sheridan PJ. Pyostomatitis vegetans as an early sign of reactivation of Crohn's disease: A case report. Journal of Periodontology. 2002;**73**:1512-1516

[41] Jones LE, Dolby AE. Desquamative gingivitis associated with psoriasis. Journal of Periodontology. 1972;**43**:35-37

[42] Yamada J, Amar S, Petrungaro P. Psoriasis-associated periodontitis: A case report. Journal of Periodontology. 1992;**63**:854-857

[43] Brice DM, Danesh-Meyer MJ. Oral lesions in patients with psoriasis: Clinical presentation and management. Journal of Periodontology. 2000;**71**:1896-1903

[44] Antunes KB, Miranda AM, Carvalho SR, Azevedo AL, Tatakis DN, Pires FR. Sarcoidosis presenting as gingival erosion in a patient under long-term clinical control. Journal of Periodontology. 2008;**79**:556-561

[45] Rees TD. Oral effects of drug abuse. Critical Reviews in Oral Biology & Medicine. 1992;**3**:163-184

[46] Endo H, Rees TD, Allen EP, et al. A stab-and-roll biopsy technique to maintain gingival epithelium for desquamative gingivitis. Journal of Periodontology. 2014;**85**:802-809. DOI: 10.1902/jop.2014.130428

[47] Sano SM, Quarracino MC, Aguas SC, et al. Sensitivity of direct immunofluorescence in oral diseases. Study of 125 cases. Medicina Oral Patologia Oral y Cirugia Bucal. 2008;**13**:E287-E291

[48] Mutasim DF, Adams BB. Immunofluorescence in dermatology. Journal of The American Academy of Dermatology. 2001;**45**:803-822; quiz 822-824

[49] Siegel MA, Balciunas BA, Kelly M, Serio FG. Diagnosis and management of commonly occurring oral vesiculoerosive disorders. Cutis. 1991;**47**:39-43

[50] Casiglia J, Woo SB, Ahmed AR. Oral involvement in autoimmune blistering diseases. Clinical Dermatology. 2001;**19**:737-741

[51] Lo Russo L, Fedele S, Guiglia R, et al. Diagnostic pathways and clinical significance of desquamative gingivitis. Journal of Periodontology. 2008;**79**:4-24

[52] Endo H, Rees TD, Niwa H, Kuyama K, Yamamoto H, Ito T. Desquamative gingivitis as an oral manifestation of mucous membrane pemphigoid: Diagnosis and treatment. In: Vega JP, editor. Advances in Dermatology Research. New York, USA: Nova Science Publishers; 2015. pp. 73-86. Available from: https://www.novapublishers.com/catalog/product_info.php?products_id=54901 [Accessed: February 9, 2017]

[53] Ingafou M, Leao JC, Porter SR, Scully C. Oral lichen planus: A retrospective study of 690 British patients. Oral Diseases. 2006;**12**:463-468

[54] Mignogna MD, Lo Russo L, Fedele S. Gingival involvement of oral lichen planus in a series of 700 patients. Journal of Clinical Periodontology. 2005;**32**:1029-1033

[55] Camacho-Alonso F, Lopez-Jornet P, Bermejo-Fenoll A. Gingival involvement of oral lichen planus. Journal of Periodontology. 2007;**78**:640-644

[56] Petruzzi M, De Benedittis M, Pastore L, Grassi FR, Serpico R. Peno-gingival lichen planus. Journal of Periodontology. 2005;**76**:2293-2298

[57] Endo H, Rees TD, Kuyama K, Matsue M, Yamamoto H. Successful treatment using occlusive steroid therapy in patients with erosive lichen planus: A report on 2 cases. Quintessence International. 2008;**39**:e162-e172

[58] Buajeeb W, Okuma N, Thanakun S, Laothumthut T. Direct immunofluorescence in oral lichen planus. Journal of Clinical and Diagnostic Research. 2015;**9**:ZC34-ZC37. DOI: 10.7860/JCDR/2015/13510.6312

[59] Ahmed AR, Hombal SM. Cicatricial pemphigoid. International Journal of Dermatology. 1986;**25**:90-96

[60] Hanson RD, Olsen KD, Rogers 3rd RS. Upper aerodigestive tract manifestations of cicatricial pemphigoid. Annals of Otology, Rhinology & Laryngology. 1988;**97**:493-499

[61] Lamey PJ, Rees TD, Binnie WH, Rankin KV. Mucous membrane pemphigoid. Treatment experience at two institutions. Oral Surgery, Oral Medicine, Oral Pathology. 1992;**74**: 50-53

[62] Chan LS, Ahmed AR, Anhalt GJ, et al. The first international consensus on mucous membrane pemphigoid: Definition, diagnostic criteria, pathogenic factors, medical treatment, and prognostic indicators. Archives of Dermatology. 2002;**138**:370-379.

[63] Endo H, Rees TD, Kuyama K, Kono Y, Yamamoto H. Clinical and diagnostic features of mucous membrane pemphigoid. Compendium of Continuing Education in Dentistry. 2006;**27**:512-516; quiz 517-518

[64] Higgins TS, Cohen JC, Sinacori JT. Laryngeal mucous membrane pemphigoid: A systematic review and pooled-data analysis. Laryngoscope. 2010;**120**:529-536

[65] Higgins GT, Allan RB, Hall R, Field EA, Kaye SB. Development of ocular disease in patients with mucous membrane pemphigoid involving the oral mucosa. British Journal of Ophthalmology. 2006;**90**:964-967

[66] Calabresi V, Carrozzo M, Cozzani E, et al. Oral pemphigoid autoantibodies preferentially target BP180 ectodomain. Journal of Clinical Immunology. 2007;**122**:207-213

[67] Bernard P, Antonicelli F, Bedane C, et al. Prevalence and clinical significance of anti-laminin 332 autoantibodies detected by a novel enzyme-linked immunosorbent assay in mucous membrane pemphigoid. JAMA Dermatology. 2013;**149**:533-540. DOI: 10.1001/jamadermatol.2013.1434

[68] Chams-Davatchi C, Valikhani M, Daneshpazhooh M, et al. Pemphigus: Analysis of 1209 cases. International Journal of Dermatology. 2005;**44**:470-476

[69] Lamey PJ, Rees TD, Binnie WH, Wright JM, Rankin KV, Simpson NB. Oral presentation of pemphigus vulgaris and its response to systemic steroid therapy. Oral Surgery, Oral Medicine, Oral Pathology. 1992;**74**:54-57

[70] Scully C, Paes De Almeida O, Porter SR, Gilkes JJ. Pemphigus vulgaris: The manifestations and long-term management of 55 patients with oral lesions. British Journal of Dermatology. 1999;**140**:84-89

[71] Sirois D, Leigh JE, Sollecito TP. Oral pemphigus vulgaris preceding cutaneous lesions: Recognition and diagnosis. Journal of the American Dental Association. 2000;**131**:1156-1160

[72] Nair PS, Moorthy PK, Yogiragan K. A study of mortality in dermatology. Indian Journal of Dermatology, Venereology and Leprology. 2005;**71**:23-25

[73] Endo H, Rees TD, Matsue M, Kuyama K, Nakadai M, Yamamoto H. Early detection and successful management of oral pemphigus vulgaris: A case report. Journal of Periodontology. 2005;**76**:154-160

[74] Endo H, Rees TD, Hallmon WW, et al. Disease progression from mucosal to mucocutaneous involvement in a patient with desquamative gingivitis associated with pemphigus vulgaris. Journal of Periodontology. 2008;**79**:369-375. DOI: 10.1902/jop.2008.070258

[75] Mignogna MD, Lo Muzio L, Bucci E. Clinical features of gingival pemphigus vulgaris. Journal of Clinical Periodontology. 2001;**28**:489-493

[76] Anhalt GJ, Labib RS, Voorhees JJ, Beals TF, Diaz LA. Induction of pemphigus in neonatal mice by passive transfer of IgG from patients with the disease. The New England Journal of Medicine. 1982;**306**:1189-1196

[77] Grando SA. Pemphigus autoimmunity: Hypotheses and realities. Autoimmunity. 2012;**45**:7-35. DOI: 10.3109/08916934.2011.606444

[78] Amagai M, Klaus-Kovtun V, Stanley JR. Autoantibodies against a novel epithelial cadherin in pemphigus vulgaris, a disease of cell adhesion. Cell. 1991;**67**:869-877

[79] Amagai M, Tsunoda K, Zillikens D, Nagai T, Nishikawa T. The clinical phenotype of pemphigus is defined by the anti-desmoglein autoantibody profile. Journal of The American Academy of Dermatology. 1999;**40**:167-170

[80] Endo H, Rees TD, Kuyama K, Matsue M, Yamamoto H. Use of oral exfoliative cytology to diagnose desquamative gingivitis: A pilot study. Quintessence International. 2008;**39**:e152-e161

[81] Endo H, Rees TD. Cinnamon products as a possible etiologic factor in orofacial granulomatosis. Medicina Oral Patologia Oral y Cirugia Bucal. 2007;**12**:E440-E444

[82] Kuttan NA, Narayana N, Moghadam BK. Desquamative stomatitis associated with routine use of oral health care products. General Dentistry. 2001;**49**:596-602

[83] Harpenau LA, Plemons JM, Rees TD. Effectiveness of a low dose of cyclosporine in the management of patients with oral erosive lichen planus. Oral Surgery, Oral Medicine, Oral Pathology, Oral Radiology, and Endodontics. 1995;**80**:161-167

[84] Stone SJ, Heasman PA, Staines KS, McCracken GI. The impact of structured plaque control for patients with gingival manifestations of oral lichen planus: A randomized controlled study. Journal of Clinical Periodontology. 2015;**42**:356-362. DOI: 10.1111/jcpe.12385

[85] Salgado DS, Jeremias F, Capela MV, Onofre MA, Massucato EM, Orrico SR. Plaque control improves the painful symptoms of oral lichen planus gingival lesions. A short-term study. Journal of Oral Pathology & Medicine. 2013;**42**:728-732. DOI: 10.1111/jop.12093

[86] Guiglia R, Di Liberto C, Pizzo G, et al. A combined treatment regimen for desquamative gingivitis in patients with oral lichen planus. Journal of Oral Pathology & Medicine. 2007;**36**:110-116

[87] Orrico SR, Navarro CM, Rosa FP, Reis FA, Salgado DS, Onofre MA. Periodontal treatment of benign mucous membrane pemphigoid. Dentistry Today. 2010;**29**:100-102; quiz 102-103

[88] Arduino PG, Lopetuso E, Carcieri P, et al. Professional oral hygiene treatment and detailed oral hygiene instructions in patients affected by mucous membrane pemphigoid with specific gingival localization: A pilot study in 12 patients. International Journal of Dental Hygiene. 2012;**10**:138-141. DOI: 10.1111/j.1601-5037.2011.00527.x

[89] Damoulis PD, Gagari E. Combined treatment of periodontal disease and benign mucous membrane pemphigoid. Case report with 8 years maintenance. Journal of Periodontology. 2000;**71**:1620-1629

[90] Akman A, Kacaroglu H, Yilmaz E, Alpsoy E. Periodontal status in patients with pemphigus vulgaris. Oral Diseases. 2008;**14**:640-643

[91] Arduino PG, Farci V, D'Aiuto F, et al. Periodontal status in oral mucous membrane pemphigoid: Initial results of a case-control study. Oral Diseases. 2011;**17**:90-94. DOI: 10.1111/j.1601-0825.2010.01709.x

[92] Tricamo MB, Rees TD, Hallmon WW, Wright JM, Cueva MA, Plemons JM. Periodontal status in patients with gingival mucous membrane pemphigoid. Journal of Periodontology. 2006;**77**:398-405

[93] Schellinck AE, Rees TD, Plemons JM, Kessler HP, Rivera-Hidalgo F, Solomon ES. A comparison of the periodontal status in patients with mucous membrane pemphigoid: A 5-year follow-up. Journal of Periodontology. 2009;**80**:1765-1773

[94] Pradeep AR, Manojkumar ST, Arjun R. Pemphigus vulgaris with significant periodontal findings: A case report. Journal of the California Dental Association. 2010;**38**:343-346

[95] Ramon-Fluixa C, Bagan-Sebastian J, Milian-Masanet M, Scully C. Periodontal status in patients with oral lichen planus: A study of 90 cases. Oral Diseases. 1999;**5**:303-306

[96] Lo Russo L, Guiglia R, Pizzo G, Fierro G, Ciavarella D, Lo Muzio L, Campisi G. Effect of desquamative gingivitis on periodontal status: A pilot study. Oral Diseases. 2010;**16**:102-107

[97] Lorenzana ER, Rees TD, Hallmon WW. Esthetic management of multiple recession defects in a patient with cicatricial pemphigoid. Journal of Periodontology. 2001;**72**:230-237

[98] Penarrocha M, Larrazabal C, Balaguer J, Serrano C, Silvestre J, Bagan JV. Restoration with implants in patients with recessive dystrophic epidermolysis bullosa and patient satisfaction with the implant-supported superstructure. The International Journal of Oral & Maxillofacial Implants. 2007;**22**:651-655

[99] Altin N, Ergun S, Katz J, Sancakli E, Koray M, Tanyeri H. Implant-supported oral rehabilitation of a patient with pemphigus vulgaris: A clinical report. Journal of Prosthodontics. 2013;**22**:581-586. DOI: 10.1111/jopr.12050

[100] Esposito SJ, Camisa C, Morgan M. Implant retained overdentures for two patients with severe lichen planus: A clinical report. Journal of Prosthetic Dentistry. 2003;**89**:6-10

[101] Toscano NJ, Holtzclaw DJ, Shumaker ND, Stokes SM, Meehan SC, Rees TD. Surgical considerations and management of patients with mucocutaneous disorders. Compendium of Continuing Education in Dentistry. 2010;**31**:344-350, 352-359; quiz 362, 364

Chapter 2

Periodontal Disease and Nuclear and Oxidative DNA Damage

Ana L. Zamora-Perez,
Guillermo M. Zúñiga-González,
Belinda C. Gómez-Meda, Blanca P. Lazalde-Ramos,
Yveth M. Ortiz-García, Gabriela Morales-Velazquez,
Celia Guerrero Velázquez and
María G. Sánchez-Parada

Additional information is available at the end of the chapter

http://dx.doi.org/10.5772/intechopen.68446

Abstract

Oral health is an important aspect of the overall health status of an individual. DNA damage has been associated with oral health and dental factors due to the increased of oxidative stress (OxS). DNA damage can produce a wide range of effects on human health. These effects could appear immediately, but others do not become evident much later. Chronic diseases have been study to understand their mechanisms, clinical implications, and the development of secondary disease such as cancer. Periodontitis is one of the most common oral diseases. It is an inflammatory chronic infectious disease, which is characterized by the loss of supporting tissues and tooth loss caused by periodontopathogens and long-term release of reactive oxygen species (ROS); thus, oxidative stress is increased during periodontitis. Oxidative stress can produce DNA damage, including the oxidation of nucleosides, which could cause DNA strand break. This oxidative damage leads the formation of micronuclei (MN) a marker of nuclear damage. Also, oxidative stress increased 8-hydroxy-2′-deoxyguanosine levels which are the most common stable product of oxidative DNA damage.

Keywords: periodontal disease, buccal mucosa, DNA damage, oxidative stress, saliva.

1. Introduction

DNA damage can generate many effects on human health and is the prime mechanism during carcinogenesis. Many of these effects could emerge directly, but others do not become evident until much later. Chronic diseases have been studied to understand their mechanisms of perpetuation of clinical complications and the development of secondary diseases such as cancer [1]. Oxidative stress (OxS) and, therefore, DNA damage has an important impact on the pathogenesis of chronic disease [2]. Periodontal diseases are inflammatory disorders characterized by gingival inflammation in which periodontopathic bacteria generate immunological inflammatory responses [3]. The OxS plays an important role in the pathogenesis of periodontitis, which can lead damage to genetic material [4]. Since periodontal disease is an example of the excess effects locally and systemically of OxS over production, the effect of periodontal disease over oxidative and nuclear DNA damage is the topic attended in this chapter.

2. Periodontitis

Moreover, dental caries, periodontal disease is one of the most prevalent oral diseases in the world and includes the major conditions gingivitis and periodontitis, which is a group of conditions affecting the supporting tissues of the teeth—the gingiva, periodontal ligament, cementum, and alveolar bone [1]. The reversible form of the disease, gingivitis, comprises inflammation of the gingival tissue without loss of alveolar bone. It is plaque induced and can be reversed with improved oral hygiene. In disease-susceptible individuals, gingivitis may develop into periodontitis, which is a chronic inflammatory condition of the gingiva causing destruction of connective tissue as well as of alveolar bone resulting in reduced support for the teeth and, ultimately, tooth loss (**Figure 1**) [5].

Periodontitis initiated by the complex interaction between the presence of periodontal pathogens (e.g., *Aggregatibacter actinomycetemcomitans, Porphyromonas gingivalis, Prevotella intermedia,* and *Fusobacterium nucleatum*) and host response [6]. Besides, the presence of periodontal pathogens associated with the progressive form of the disease, microbial by-products, the host immune response, environmental and behavior factors, and genetics may contribute the risk for developing periodontal disease [7].

Two main forms of periodontitis have been identified, chronic or aggressive, and are characterized by gingival inflammation and bleeding, periodontal pocket formation, destruction of

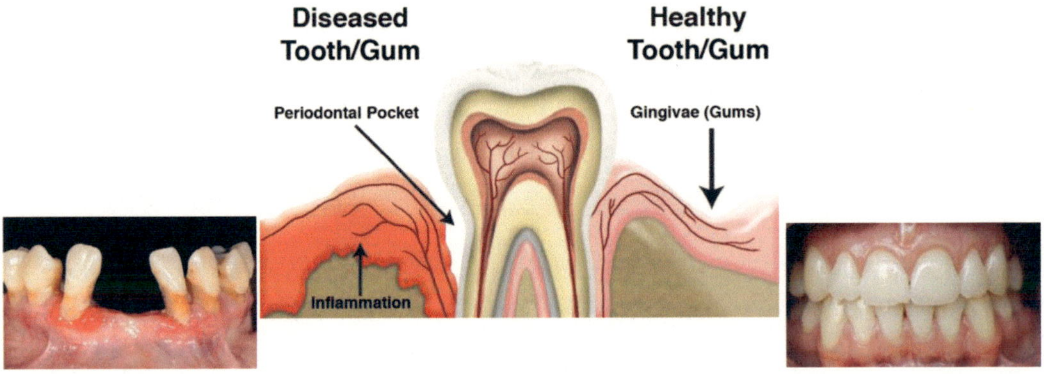

Figure 1. Characteristics of periodontitis. Healthy periodontal tissue (right) and periodontitis (left). Periodontitis is characterized by progressive and irreversible alveolar bone loss, and, ultimately, loosening and loss of teeth.

http://dx.doi.org/10.5772/intechopen.68446

connected tissues attachment, and alveolar bone loss. But, loss of connective tissue attachment is faster in aggressive periodontitis than in chronic periodontitis [8].

Moreover, the pathogenesis of periodontal diseases is mediated by the inflammatory response to bacteria in the dental biofilm. The inflammatory reaction that characterizes periodontitis is the complex interaction between periodontopathic bacteria and the host defense system, and its purpose is to protect the tissues from bacterial attack [6]. In periodontitis, neutrophil plays an important role in the initial host inflammation. Exaggerated neutrophil activity is the biological features characteristic of the periodontitis phenotype in agreement with a hyper-inflammatory host response. Thus, reactive oxygen species (ROS) produced from neutrophil are implicated in the destruction of periodontal tissue; therefore, oxidative stress (OxS) is enhanced during periodontitis [9].

3. Free radicals (FR) and oxidative stress

A free radical (FR) is any molecular species that contains at least one unpaired electron. The unpaired electron increased the chemical reactivity of an atom or molecule that generates a high instability. Due to the increase in FR, oxidative stress (OxS) arises. The OxS has been defined as a disturbance in the balance between the production of reactive oxygen/nitrogen species (ROS/RNS; FR) and the antioxidant defense system capacity to counteract their action [10]. The OxS occurs from an improved ROS/RNS generation or from a deterioration of the antioxidant protective ability. This process leads to the oxidation of biomolecules with consequent loss of its biological functions, whose manifestation is the potential oxidative damage to cells and tissues. Accumulation of ROS/RNS can result in several adverse effects such as lipid peroxidation, protein oxidation, and DNA damage (**Figure 2**) [11].

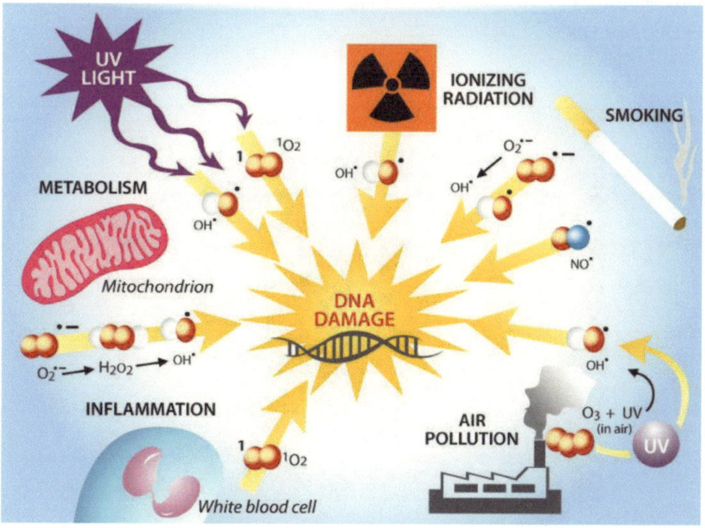

Figure 2. Sources of free radicals that arise oxidative stress.

4. Nuclear and oxidative DNA damage

DNA is chemically unstable and vulnerable to oxidation, due to its susceptibility to endogenous and exogenous damage. The endogenous genotoxic agents are mainly produced by cellular metabolism and composed of ROS and RNS, estrogen metabolites, and aldehydes produced by lipid peroxidation [12, 13]. The OxS leads to different lesions in DNA, including direct modification of nucleotide bases, training sites a purinic/a pyrimidinic, single strand break, the oxidation of nucleosides, which could cause DNA strand breaks; this type of damage could have teratogenic or carcinogenic consequences [14].

One method for measuring DNA nuclear damage is the micronuclei (MN) assay [15–17]. MN are extranuclear bodies originated from chromosome fragments or whole chromosome that spontaneously or because of clastogenic (agents who broke chromosome) or aneuploidogenic (disrupted the spindle apparatus) agents that were not incorporated into the nucleus after cell division (**Figure 3**) [18]. The MN formation leads to cell death, genomic instability, or cancer development. Therefore, the increased in MN frequency is linking to environmental and occupational exposure to genotoxic agents, lifestyle, genetic profile cancer, and occurrence of other diseases, and MN screening is considered as a biomarker of DNA nuclear damage [19].

On the other hand, different markers of oxidative DNA damage have been identified. The most popular markers were designed for lipid peroxidation, such as malondialdehye (MDA), oxidized low-density lipoprotein (LDL), MDA-modified LDL, among other. In recent years, 8-hydroxy-2′-deoxyguanosine (8-OHdG or 8-oxodG) has appeared as a marker of oxidative stress in body fluids [20]. The 8-OHdG is the most common stable product of oxidative DNA damage caused by ROS. Among all purine and pyridine bases, guanine is most susceptible to oxidation. Hydroxyl radical addition to the eighth position of the molecule leads to the formation of guanine-modified product 8-OHdG (**Figure 4**) [21]. Oxidative-modified DNA in the form of 8-OHdG can be quantified to indicate the extent damage to genetic material is the most frequent and most mutagenic lesion in nuclear DNA and is important in mutagenesis and carcinogenesis processes [22].

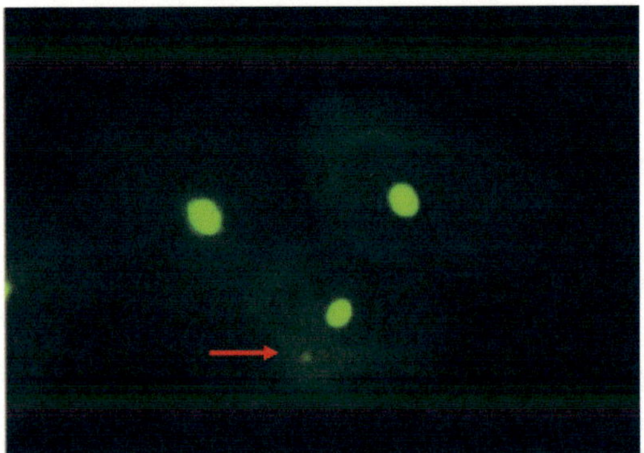

Figure 3. MN in buccal mucosa cells (oil-immersion objective 60x, acridine orange stain).

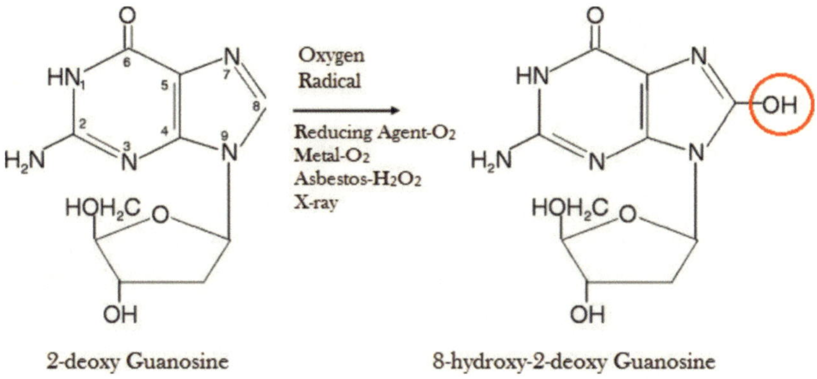

Figure 4. 8-OHdG formation by oxygen radicals.

5. Periodontitis and OxS: nuclear and oxidative DNA damage

The OxS plays an important role in the pathology of several diseases, including arthritis, Alzheimer's disease, diabetes, Parkinson's disease, and more recently periodontitis. The OxS is a phenomenon that occurs within the periodontal disease and has been linked with both onset of periodontal tissue destruction [23] and systemic inflammation [24]. Inflammatory periodontal disease resulting in tissue damage is mediated by ROS which are formed during the phagocytosis of periodontopathic bacteria by polymorphonuclear leukocytes. ROS generation can occur through different mechanisms such as protein disruption, lipid peroxidation, induction of proinflammatory cytokines, and DNA damage [22]. Therefore, periodontitis is associated with OxS which in turn can lead to nuclear and oxidative DNA damage and thus the formation of MN and 8-OHdG [25].

Some authors have been demonstrated that individual with periodontal disease exhibited an increase in the frequency of MN, which is directly related to DNA damage [25–27]. Similarly, elevated MN frequency has been reported in patients with cancer [28], rheumatoid arthritis [29], autoimmune diseases [30], and premature aging syndrome [31]. The presence of MN in a cell is an indicator of DNA damage and genetic instability, and it could be associated with the collateral complications in these patients and with future risk of cancer development in humans.

On the other hand, 8-OHdG level has been studies in oral pathologies, including periodontal disease [25, 32–35] and oral cancer [36]. As described above, in periodontitis OxS because of the formation of ROS, which is stimulated by neutrophils, produce damage of the bone-supporting tissues. The exceeds of ROS levels, the reduction of antioxidant enzyme activity, and defects in DNA reparation mechanism led to increased oxidative DNA damage [35].

8-OHdG is used as a standard biomarker of oxidative-induced DNA damage mainly because of its reliable detectability. Elevated levels of 8-OHdG from cancer patients compared with healthy subjects have been observed in lung cancer [37], basal cell carcinoma [38], colorectal cancer [39], bladder cancer [40], and renal cell carcinoma [41]. With respect to periodontitis, published data on oxidative damage to DNA have been reported by many authors around the world who investigated 8-OHdG levels in the saliva of periodontitis patients [4, 25, 33, 34]. These studies demonstrated that salivary levels of 8-OHdG in samples from periodontitis patients were significantly higher than those from periodontally healthy controls and indicated that salivary 8-OHdG levels may be a useful marker for disease activity and may be indirectly reflect disease severity parameters [4, 25, 33, 34].

Also, a study report significant positive correlation between MN frequency (a marker of nuclear damage) and 8-OHdG enzyme levels in subjects with periodontitis. This finding could suggest that these variables are associated and can be hypothesized that they could be linked in the development of periodontal disease [25]. The augmented 8-OHdG levels might indicate early oxidative mitochondrial DNA damage [33], and mitochondrial DNA undertakes OxS early than nuclear DNA [42].

6. Conclusion

Periodontal diseases are prevalent in human populations and represent a significant public health problem [43], and oxidative damage plays an important function in the pathogeny of the disease [9]. Nuclear and oxidative DNA damage area increased in subjects with periodontal disease, and genetic damage is a critical event not only in the initiation phase but also in the promotion and progression phases, which could be related to carcinogenesis events. Moreover, recent studies have associated periodontitis with some cancer including head and neck cancer [44], pancreatic cancer [45], colon cancer [46], and orodigestive cancers [47], which are relevant to the control of this disease and to promote the importance of good oral health.

Author details

Ana L. Zamora-Perez[1]*, Guillermo M. Zúñiga-González[2], Belinda C. Gómez-Meda[3], Blanca P. Lazalde-Ramos[4], Yveth M. Ortiz-García[1], Gabriela Morales-Velazquez[1], Celia Guerrero Velázquez[1] and María G. Sánchez-Parada[5]

*Address all correspondence to: anazamora@gmail.com

1 Institute of Dentistry Research, University Center for Health Science, University of Guadalajara, Guadalajara, Jalisco, Mexico

2 Mutagenesis Laboratory, Western Biomedical Research Center, Mexican Institute of Social Security, Guadalajara, Jalisco, Mexico

3 Department of Molecular Biology and Genomics, Institute of Molecular Biology in Medicine and Gene Therapy, University Center of Health Sciences, University of Guadalajara, Guadalajara, Jalisco, Mexico

4 Academic Unit of Chemical Sciences, Autonomous University of Zacatecas, Zacatecas, Mexico

5 Health Science Department, University Center of Tonalá, Tonalá, Jalisco, Mexico

References

[1] Yfjord JE, Bodvarsdottir SK. Genomic instability and cancer: Networks involved in response to DNA damage. Mutation Research. 2005;**592**:18-28. DOI:10.1016/j.mrfmmm.2005.05.010

[2] Wu LL, Chiou CC, Chang PY, Wu JT. Urinary 8-OHdG: A marker of oxidative stress to DNA and a risk factor for cancer, atherosclerosis and diabetics. Clinical Chimica Acta. 2004;**339**:1-9. DOI: 10.1016/j.cccn.2003.09.010

[3] Papapanou PN. Epidemiology of periodontal diseases: An update. International Academy of Periodontology. 1999;**1**:110-116.

[4] Sezer U, Ciçek Y, Canakçi CF. Increased salivary levels of 8-hydroxydeoxyguanosine may be a marker for disease activity for periodontitis. Disease Markers. 2012;**32**:165-172. DOI:10.3233/DMA-2011-0876

[5] Yucel-Lindberg T, Båge T. Inflammatory mediators in the pathogenesis of periodontitis. Expert Reviews in Molecular Medicine. 2013;**5**:15:e7. DOI:10.1017/erm.2013.8

[6] Kornman KS. Mapping the pathogenesis of periodontitis: A new look. Journal of Periodontology. 2008;**79:**1560-1568. DOI: 10.1902/jop.2008.080213

[7] Seymour GJ. Possible mechanisms involved in the immunoregulation of chronic inflammatory periodontal disease. Journal of Dental Research. 1987;**66**:2-9. DOI: 10.1177/00220345870660010401

[8] Savage A, Eaton KA, Moles DR, Needleman I. A systematic review of definitions of periodontitis and methods that have been used to identify this disease. Journal of Clinical Periodontology. 2009;**36**:458-467. DOI: 10.1111/j.1600-051X.2009.01408.x

[9] Chapple IL, Matthews JB. The role of reactive oxygen and antioxidant species in periodontal tissue destruction. Periodontology. 2000. 2007;**43**:160-232. DOI: 10.1111/j.1600-0757.2006.00178.x

[10] Betteridge DJ. What is oxidative stress? Metabolism. 2000;**49**:3-8.

[11] Lafleur MV, Retel J. Contrasting effects of SH-compounds on oxidative DNA damage: Repair and increase of damage. Mutation Research. 1993;**295**:1-10. DOI:10.1016/0921-8734(93)90006-O

[12] De Bont R, van Larebeke N. Endogenous DNA damage in humans: A review of quantitative data. Mutagenesis. 2004;**19**:169-185.

[13] Pisoschi AM, Pop A. The role of antioxidants in the chemistry of oxidative stress: A review. European Journal of Medicinal Chemistry 2015;**97**:55-74. DOI: 10.1016/j.ejmech.2015.04.040

[14] Yfjord JE, Bodvarsdottir SK. Genomic instability and cancer: Networks involved in response to DNA damage. Mutation Research. 2005;**592**:18-28. DOI:10.1016/j.mrfmmm.2005.05.010

[15] Torres-Bugarın O, Covarrubias-Bugarın R, Zamora-Perez AL, Torres-Mendoza BM, García-Ulloa M, Martínez-Sandoval FG. Anabolic androgenic steroids induce micronuclei in buccal mucosa cells of bodybuilders. British Journal of Sports Medicine. 2007;**41**:592-596. DOI: 10.1136/bjsm.2006.032474

[16] Zúñiga-González GM, Batista-González CM, Gómez-Meda BC Zamora-Perez AL, Muñoz-Magallanes T, Ramos-Valdés C, Gallegos-Arreola MP. Micronuclei in diabetes: Folate supplementation diminishes micronuclei in diabetic patients but not in an animal model. Mutation Research. 2007;**634**:126-134. DOI:10.1016/j.mrgentox.2007.06.006

[17] Zamora-Perez AL, Mariaud-Schmidt RP, Fuentes-Lerma MG, Guerrero-Velázquez C, Gómez-Meda BC, López-Verdín S, Zúñiga-González GM. Increased number of micronuclei and nuclear anomalies in buccal mucosa cells from people exposed to alcohol-containing mouthwash. Drug and Chemical Toxicology. 2013;**36**:255-260. DOI: 10.3109/01480545.2012.737804

[18] Heddle JA, Cimino MC, Hayashi M, Romagna F, Shelby MD, Tucker JD, Vanparys P, MacGregor JT. Micronuclei as an index of cytogenetic damage: Past, present and future. Environmental and Molecular Mutagenesis. 1991;**18**:227-291.

[19] Bonassi S, Ugolini D, Kirsch-Volders M, Strömberg U, Vermeulen R, Tucker JD. Human population studies with cytogenetic biomarkers: Review of the literature and future prospectives. Environmental and Molecular Mutagenesis. 2005;**45**:258-270.

[20] Sosa V, Moline T, Somoza R, Paciucci R, Kondoh H, LLeonart ME. Oxidative stress and cancer: An overview. Ageing Research Reviews. 2013;**12**:376-390. DOI: 10.1016/j.arr.2012.10.004

[21] Di Minno A, Turnu L, Porro B, Squellerio I, Cavalca V, Tremoli E, Di Minno MN. 8-Hydroxy-2-deoxyguanosine levels and heart failure: A systematic review and meta-analysis of the literature. Nutrition, Metabolism & Cardiovascular Diseases. 2016;**16**:30194-30196. DOI: 10.1016/j.numecd.2016.10.009

[22] Evans MD, Cooke MS. Factors contributing to the outcome of oxidative damage to nucleic acids. Bioessays. 2004;**26**:533-542. DOI: 10.1002/bies.20027

[23] Chapple IL, Matthews JB. The role of reactive oxygen and antioxidant species in periodontal tissue destruction. Periodontology. 2000. 2007;**43**:160-232. DOI: 10.1111/j.1600-0757.2006.00178.x

[24] Lamster IB, Pagan M. Periodontal disease and the metabolic syndrome. International Dental Journal. 2016;**67**:67-77. DOI: 10.1111/idj.12264

[25] Zamora-Perez AL, Ortiz-García YM, Lazalde-Ramos BP, Guerrero-Velázquez C, Gómez-Meda BC, Ramírez-Aguilar MÁ, Zúñiga-González GM. Increased micronuclei and nuclear abnormalities in buccal mucosa and oxidative damage in saliva from patients with chronic and aggressive periodontal diseases. Journal of Periodontology Research. 2015;**50**:28-36. DOI: 10.1111/jre.12175

[26] Bastos-Aires D, Azevedo A, Pereira ML, Perez-Mongiovi D, Teixeira A. Preliminary study of micronuclei levels in oral exfoliated cells from patients with periodontitis. Journal of Dental Sciences. 2013;**8**:200-204. DOI:10.1016/j.jds.2012.12.007

[27] D'Agostini F, Calcagno E, Micale RT, La Maestra S, De Flora S, Cingano L. Cytogenetic analysis of gingival epithelial cells, as related to smoking habits and occurrence of periodontal disease. International Journal of Hygiene and Environmental Health. 2013;**216**:71-75. DOI: 10.1016/j.ijheh.2012.01.005

[28] Duffaud F, Orsière T, Villani P, Pelissier AL, Volot F, Favre R, Botta A. Comparison between micronucleated lymphocyte rates observed in healthy subjects and cancer patients. Mutagenesis. 1997;**12**:227-231.

[29] Ramos-Remus C, Dorazco-Barragan G, Aceves-Avila FJ, Alcaraz-Lopez F, Fuentes-Ramirez F, Michel-Diaz J, Torres-Bugarin O, Ventura-Aguilar A, Zuñiga-González G. Genotoxicity assessment using micronuclei assay in rheumatoid arthritis patients. Clinical and Experimental Rheumatology. 2002;**20**:208-212.

[30] Milenkova M, Milanov I, Kmetska K, Deleva S, Popova L, Hadjidekova V, Groudeva V, Hadjidekova S, Domínguez I. Chromosomal radiosensitivity in patients with multiple sclerosis. Mutation Research. 2013;**749**:3-8. DOI: 10.1016/j.mrfmmm.2013.08.004

[31] Weirich-Schwaiger H, Weirich HG, Gruber B, Schweiger M, Hirsch-Kauffmann M. Correlation between senescence and DNA repair in cells from young and old individuals and in premature aging syndromes. Mutation Research. 1994;**316**:37-48. DOI:10.1016/0921-8734(94)90006-X

[32] Akalın FA, Baltacıoglu E, Alver A, Karabulut E. Lipid peroxidation levels and total oxidant status in serum, saliva and gingival crevicular fluid in patients with chronic periodontitis. Journal of Clinical Periodontology. 2007;**34**:558-565. DOI: 10.1111/j.1600-051X.2007.01091.x

[33] Takane M, Sugano N, Iwasaki H. New biomarker evidence of oxidative DNA damage in whole saliva from clinically healthy and periodontally diseased individuals. Journal of Periodontology. 2002;**73**:551-554. DOI: 10.1902/jop.2002.73.5.551

[34] Canakçi CF, Canakçi V, Tatar A, Eltas A, Sezer U, Ciçek Y, Oztas S. Increased salivary level of 8-hydroxydeoxyguanosine is a marker of premature oxidative mitochondrial DNA damage in gingival tissue of patients with periodontitis. Archivum Immunologiae et Therapiae Experimentalis (Warsz). 2009;**57**:205-211. DOI: 10.1007/s00005-009-0026-9

[35] Su H, Gornitsky M, Velly AM, Yu H, Benarroch M, Schipper HM. Salivary DNA, lipid, and protein oxidation in nonsmokers with periodontal disease. Free Radical Biology and Medicine. 2009;**46**:914-921.

[36] Bahar G, Feinmesser R, Shpitzer T, Popovtzer A, Nagler RM. Salivary analysis in oral cancer patients: DNA and protein oxidation, reactive nitrogen species, and antioxidant profile. Cancer. 2007;**109**:54-59. DOI: 10.1002/cncr.22386

[37] Erhola M, Toyokuni S, Okada K, Tanaka T, Hiai H, Ochi H, Uchida K, Osawa T, Nieminen MM, Alho H, Kellokumpu-Lehtinen P. Biomarker evidence of DNA oxidation in lung cancer patients: Association of urinary 8-hydroxy-2'-deoxyguanosine excretion with radiotherapy, chemotherapy, and response to treatment. FEBS Letter. 1997;**409**:287-291. DOI: 10.1016/S0014-5793(97)00523-1

[38] Kinoshita A, Wanibuchi H, Morimura K, Wei M, Shen J, Imaoka S, Funae Y, Fukushima S. Phenobarbital at low dose exerts hormesis in rat hepatocarcinogenesis by reducing oxidative DNA damage, altering cell proliferation, apoptosis and gene expression. Carcinogenesis. 2003;**24**:1389-1399. DOI: 10.1093/carcin/bgg079

[39] Sato T, Takeda H, Otake S, Yokozawa J, Nishise S, Fujishima S, Orii T, Fukui T, Takano J, Sasaki Y, Nagino K, Iwano D, Yaoita T, Kawata S. Increased plasma levels of 8-hydroxy-deoxyguanosine are associated with development of colorectal tumors. Journal of Clinical Biochemistry and Nutrition. 2010;**47**:59-63. DOI: 10.3164/jcbn.10-12

[40] Chiou CC, Chang PY, Chan EC, Wu TL, Tsao KC, Wu JT. Urinary 8-hydroxydeoxyguanosine and its analogs as DNA marker of oxidative stress: Development of an ELISA and measurement in both bladder and prostate cancers. Clinical Chimica Acta. 2003;**334**:87-94. DOI: 10.1016/S0009-8981(03)00191-8

[41] Wada T, Tanji N, Ozawa A, Wang J, Shimamoto K, Sakayama K, Yokoyama M. Mitochondrial DNA mutations and 8-hydroxy-2'-deoxyguanosine Content in Japanese patients with urinary bladder and renal cancers. Anticancer Research. 2006;**26**:3403-3408

[42] Nomoto K, Tsuneyama K, Takahashi H, Murai Y, Takano Y. Cytoplasmic fine granular expression of 8-hydroxydeoxyguanosine reflects early mitochondrial oxidative DNA damage in nonalcoholic fatty liver disease. Applied Immunohistochemistry & Molecular Morphology. 2008;**16**:71-75. DOI: 10.1097/PAI.0b013e31803156d5

[43] Bloching M, Reich W, Schubert J, Grummt T, Sandner A. The influence of oral hygiene on salivary quality in the Ames Test, as a marker for genotoxic effects. Oral Oncology 2007;**43**:933-939. DOI: 10.1016/j.oraloncology.2006.11.006

[44] Gondivkar SM, Gondivkar RS, Gadbail AR, Chole R, Mankar M, Yuwanati M. Chronic periodontitis and the risk of head and neck squamous cell carcinoma: Facts and figures. Experimental Oncology. 2013;**35**:163-167.

[45] Michaud DS, Joshipura K, Giovannucci E, Fuchs CS. A prospective study of periodontal disease and pancreatic cancer in US male health professionals. Journal of National Cancer Institute. 2007;**99**:171-175. DOI: 10.1093/jnci/djk021

[46] Kostic AD, Gevers D, Pedamallu CS, Michaud M, Duke F, Earl AM, Ojesina AI, Jung J, Bass AJ, Tabernero J, Baselga J, Liu C, Shivdasani RA, Ogino S, Birren BW, Huttenhower C, Garrett WS, Meyerson M. Genomic analysis identifies association of Fusobacterium with colorectal carcinoma. Genome Research. 2012;**22**:292-298. DOI: 10.1101/gr.126573.111

[47] Ahn J, Segers S, Hayes RB. Periodontal disease, porphyromonas gingivalis serum antibody levels and orodigestive cancer mortality. Carcinogenesis. 2012;**33**:1055-1058. DOI: 10.1093/carcin/bgs112

Chapter 3

Oral and Periodontal Diseases in Consanguineous Marriages

Metin Çalisir

Additional information is available at the end of the chapter

http://dx.doi.org/10.5772/intechopen.68801

Abstract

Periodontitis is defined as an inflammatory disease of supporting tissues of teeth characterized by progressive destruction of the periodontal ligament and alveolar bone. Periodontal manifestations of these genetic disorders or syndromes, such as familial and cyclic neutropenias, granulomatous disease, agranulocytosis, Langerhans' cell disease, glycogen storage disease, hypophosphatasia, leucocyte adhesion deficiency, and Papillon-Lefèvre, Chédiak-Higashi, Cohen, Ehlers-Danlos, Marfan, Down, Haim-Munk, and Kindlers syndromes, imitate some types of periodontal diseases. Most of these syndromes have autosomal-recessive characterization and can be seen commonly in consanguineous marriages. Therefore, consanguineous marriages have generally been accepted as having important detrimental effects on offspring. There is a lot of genetic research about consanguineous marriage and its detrimental effects on offspring. Although consanguineous marriages are common in the world, the relationship with oral and periodontal diseases has not been thoroughly investigated. We do not have enough of an understanding of the effects of consanguineous marriage on oral and periodontal diseases. In this chapter, previous studies in the literature related to this subject will be investigated and evaluated, and then this research will be related to oral and periodontal diseases. Therefore, this chapter will guide further research. The aim of this chapter is to show the relation between consanguineous marriages and oral-periodontal diseases.

Keywords: periodontal diseases, genetic disorders related with periodontitis, consanguinity

1. Introduction

1.1. Oral and periodontal health

Etymologically, the word "health" was reproduced from the Old English "hale" and means wholesome, sound, or well-being [1]. Although there is significant improvement in oral health in developed countries, oral disease still persists as a global problem, especially among underprivileged groups in both developing and developed countries [2]. The global public health problems associated with oral disease are a serious burden on governments [3]. In the Preamble to the Constitution of the World Health Organization (WHO) [4, 5], health was described as "a state of complete physical, mental and social well-being and not merely the absence of disease or infirmity." Moreover, the Preamble proposes: "The enjoyment of the highest attainable standard of health is one of the fundamental rights of every human being without distinction of race, religion, political belief, economic or social condition." Therefore, the WHO suggests that complete health should be an endpoint that people and society should struggle to achieve. At the Ottawa Charter for Health Promotion (1986), the WHO added that "health is a resource for everyday life, not the objective of living." This means that health is a necessity for people's daily lives. "Health promotion is the process of enabling people to increase control over, and to improve, their health." For this purpose, government and health care workers have important duties to extend health services for people. What is "complete physical and mental health" and "absence of disease or infirmity"? Unfortunately, these questions have not been—and probably never will be—answered satisfactorily [1].

Tooth caries, periodontal diseases, loss of teeth, oral mucosal lesions, and cancers are some of the major oral health problems that the public face. Pain and trouble with eating, chewing, smiling, speaking, and communication due to discolored, rotten, or missing teeth are factors that adversely affect people's everyday lives [6]. Periodontal diseases have historically been considered one of the most important global oral health burdens for governments [7, 8].

Periodontal health means the absence of any clinical signs and symptoms of current or past periodontal disease [1]. For many patients, healthy periodontium is comfortable and free of functional and aesthetic problems [9]. The American Academy of Periodontology (AAP) has defined health as "the condition of a patient when there is function without evidence of disease or abnormality" (AAP 2001). It could be said one has periodontal health if there are no disease signs and symptoms of periodontal tissues. The diagnosis of periodontal disease is usually documented by the presence of bleeding on probing (BOP), probing pocket depth (PPD), and clinical attachment level (CAL) loss. However, other symptoms of periodontal disease include the results of chronic gingival inflammation and the destruction of tooth-supporting tissues, such as redness, bleeding on brushing, loosening of affected teeth, and persistent bad breath [10]. These symptoms affect the quality of daily life of people.

2. Classification system for periodontal diseases and conditions

The most commonly accepted systems of classification of periodontal disease have been offered by the American Academy of Periodontology (AAP). (*International Workshop for Classification of Periodontal Diseases in 1999*) [11].

Partial list of periodontal disease which may be associated with genetic conditions has been given below [11].

(1) **Gingival lesions of genetic origin**

   (a) Hereditary gingival fibromatosis

   (b) Other

(2) **Chronic periodontitis**

   (a) Localized chronic periodontitis

   (b) Generalized chronic periodontitis

(3) **Aggressive periodontitis**

   (a) Localized aggressive periodontitis

   (b) Generalized aggressive periodontitis

(4) **Periodontitis as a manifestation of systemic diseases**

   (a) **Associated with hematologic disorders**

   - Acquired neutropenia
   - Leukemias
   - Other

   (b) **Associated with genetic disorders**

   - Familial and cyclic neutropenia
   - Down's syndrome
   - Leukocyte adhesion deficiency syndromes
   - Papillon-Lefévre syndrome
   - Chediak-Higashi syndrome

- Langerhans cell disease (histiocytosis syndromes)
- Glycogen storage disease
- Chronic granulomatous disease
- Infantile genetic agranulocytosis
- Cohen syndrome
- Ehlers-Danlos syndrome (types IV and VIII)
- Hypophosphatasia
- Crohn disease (inflammatory bowel disease)
- Marfan syndrome
- Other

(c) **Not otherwise specified (NOS)**

2.1. Periodontitis

Periodontal diseases are major global oral health problems that occur on teeth and tissues around the teeth. One of the most common periodontal disease is periodontitis. Periodontitis starts first on gingiva and progresses to periodontal ligament and alveolar bone, which causes the degradation of supporting tissues of teeth and eventually leads to loss of teeth [12]. Periodontitis is primarily caused by pathogenic microorganisms in the biofilm. The other predisposing factors are genetic and environmental factors [13].

The shifting of the nucleotides in the genes can lead to periodontitis. Susceptibility to periodontitis among patients is different [14]. The correlation between genetic composition and periodontal diseases is complex and not clearly explained [11]. Only a special gene is not correlated with the all mechanisms of the disease [14]. Family history is a criterion for periodontal diseases that must be taken into consideration [11]. Although the family aggregation may be affected by both genetic and environmental factors, studies on twins reared apart have shown that genetic factors are effective parameters for diseases [15].

According to the studies on monozygotic and dizygotic twins, 50% of variance in periodontal disease has been associated with genetic factors [16]. Also, genetic factors have an important role on the balance between protective and destructive chemical mediators [17, 18]. Genetic components may determine the roles of the immune system, host response, and cytokines in periodontal disease [19]. Researchers who have investigated the genetic effect on periodontal diseases have focused on familial aggregation and genetic components of aggressive periodontitis (AP) [20], periodontitis associated with Mendelian-inherited diseases [20], twin research [15, 21], and segregation analysis and linkage studies [22, 23].

2.1.1. Genetic studies on chronic periodontitis and aggressive periodontitis

Chronic periodontitis (CP) is the most common type of periodontitis and shows a slow rate of progression. It can begin in adolescence but usually does not become clinically significant until 35 years of age [24, 25]. There is no proven genetic determinant for patients with chronic periodontitis in any research. To determine the role of genetic factors in chronic periodontitis, twin and family studies are the optimal methods [26].

In a study, chronic periodontitis was shown to be 50% of heritable [16]. Chronic periodontitis has shown familial heredity in a Dutch population epidemiological study [27]. Also, there is some evidence that shows a correlation between IL-1, IL-6, IL-10, VDR, and CD14 genes and chronic periodontitis susceptibility [26]. IL-1 polymorphisms have been associated with severity of periodontitis [28, 29].

Aggressive periodontitis (AP) is a type of periodontitis that is characterized by destruction of periodontal tissues and alveolar bone, despite the presence of a small amount of dental plaque. It occurs in systemically healthy individuals who are generally younger in age, but patients may be older [11]. There are two types of aggressive periodontitis. Generalized and localized forms of aggressive periodontitis are rare types of periodontal disease that first occur with rapid attachment and bone loss and tend to appear in the families [30]. The prevalence of localized aggressive periodontitis (LAP) is less than 1% and that of generalized aggressive periodontitis (GAP) is 0.13%. Black populations are at higher risk than whites; male population is at higher risk of GAP than females [31].

Both genetic and environmental factors have crucial roles in the occurrence of these diseases. Chronic periodontitis and aggressive periodontitis are also affected by the combined effects of environmental and genetic factors [32, 33].

Although the familial aggregation of aggressive periodontitis is known, the mode of inheritance is still unclear. Family linkage studies have informed different modes of inheritance such as X-linked-dominant [34], autosomal-dominant [23], autosomal-recessive [22], or both X-linked-dominant and autosomal-dominant [35].

Polymorphisms in the cytokine genes, such as interleukin-1 receptor antagonist (*IL-1RN*) and interleukin-4 (*IL-4*), have been found to be positively correlated with aggressive periodontitis [36, 37]. A combination of two alleles of interleukin, *IL-1A*$^{-889}$ and *IL-1B*$^{+3954}$, have been found associated with aggressive periodontitis [38–40]. *IL-4-590* T/T, *IL-4-34* T/T genotype, *IL-6-174*G allele, and *IL-6-572* C/G polymorphism are associated with aggressive periodontitis [41, 42]. A relationship between *IL-6-1363,-1480* polymorphism and LAP susceptibility has been found [43].

IL-10 promoter polymorphisms at positions −1082 G-A, −819C-T, and −590C-A [44] and FPR348 T-C gene polymorphism in African-American people [45] are potential risk indicators for GAP. It is said that Fc gamma RIIIb-NA2 allele and Fc gamma RIIIb-NA2/NA2 genotype, composite genotype FcaRIIIb-NA2/NA2, FCgammaRIIIa-H/H131 [46], and FCgamma polymorphisms [47] may lead to aggressive periodontitis. IL-1 (IL-1α and IL-1β) genes genotype-positive individuals have higher levels of virulent bacterial complexes. The number of virulent bacterial species in deep pockets is seen at higher levels in IL-1 genes genotype-positive people than genotype-negative people [48].

Angiotensinogen, cathepsin C, E-selectin, formyl peptide receptor, NADPH oxidase, plasminogen activator inhibitor 1, calprotectin, tissue inhibitor of matrix metalloproteinase 2, and tissue plasminogen activator have been correlated with aggressive periodontitis [49]. TLR-4 399 Ile polymorphism has shown a protective effect against aggressive periodontitis in contrast to chronic periodontitis [50]. HLA-DR4 gene polymorphism is found in higher frequency in rapidly progressive periodontitis patients, and HLA-A9, B-15 gene polymorphisms are found to be significantly elevated [51, 52]. HLA-DQB1 plays a crucial role in pathogenesis of aggressive periodontitis [53].

2.1.2. Role of genetic factors in periodontitis as a manifestation of systemic diseases

Periodontal diseases include a wider spectrum of diseases than just periodontitis. Some periodontal diseases are affected by genetic variations. Thus, it could be said that genetic factors play a crucial role in periodontal health and disease (**Table 1**) [16, 54].

Syndrome	Mutated gene	Chromosome region
Ehlers-Danlos syndrome	Collagen alpha-1(V) gene (COL5A1) or the collagen alpha-2(V) gene (COL5A2) Type III collagen for EDS type IV, unknown for EDS type VIII	9q34, 2q31
Papillon-Lefévre syndrome and Haim-Munk syndrome	Cathepsin C (CTSC gene) (dipeptidyl aminopeptidase)	11q14.1–q14.3
Hypophosphatasia	ALPL, tissue non-specific alkaline phosphatase	1p36.12
Chediak-Higashi syndrome	Lysosomal trafficking regulator CHS1/LYST, abnormal transport of vesicles to and from neutrophil lysozyme caused by mutations in lysosomal trafficking regulator gene (LYST)	1q42.1–q42.2
Leukocyte adhesion deficiency type I	Beta-2 integrin chain	21q22.3
Leukocyte adhesion deficiency type II	GDP-fucose transporter-1	11p11.2
Congenital and cyclic neutropenia	ELANE	19p13.3
Glycogen storage disease	SLC37A4	11q23.3
Down syndrome	Multiple, vertical trisomic regions at least 5Mb (megabase) long	Trisomy 21

Table 1. Some syndromes with clinical manifestations of severe periodontitis.

http://dx.doi.org/10.5772/intechopen.68801

3. Consanguineous marriages

Linguistically, the word "consanguinity" is reproduced from two Latin words: "con" meaning common or shared and "sanguineus" meaning blood. The meaning of consanguineous marriage is a relationship between biologically related individuals. As a clinical genetic term, "a consanguineous marriage" is a union between couples who are related as second cousins or closer [55–57]. The terms of inbreeding and consanguinity are used to define relations between couples who have at least one common ancestor [58, 59]. It is estimated that more than one billion of the global population who live in different communities and countries prefer consanguineous marriage [56, 60]. At present, this rate corresponds about 20% of world populations [56]. Categories of consanguineous marriages are different (**Figure 1**).

Consanguinity rates differ in communities depending on religion, culture, and geography. The prevalence is high among Middle Eastern and Arab citizens [61]. The highest rates of consanguineous marriages in the world are seen in many Arab countries where 20–50% of all marriages include consanguineous marriages, especially first cousin marriages [62]. In developed countries, the rate of consanguineous marriage has decreased to a low level but includes different ethnic groups, some of which continue to practice their traditional cultural habits [63]. It is commonly accepted that consanguinity is more prevalent among underprivileged persons in poor communities [64–66]. Education level and socio-economic status of the persons may have a potential effect on consanguinity [67].

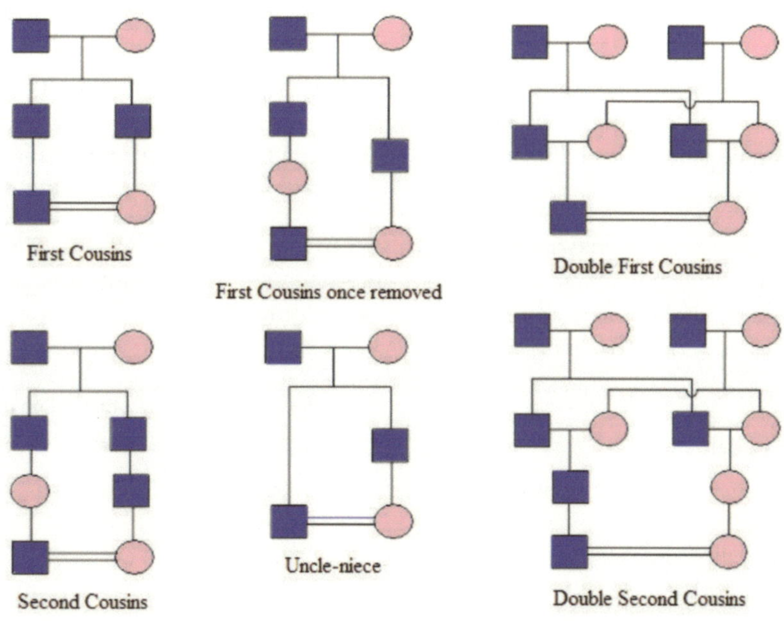

Figure 1. Categories of consanguineous marriages.

Studies of consanguineous marriage and genetic disorders have yielded conflicting results [68, 69]. The correlation between relationship and proportion of genes is as follows [70] (**Table 2**).

Research on the association between consanguinity and the different parameters of oral and periodontal health is limited, both in quantity and in quality [71].

Consanguineous marriage leads to increased genetic homogeneity of inbred individuals. Inbred individuals have similar paternal and maternal genetic materials. The detrimental effects of inbreeding are the result of homozygosity of harmful genes [58].

Consanguineous marriages have generally been accepted as having important detrimental effects on offspring [72, 73]. Some of the rare autosomal-recessive diseases can commonly be seen in consanguineous marriages. Health workers should be aware of these conditions and should inform patients about possible syndromes [73, 74].

The high consanguinity rates in communities could induce the expression of autosomal-recessive diseases. These include very rare or new syndromes. Therefore, health workers must be aware of the risks associated with consanguineous marriages. Currently, many young consanguineous couples planning to have children are afraid of the consequences of consanguinity for their offspring [74].

If there is a closer biological relationship between parents, identical copies of one or more detrimental recessive gene will be transferred to their offspring [73]. If one of the parents is affected, in general, consanguineous marriage does not increase the risk for autosomal-dominant conditions in offspring [75].

If parents are not related, their offspring have a 2–3% possibility of inheriting detrimental genes. If parents are first cousins, their offspring have up to 5–6% possibility of inheriting detrimental genes because they will both transport the same autosomal-recessive mutation. If parents are consanguineous, no increased rate is observed for X-linked or autosomal-dominant genes [70].

Although consanguineous marriages are common in the world, the effects on oral diseases have not been thoroughly investigated. We do not have enough of an understanding of the effects of consanguineous marriage on oral and periodontal diseases.

Relationship	**Relationship degree**	**Proportion of genes**
Identical (monozygotic) twins		100%
Brothers and sisters, non-identical (dizygotic) twins, parents and children	First degree (1°)	½, 50%
Uncles and aunts, nephews and nieces, grandparents and half-brothers and half-sisters	Second degree (2°)	¼, 25%
First cousins, half-uncles and aunts and half-nephews and nieces	Third degree (3°)	1/8, 12.5%

Table 2. Proportion of genes among the relatives [70].

4. Genetic disorders with periodontal manifestations and consanguinity

Genetic disorders with periodontal manifestations are as follows: familial and cyclic neutropenias (CyN); Crohn disease; chronic granulomatous disease (CGD); agranulocytosis; Langerhans' cell disease; glycogen storage disease; hypophosphatasia; and leucocyte adhesion deficiency, Papillon-Lefèvre, Chédiak-Higashi, Cohen, Ehlers-Danlos (types 4 and 8), Marfan, Down, Haim-Munk, and Kindlers syndromes [13].

Familial gingival fibromatosis is a rare hereditary condition that causes aesthetic, functional, psychological, and masticatory problems for patients [76]. It may manifest as an autosomal-dominant and autosomal-recessive mode of inheritance [77, 78]. Consanguinity has been observed in the recessive mode of familial gingival fibromatosis [79, 80].

Leukocyte adhesion deficiency (LAD) type I is caused by the combined loss of expression on the surface of leukocytes of the leukocyte integrins LFA-1, Mac-1, and pl50, 95. It is a rare, inherited, autosomal-recessive, immunodeficiency disease [81]. Leukocyte adhesion deficiency type II is a disease with impaired fucosylation leading to an abnormal sialyl-lewis X (CD15). It is characterized by recurrent infections, persistent leukocytosis, and severe mental and growth retardation [82]. Leukocyte adhesion deficiency II was first described in two nonrelated children who have consanguineous parents [83, 84]. In a study, consanguinity has been found as a major factor for the distribution of LAD [85].

Langerhans-cell histiocytosis (LCH), once known as histiocytosis X, is considered a rare and non-hereditary disorder that includes a variety of diseases characterized by the dysregulated proliferation of Langerhans cells and infiltration of organs by pathological Langerhans cells [86]. Research on the relationship between periodontitis and consanguineous marriage is limited [87].

Glycogen storage disease type 1 (GSD-1) is a autosomal-recessive disorder that is caused by a deficiency in microsomal glucose-6-phosphatase activity [88]. Because of neutrophil dysfunction and neutropenia, there is an increased susceptibility to bacterial infection. This leads to symptoms of periodontitis [89, 90]. In a linkage analysis, consanguineous marriages and glycogen storage disease type 1 have been found to be related to each other [88].

Chronic granulomatous disease (CGD) is a rare inherited disease of the innate immune system that is characterized by impaired phagocyte microbicidal activity. It is caused by genetic defects in the superoxide-generating NADPH oxidase of phagocytes [91]. In a retrospective study, 14 patients with CGD were investigated. According to results of this study, a high consanguinity rate (75%) was observed [92].

Infantile genetic agranulocytosis is rare, inherited as an autosomal-recessive pattern, and characterized by severe neutropenia [93]. Patients may suffer from recurrent gingivitis and even severe periodontitis [94]. To have a family history of consanguineous parenthood may be a predisposing factor for infantile genetic agranulocytosis [95].

Some rare syndromes affecting phagocytes, epithelia, connective tissue, and teeth may cause severe periodontal conditions. Some genes that were responsible for these syndromes were identified. Haim-Munk and Papillon-Lefèvre syndromes (PLS) are rare autosomal-recessive disorders associated with periodontitis onset at early stage of the life. At childhood, both deciduous and permanent teeth are lost early. Mutations in the cathepsin gene (CTSC) on chromosome 11q 14–21 are the cause of PLS [96–98]. Papillon-Lefèvre syndrome is an autosomal-recessive disorder, and consanguinity in 20–40% of patients has been demonstrated in some studies [99, 100]. Consanguineously married parents may have offspring with PLS [101, 102]. In patients with PLS, deciduous teeth are lost early, but gingiva remains healthy. When permanent teeth erupt, gingivitis and periodontitis occur and all permanent teeth except the third molars are lost in a short time [103].

Ehler-Danlos syndrome is a group of autosomal-recessive disorders that affect the connective tissues such as skin, blood vessels, joints, etc. [104, 105]. In a case study, a patient with third-degree consanguineous parents has been described as having the appearance of old age, hypermobile joints, and skin laxity [106].

Once a patient's host response or immune system is impaired, severe periodontal disease and loss of periodontal tissues are often seen. Various systemic diseases such as leukemia, thrombocytopenia, and leucocyte disorders, such as agranulocytosis, cyclic neutropenia, and leucocyte adhesion deficiency, could result in increased severity of periodontal disease [13].

Cyclic neutropenia (CyN) is defined as an absolute neutrophil count (ANC) less than 0.5 × 109/L for at least 3–5 days per approximately 21-day cycles [107]. Neutrophil elastase (NE) gene (ELANE, formerly known as ELA2) located on chromosome 19p13.3 is the suspected gene that is the only known genetic defect in patients with CyN. This condition shows an autosomal-dominant transmission [108, 109]. Alangari et al. [110] have investigated both cyclic neutropenia and severe congenital neutropenia (SCN) phenotypes in an extended consanguineous multiplex family. According to results of this study, they have shown for the first time that a G6PC3 homozygous mutation resulted in a phenotype that is compatible with CyN in addition to the classical phenotype of SCN. They have reported that mutations in that gene could be said to have an autosomal-recessive pattern of inheritance in patients with CyN.

Chediak-Higashi syndrome (CHS) is a severe autosomal-recessive disease. It is characterized by partial oculocutaneous albinism, a predisposition to infections, the presence of abnormally large granules in many different cell types, and insufficient natural killer cell activity [111–113]. In consanguineous families, patients with Chediak-Higashi syndrome were found to have homozygous for the haplotype defined by the markers DIS235 and DIS2649 [111].

Cohen syndrome is a rare autosomal-recessive syndrome [114]. Diagnosis of Cohen syndrome is determined as the presence of at least seven of the following clinical symptoms as originally reported by Cohen et al. [114] and further described by Norio et al. [115]: mental retardation, microcephaly, characteristic facial appearance, slim tapering extremities with relative truncal obesity, hypotonia, joint hyperextensibility, benign neutropenia, and ophthalmic abnormalities such as myopia and retinal dystrophy. Cohen syndrome has been shown to be related with consanguinity [116].

Down syndrome is one of the most common human chromosomal disorders. Incidence of Down syndrome is quite high about 1 in 700 live births [117]. It is a result of an extra copy of the human chromosome 21 (trisomy 21) [118], and it is the most frequent genetic cause of mental retardation [117]. Studies investigating the relationship between Down syndrome and consanguineous marriage are contradictory [119–121].

Marfan syndrome is an autosomal-dominant disorder and a heritable disorder of fibrous connective tissue. The main symptoms occur in three systems: skeletal, ocular, and cardiovascular [122]. It appears to be due to heterozygous mutation in the fibrillin-1 gene on chromosome 15q21. De Vries et al. [123] described Marfan syndrome in two cousins from a consanguineous Turkish family.

Inflammatory bowel diseases (IBD) in the form of Crohn disease and ulcerative colitis result from a dysregulated immune response to environmental factors in genetically susceptible people [124]. In a study, Crohn disease was found to be related with consanguinity [125].

Kindler syndrome, a rare subtype of inherited epidermolysis bullosa, shows oral symptoms such as gingivitis, periodontitis, and loss of teeth. Kindler syndrome is reported more frequently in populations with high rates of consanguinity [126].

5. Conclusion

There does not seem to exist sufficient research on periodontal diseases related to the genetic disorders. Moreover, further research is needed on periodontal diseases in relation to consanguineous marriages.

Author details

Metin Çalisir

Address all correspondence to: metincalisir@adiyaman.edu.tr

Department of Periodontology, Faculty of Dentistry, Adiyaman University, Adiyaman, Turkey

References

[1] Mariotti A, Hefti AF. Defining periodontal health. BMC Oral Health. 2015;**15**:S6. DOI: 10.1186/1472-6831-15-S1-S6

[2] Petersen PE. The World Oral Health Report 2003: Continuous improvement of oral health in the 21st century—The approach of the WHO Global Oral Health Programme. Community Dentistry and Oral Epidemiology. 2003;**31**:3-24. DOI: 10.1046/j.2003.com122.x

[3] Petersen PE, Kandelman D, Arpin S, Ogawa H. Global oral health of older people—Call for public health action. Community Dental Health. 2010;**27**:257-268. DOI: 10.1922/CDH_2711Petersen11

[4] WHO. Preamble to the Constitution of the World Health Organization as adopted by the International Health Conference, New York: WHO; 1946

[5] WHO. Constitution of the World Health Organization. Chronicle World Health Organization. 1947;**1**:29-43. PMID:20267861

[6] Petersen PE, Bourgeois D, Ogawa H, Estupinan-Day S, Ndiaye C. The global burden of oral diseases and risks to oral health. Bulletin of the World Health Organization. 2005;**83**:661-669. DOI: /S0042-96862005000900011

[7] Petersen PE. Challenges to improvement of oral health in the 21st century—The approach of the WHO Global Oral Health Programme. International Dental Journal. 2004;**54**:329-343. DOI: 0020-6539/04/06329-15

[8] WHO. WHO Oral Health Country/Area Profile. Geneva: World Health Organization. 2005. Available from: http://www.whocollab.od.mah.se/index.html

[9] Armitage GC. Periodontal diagnoses and classification of periodontal diseases. Periodontology 2000. 2004;**34**:9-21. DOI: 10.1046/j.0906-6713.2002.003421.x

[10] Sam KSNg, Keung Leung W. Oral health-related quality of life and periodontal status. Community Dentistry and Oral Epidemiology. 2006;**34**:114-122. DOI: 10.1111/j.1600-0528.2006.00267.x

[11] Armitage GC. Development of a classification system for periodontal diseases and conditions. Annals of Periodontology. 1999;**4**:1-6. DOI: 10.1902/annals.1999.4.1.1

[12] Kinane DF, Attström R. Advances in the pathogenesis of periodontitis. Journal of Clinical Periodontology. 2005;**32**:130-131. DOI: 10.1111/j.1600-051X.2005.00823.x

[13] Pihlstrom BL, Michalowicz BS, Johnson NW. Periodontal diseases. Lancet. 2005;**366**:1809-1820. DOI: 10.1016/S0140-6736(05)67728-8

[14] Tarannum F, Faizuddin M. Effect of gene polymorphisms on periodontal diseases. Indian Journal of Human Genetics. 2012;**18**:9-19. DOI: 10.4103/0971-6866.96638

[15] Michalowicz BS, Aeppli D, Virag JG, Klump DG, Hinrichs JE, Seqal NL, Bouchard Jr TJ, Pihlstrom BL. Periodontal findings in adult twins. Journal of Periodontology. 1991;**62**:293-299. DOI: 10.1902/jop.1991.62.5.293

[16] Michalowicz BS, Diehl SR, Gunsolley JC, Sparks BS, Brooks CN, Koertge TE, Califano JV, Burmeister JA, Schenkein HA. Evidence of a substantial genetic basis for risk of adult periodontitis. Journal of Periodontology. 2000;**71**:1699-1707. DOI: 10.1902/jop.2000.71.11.1699

[17] Barksby HE, Nile CJ, Jaedicke KM, Taylor JJ, Preshaw PM. Differential expression of immunoregulatory genes in monocytes in response to *Porphyromonas gingivalis* and *Escherichia coli* lipopolysaccharide. Clinical and Experimental Immunology. 2009;**156**:479-487. DOİ: 10.1111/j.1365-2249.2009.03920.x

[18] Garlet GP, Cardoso CR, Silva TA, Ferreira BR, Avila-Campos MJ, Cunha FQ, Silva JS. Cytokine pattern determines the progression of experimental periodontal disease induced

by *Actinobacillus actinomycetemcomitans* through the modulation of MMPs, RANKL, and their physiological inhibitors. Oral Microbiology and Immunology. 2006;**21**:12-20. DOI: 10.1111/j.1399-302X.2005.00245.x

[19] Yoshie H, Kobayashi T, Tai H, Galicia JC. The role of genetic polymorphisms in periodontitis. Periodontology 2000. 2007;**43**:102-132. DOI: 10.1111/j.1600-0757.2006.00164.x

[20] Kinane DF, Hart TC. Genes and gene polymorphisms associated with periodontal disease. Critical Reviews in Oral Biology and Medicine. 2003;**14**:430-449. PMID:14656898

[21] Corey LA, Nance WE, Hofstede P, Schenkein HA. Self-reported periodontal disease in a Virginia twin population. Journal of Periodontology. 1993;**64**:1205-1208. DOI: 10.1902/jop.1993.64.12.1205

[22] Beaty TH, Boughman JA, Yang P, Astemborski JA, Suzuki JB. Genetic analysis of juvenile periodontitis in families ascertained through an affected proband. American Journal of Human Genetics. 1987;**40**:443-452. PMID:3578282

[23] Marazita ML, Burmeister JA, Gunsolley JC, Koertge TE, Lake K, Schenkein HA. Evidence for autosomal dominant inheritance and race-specific heterogeneity in early-onset periodontitis. Journal of Periodontology. 1994;**65**:623-630. DOI: 10.1902/jop. 1994.65.6.623 DOI:10.1902/jop.1994.65.6.623

[24] Williams RC. Periodontal disease. The New England Journal of Medicine. 1990;**322**:373-382. DOI: 10.1056/NEJM199002083220606

[25] Loesche WJ, Grossman NS. Periodontal disease as a specific, albeit chronic, infection: Diagnosis and treatment. Clinical Microbiology Reviews. 2001;**14**:727-752. DOI: 10.1128/CMR.14.4.727-752.2001; DOI:10.1128%2FCMR.14.4.727-752.2001#pmc_ext

[26] Laine ML, Loos BG, Crielaard W. Gene polymorphisms in chronic periodontitis. International Journal of Dentistry. 2010;**2010**:22. Article ID 324719; DOI: 10.1155/2010/324719

[27] Petit MD, van Steenbergen TJ, Timmerman MF, de Graaff J, van der Velden U. Prevalence of periodontitis and suspected periodontal pathogens in families of adult periodontitis patients. Journal of Clinical Periodontology. 1994;**21**:76-85. DOI: 10.1111/j.1600-051X.1994.tb00283.x

[28] Papapanou PN, Neiderud AM, Sandros J, Dahlén G. Interleukin-1 gene polymorphism and periodontal status. A case-control study. Journal of Clinical Periodontology. 2001;**28**:389-396. DOI: 10.1034/j.1600-051x.2001.028005389.x

[29] McDevitt MJ, Wang HY, Knobelman C, Newman MG, di Giovine FS, Timms J, Duff GW, Kornman KS. Interleukin-1 genetic association with periodontitis in clinical practice. Journal of Periodontology. 2000;**71**:156-163. DOI: 10.1902/jop.2000. 71.2.156 DOI:10.1902/jop.2000.71.2.156

[30] Llorente MA, Griffiths GS. Periodontal status among relatives of aggressive periodontitis patients and reliability of family history report. Journal of Clinical Periodontology. 2006;**33**:121-125. DOI: 10.1111/j.1600-051X.2005.00887.x

[31] Susin C, Haas AN, Albandar JM. Epidemiology and demographics of aggressive periodontitis. Periodontology 2000. 2014;**65**:27-45. DOI: 10.1111/prd.12019

[32] Vieira AR, Albandar JM. Role of genetic factors in the pathogenesis of aggressive periodontitis. Periodontology 2000. 2014;**65**:92-106. DOI: 10.1111/prd.12021

[33] Loos BG, John RP, Laine ML. Identification of genetic risk factors for periodontitis and possible mechanisms of action. Journal of Clinical Periodontology. 2005;**32**:159-179. DOI: 10.1111/j.1600-051X.2005.00806

[34] Page RC, Vandersteen GE, Ebersole JL, Williams BL, Dixon IL, Altman LC. Clinical and laboratory studies of a family with high prevalence of juvenile periodontitis. Journal of Periodontology. 1985;**56**:602-610. DOI: 10.1902/jop.1985.56.10.602

[35] Hodge PJ, Teaque PW, Wright AF, Kiane DF. Clinical and genetic analysis of a large north European Caucasian family affected by early-onset periodontitis. Journal of Dental Research. 2000;**79**:857-863. PMID:10765960

[36] Tai H, Endo M, Shimada Y, Gou E, Kobayashi T, Yamazaki K, Yoshie H. Association of interleukin-1 receptor antagonist gene polymorphisms with early onset periodontitis in Japanese. Journal of Clinical Periodontology. 2002;**29**:882-888. DOI: 10.1034/j.1600-051X .2002.291002.x

[37] Michel J, Gonzáles JR, Wunderlich D, Diete A, Herrmann JM, Meyle J. Interlekin-4 polymorphisms in early-onset periodontitis. Journal of Clinical Periodontology. 2001;**28**:483-488. DOI: 10.1034/j.1600-051x.2001.028005483.x

[38] Kornman KS, Crane A, Wang HY, di Giovine FS, Newman MG, Pirk FW, Wilson Jr TG, Higginbottom FL, Duff GW. The interleukin-1 genotype as a severity factor in adult periodontitis. Journal of Clinical Periodontology. 1997;**24**:72-77. DOI: 10.1111/j.1600-051X.1997.tb01187.x

[39] Quappe L, Jara L, Lopez NY. Association of interleukin 1 polymorphism with aggressive periodontitis. Journal of Periodontology. 2004;**75**:1509-1515. DOI: 10.1902/jop.2004. 75.11.1509

[40] Müller HP, Barrieshi-Nusair KM. A combination of alleles 2 of interleukin (IL)-1A^{-889} and IL-1B^{+3954} is associated with lower gingival bleeding tendency in plaque-induced gingivitis in young adults of Arabic heritage. Clinical Oral Investigations. 2007;**11**:297-302. DOI: 10.1007/s00784-007-0120-5

[41] Gonzales JR, Mann M, Stelzig J, Bödeker RH, Meyle J. Single nucleotide polymorphisms in the IL-4 and IL-13 promoter region in aggressive periodontitis. Journal of Clinical Periodontology. 2007;**34**:473-479. DOI: 10.1111/j.1600-051X. 2007.01086.x DOI:10.1111/ j.1600-051X.2007.01086.x

[42] Shao MY, Huang P, Cheng R, Hu T. Interleukin-6 polymorphisms modify the risk of periodontitis: A systematic review and metaanalysis. Journal of Zhejiang University. Science B. 2009;**10**:920-927. DOI: 10.1631/jzus.B0920279.

[43] Nibali L, Griffiths GS, Donos N, Parkar M, D'Aiuto F, Tonetti MS, Brett PM. Association between interleukin-6 promoter haplotypes and aggressive periodontitis. Journal of Clinical Periodontology. 2008;**35**:193-198. DOI: 10.1111/j.1600-051X.2007.01188.x

[44] Reichert S, Machulla HK, Klapproth J, Zimmermann U, Reichert Y, Gläser CH, Schaller HG, Stein J, Schulz S. The interleukin-10 gene promoter haplotype ATA is a putative risk factor for aggressive periodontitis. Journal of Periodontal Research. 2008;**43**:40-47. DOI: 10.1111/j.1600-0765.2007.00992.x.

[45] Maney P, Emecen P, Mills JS, Walters JD. Neutrophil formylpeptide receptor single nucleotide polymorphism 348T>C in aggressive periodontitis. Journal of Periodontology. 2009;**80**:492-498. DOI:10.1902/jop.2009.080225;DOI:10.1902%2Fjop.2009.080225#pmc_ext

[46] de Souza RC, Colombo AP. Distribution of FcgammaRIIa and FcgammaRIIIb genotypes in patients with generalized aggressive periodontitis. Journal of Periodontology. 2006;**77**:1120-1128. DOI: 10.1902/jop.2006.050305

[47] Nibali L, Parkar M, Brett P, Knight J, Tonetti MS, Griffiths GS. NADPH oxidase and FcgammaR polymorphisms as risk factors for aggressive periodontitis: A case control association study. Journal of Clinical Periodontology. 2006;**33**:529-539. DOI: 10.1111/j.1600-051X.2006.00952.x

[48] Socransky SS, Haffajee AD, Smith C, Duff GW. Microbiological parameters associated with IL-1 gene polymorphisms in periodontitis patients. Journal of Clinical Periodontology. 2000;**27**:810-818. DOI: 10.1034/j.1600-051x.2000.027011810.x

[49] Joshipura V, Yadalam U, Brahmavar B. Aggressive periodontitis: A review. Journal of International Clinical Dental Research Organization. 2015;**7**:11-17. DOI: 10.4103/2231-0754.153489

[50] Ozturk A, Vieira AR. TLR4 as risk factor for periodontal disease: A reappraisal. Journal of Clinical Periodontology. 2009;**36**:279-286. DOI: 10.1111/j.1600-051X.2009.01370.x

[51] Katz J, Goultschin J, Benoliel R, Brautbar C. Human leukocyte antigen (HLA) DR4: Positive association with rapidly progressing periodontitis. Journal of Periodontology. 1987;**58**;607-610. DOI: 10.1902/jop.1987.58.9.607

[52] Shapira L, Eizenberg S, Sela MN, Soskolne A, Brautbar H. HLA A9 and B15 are associated with the generalized form, but not the localized form, of early-onset periodontal diseases. Journal of Periodontology. 1994;**65**:219-223. DOI: 10.1902/jop. 1994.65.3.219

[53] Ohyama H, Takashiba S, Oyaizu K, Nagai A, Naruse T, Inoko H, Kurihara H, Murayama Y. HLA class II genotypes associated with early onset periodontitis: DQB1 molecule primarily confers susceptibility to the disease. Journal of Periodontology. 1996;**67**:888-894. DOI: 10.1902/jop.1996.67.9.888

[54] Hart TC, Atkinson JC. Mendelian forms of periodontitis. Periodontology 2000. 2007;**45**: 95-112. DOI: 10.1111/j.1600-0757.2007.00233.x

[55] Alwan A, Modell B. Community control of genetic and congenital disorders. EMRO Technical Publication Series 24. Egypt: WHO Regional Office for the Eastern Mediterranean Region; 1997

[56] Modell B, Darr A. Science and society: Genetic counselling and customary consanguineous marriage. Nature Reviews. Genetics. 2002;**3**:225-229. DOI: 10.1038/nrg754

[57] Bittles A. Consanguinity and its relevance to clinical genetics. Clinical Genetics. 2001;**60**:89-98. DOI: 10.1034/j.1399-0004.2001.600201.x

[58] Abdalla B, Zaher A. Consanguineous marriages in the Middle East: Nature versus nurture. The Open Complementary Medicine Journal. 2013;**5**:1-10

[59] Shawky RM, Elsayed SM, Zaki ME, Nour El-Din SM, Kamal FM. Consanguinity and its relevance to clinical genetics. The Egyptian Journal of Medical Human Genetics. 2013;**14**:157-164. DOI: http://dx.doi.org/10.1016/j.ejmhg.2013.01.002; DOI: 10.1016/j.ejmhg.2013.01.002#doilink

[60] Bittles AH, Black ML. Evolution in health and medicine Sackler colloquium: Consanguinity, human evolution, and complex diseases. Proceedings of the National Academy of Sciences of the USA. 2010;**107**:1779-1786. DOI: 10.1073/pnas. 0906079106

[61] Bener A, Hussain R. Consanguineous unions and child health in the State of Qatar. Paediatric and Perinatal Epidemiology. 2006;**20**:372-378. DOI: 10.1111/j.1365-3016.2006.00750.x

[62] Tadmouri GO. Genetic disorders in Arab populations: A 2008 update. In: Tadmouri GO, Taleb Al Ali M, Al Khaja N, editors. Genetic Disorders in the Arab World. Oman. Dubai; 2008. pp. 8-43

[63] Bundey S, Alam H, Kaur A, Mir S, Lancashire RJ. Race, consanguinity and social features in Birmingham babies: A basis for prospective study. Journal of Epidemiology & Community Health. 1990;**44**:130-135. DOI: 10.1136/jech.44.2.130

[64] Fuster V, Colantonio SE. Socioeconomic, demographic, and geographic variables affecting the diverse degrees of consanguineous marriages in Spain. Human Biology. 2004;**76**: 1-14. DOI: 10.1353/hub.2004.0021

[65] Hussain R, Bittles AH. Sociodemographic correlates of consanguineous marriage in the Muslim population of India. Journal of Biosocial Science. 2000;**32**:433-442. DOI: 10.1017/S0021932000004338

[66] Liascovich R, Rittler M, Castilla EE. Consanguinity in South America: Demographic aspects. Human Heredity. 2001;**51**:27-34. DOI: 10.1159/000022956

[67] Kerkeni E, Monastiri K, Saket B, Rudan D, Zgaga L, Ben Cheikh H. Association among education level, occupation status, and consanguinity in Tunisia and Croatia. Croatian Medical Journal. 2006;**47**:656-661. PMID:16912991

[68] Jaouad IC, Elalaoui SC, Sbiti A, Elkerh F, Belmahi L, Sefiani A. Consanguineous marriages in Morocco and the consequence for the incidence of autosomal recessive disorders. Journal of Biosocial Science. 2009;**41**:575-581. DOI: 10.1017/ S0021932009003393

[69] El Mouzan MI, Al Salloum AA, Al Herbish AS, Qurachi MM, Al Omar AA. Consanguinity and major genetic disorders in Saudi children: A community-based cross-sectional study. Annals of Saudi Medicine. 2008;**28**:169-173. DOI: 10.4103/ 0256-4947.51726

[70] When Parents Are Related—Consanguinity. Centre for genetic education. Fact Sheet 18 [Internet]. 2016, pp. 1-3. Available from: www.genetics.edu.au

[71] Tadmouri GO, Nair P, Obeid T, Al Ali MT, Al Khaja N, Hamamy HA. Consanguinity and reproductive health among Arabs. Reproductive Health. 2009;**6**:17. DOI: 10.1186/1742-4755-6-17

[72] Sibert JR, Jadhav M, Inbaraj SG. Fetal growth and parental consanguinity. Archives of Disease in Childhood. 1979;**54**:317-319. DOI: 10.1136/adc.54.4.317

[73] Bennett RL, Motulsky AG, Bittles A, Hudgins L, Uhrich S, Doyle DL, Silvey K, Scott CR, Cheng E, McGillivray B, Steiner RD, Olson D. Genetic counseling and screening of consanguineous couples and their offspring: Recommendations of the national society of genetic counselors. Journal of Genetic Counseling. 2002;**11**:97-119. DOI: 10.1023/A:1014593404915

[74] Hamamy H. Consanguineous marriages. Preconception consultation in primary health care settings. Journal of Community Genetics. 2012;**3**:185-192. DOİ: 10.1007/s12687-011-0072-y

[75] Hamamy HA, Masri AT, Al-Hadidy AM, Ajlouni KM. Consanguinity and genetic disorders. Profile from Jordan. Saudi Medical Journal. 2007;**28**:1015-1017. PMID: 17603701

[76] Carranza FA, Hogan EL. Gingival enlargement. In: Newman, Takei HH, Carranza FA, editors. Clinical Periodontology. 9th ed. Philadelphia, PA: Saunders; 2002. pp. 279-296

[77] Bozzo L, de Almedia OP, Scully C, Aldred MJ. Hereditary gingival fibromatosis. Report of an extensive four-generation pedigree. Oral Surgery Oral Medicine Oral Pathology. 1994;**78**:452-454. DOI: 10.1016/0030-4220(94)90037-X; DOI: 10.1016/0030-4220(94)90037-X#_blank#Persistent link using digital object identifier

[78] Martelli-Junior H, Lemos DP, Silva CO, Graner E, Coletta RD. Hereditary gingival fibromatosis: Report of a five generation family using cellular proliferation analysis. Journal of Periodontology. 2005;**76**:2299-2305. DOI: 10.1902/jop.2005. 76.12.2299

[79] Sharma S, Goyal D, Shah G, Ray A. Familial gingival fibromatosis: A rare case report. Contemporary Clinical Dentistry. 2012;**3**:63-66. DOI: 10.4103/0976-237X. 95108; DOI: 10.4103%2F0976-237X.95108#pmc_ext

[80] Kharbanda P, Sidhu SS, Panda SK, Deshmukh R. Gingival fibromatosis: Study of three generations with consanguinity. Quintessence International. 1993;**24**:161-164. PMID: 8511274

[81] Wardlaw AJ, Hibbs ML, Stacker SA, Springer TA. Distinct mutations in two patients with leukocyte adhesion deficiency and their functional correlates. The Journal of Experimental Medicine. 1990;**172**:335-345. DOI: 10.1084/jem.172.1.335

[82] Wild MK, Luhn K, Marquardt T, Vestweber D. Leukocyte adhesion deficiency II: Therapy and genetic defect. Cells Tissues Organs. 2002;**172**:161-173. DOI: 10.1159/000066968

[83] Etzioni A, Frydman M, Pollack S, Avidor I, Phillips ML, Paulson JC, Gershoni-Baruch R. Brief report: Recurrent severe infections caused by a novel leukocyte adhesion deficiency. The New England Journal of Medicine. 1992;**327**:1789-1792. DOI: 10.1056/NEJM199212173272505

[84] Frydman M, Etzioni A, Eidlitz-Markus T, Avidor I, Varsano I, Shechter Y, Orlin JB, Gershoni-Baruch R. Rambam-Hasharon syndrome of psychomotor retardation, short stature, defective neutrophil motility, and Bombay phenotype. American Journal of Medical Genetics. 1992;**44**:297-302. DOI: 10.1002/ajmg.1320440307

[85] Movahedi M, Entezari N, Pourpak Z, Mamishi S, Chavoshzadeh Z, Gharagozlou M, Mir-Saeeid-Ghazi B, Fazlollahi MR, Zandieh F, Bemanian MH, Farhoudi A, Aghamohammadi A. Clinical and laboratory findings in Iranian patients with leukocyte adhesion deficiency (Study of 15 Cases). Journal of Clinical Immunology. 2007;**27**:302-307. DOI: 10.1007/s10875-006-9069-4

[86] Nezelof C, Frileux-Herbet F, Cronier-Sachot J. Disseminated histiocytosis X: Analysis of prognostic factors based on a retrospective study of 50 cases. Cancer 1979;**44**:1824-1838. DOI: 10.1002/1097-0142(197911)44:5<1824:: AIDCNCR 2820440542> 3.0.CO;2-J

[87] Hanapiah F, Yaacob H, Ghani KS, Hussin AS. Histiocytosis X: Evidence for a genetic etiology. Journal of the Nihon University School of Dentistry. 1993;**35**:171-174. PMID: 8246038

[88] Annabi B, Hiraiwa H, Mansfield BC, Lei KJ, Ubagai T, Polymeropoulos MH, Moses SW, Parvari R, Hershkovitz E, Mandel H, Fryman M, Chou JY. The gene for Glycogen-Storage disease Type 1b maps to chromosome 11q23. The American Journal of Human Genetics. 1998;**62**:400-405. DOI: 10.1086/301727 DOI: 10.1086%2F301727#pmc_ext

[89] Gallin JI. Disorders of phagocytic cells. In: Gallin JI, Goldstein IM, Snyderman R, editors. Inflammation: Basic Principles and Clinical Correlates. 2nd ed. New York: Raven Press; 1992. pp. 859-874

[90] Anderson DC, Kishimoto TK, Smith CW. Leukocyte adhesion deficiency and other disorders of leukocyte adherence and mobility. In: Scriver CR, Beaudet AL, Sly WS, Valle D, editors. The Metabolic and Molecular Bases of Inherited Disease. 7th ed. New York: McGraw-Hill; 1995. pp 3955-3994

[91] Dinauer MC, Orkin SH. Chronic granulomatous disease. Annual Review of Medicine. 1992;**43**:117-124. DOI: 10.1146/annurev.me.43.020192.001001

[92] Barbouche MR, Sghiri R, Mellouli F, Boukhdir Y, Dellagi K, Bejaoui M. Chronic septic granulomatous disease: 14 cases. Presse Medicale. 1999;**28**:2034-2036. PMID: 10605470

[93] Aytekin C, Germeshausen M, Tuygun N, Tanir G, Dogu F, Ikinciogullari A. Eponym kostmann disease. European Journal of Pediatrics. 2010;**169**:657-660. DOI: 10.1007/s00431-010-1149-z DOI:10.1007/s00431-010-1149-z#_blank

[94] Carlsson G, Wahlin YB, Johansson A, Olsson A, Eriksson T, Claesson R, Hänström L, Henter JI. Periodontal disease in patients from the original Kostmann family with severe congenital neutropenia. Journal of Periodontology. 2006;**77**:744-751. DOI: 10.1902/jop.2006.050191

[95] Zeidler C, Germeshausen M, Klein C, Welte K. Clinical implications of ELA2-, HAX1-, and G-CSF-receptor (CSF3R) mutations in severe congenital neutropenia. British Journal of Haematology. 2009;**144**:459-467. DOI: 10.1111/j.1365-2141. 2008.07425.x

[96] Hart TC, Hart PS, Bowden DW, Michalec MD, Callison SA, Walker SJ, Zhang Y, Firatli E. Mutations of the cathepsin C gene are responsible for Papillon-Lefevre syndrome. Journal of Medical Genetics. 1999;**36**:881-887. DOI: 10.1136/jmg.36.12.881 DOI: 10.1136/jmg.36.12.881#_new

[97] Toomes C, James J, Wood AJ, Wu CL, McCormick D, Lench N, Hewitt C, Moynihan L, Roberts E, Woods CG, Markham A, Wong M, Widmer R, Ghaffar KA, Pemberton M, Hussein IR, Temtamy SA, Davies R, Read AP, Sloan P, Dixon MJ, Thakker NS. Loss-of-function mutations in the cathepsin C gene result in periodontal disease and palmoplantar keratosis. Nature Genetics. 1999;**23**:421-424. DOI: 10.1038/70525

[98] Hart TC, Hart PS, Michalec MD, Zhang Y, Firatli E, Van Dyke TE, Stabholz A, Zlotogorski A, Shapira L, Soskolne WA. Haim-Munk syndrome and Papillon-Lefevre syndrome are allelic mutations in cathepsin C. Journal of Medical Genetics. 2000;**37**:88-94. DOI: 10.1136/jmg.37.2.88 DOI: 10.1136%2Fjmg.37.2.88#pmc_ext

[99] Kaya FA, Polat ZS, Baran EA, Tekin GG. Papillon-Lefevre syndrome-3 years follow up: A case report. International Dental and Medicine Disorders. 2008;**1**:24-28

[100] Zhang Y, Lundgren T, Renvert S, Tatakis DN, Firatli E, Uygur C, Hart PS, Gorry MC, Marks JJ, Hart TC. Evidence of a founder effect for four cathepsin C gene mutations in Papillon–Lefèvre syndrome patients. Journal of Medical Genetics. 2001;**38**:96-101. DOI: 10.1136/jmg.38.2.96 DOI: 10.1136%2Fjmg.38.2.96#pmc_ext

[101] Khan FY, Jan SM, Mushtaq M. Papillon–Lefèvre syndrome: Case report and review of the literature. Journal of Indian Society of Periodontology. 2012;**16**:261-265. DOI: 10.4103/0972-124X.99273 DOI: 10.4103%2F0972-124X.99273#pmc_ext

[102] Rathod VJ, Joshi NV. Papillon–Lefevre syndrome: A report of two cases. Journal of Indian Society of Periodontology. 2010;**14**:275-278. DOI: 10.4103/0972-124X.76934 DOI:10.4103%2F0972-124X.76934#pmc_ext

[103] Shah AF, Tandage P, Agarwal S. Papillon-Lefevre syndrome: Reporting consanguinity as a risk factor. The Saudi Dental Journal. 2014;**26**:126-131. DOI: 10.1016/j.sdentj.2014.02.004 DOI: 10.1016%2Fj.sdentj.2014.02.004#pmc_ext

[104] Kresse H, Rosthøj S, Quentin E, Hollmann J, Glössl J, Okada S, Tønnesen T. Glycosaminoglycan-free small proteoglycan core protein is secreted by fibroblasts from a patient with a syndrome resembling progeroid. American Journal of Human Genetics. 1987;**41**:436-453. PMID: 3631078

[105] Urmil MAK. Ehlers-Danlos Syndrome Type V. Medical Journal Armed Forces India. 2004;**60**:81-83. DOI: 10.1016/S0377-1237(04)80171-0; DOI: 10.1016%2FS0377-1237(04)80171-0#pmc_ext

[106] Anitha GFS, Shanmugam VK, Rajendran VV. A rare case of Ehler Danlos syndrome - Progeroid type: A case report. International Journal of Contemporary Pediatrics. 2017;**4**:261-263. DOI: 10.18203/2349-3291.ijcp20164614

[107] Haurie C, Dale DC, Mackey MC. Cyclical neutropenia and other periodic hematological disorders: A review of mechanisms and mathematical models. Blood. 1998;**92**:2629-2640. PMID: 9763544

[108] Horwitz M, Benson KF, Person RE, Aprikyan AG, Dale DC. Mutations in ELA2, encoding neutrophil elastase, define a 21-day biological clock in cyclic haematopoiesis. Nature Genetics. 1999;**23**:433-436. DOİ: 10.1038/70544.

[109] Horwitz MS, Duan Z, Korkmaz B, Lee HH, Mealiffe ME, Salipante SJ. Neutrophil elastase in cyclic and severe congenital neutropenia. Blood. 2007;**109**:1817-1824. DOİ: 10.1182/blood-2006-08-019166.

[110] Alangari AA, Alsultan A, Osman ME, Anazi S, Alkuraya FS. A novel homozygous mutation in G6PC3 presenting as cyclic neutropenia and severe congenital neutropenia in the same family. Journal of Clinical Immunology. 2013;**33**:1403-1406. DOI: 10.1007/s10875-013-9945-7

[111] Barrat FJ, Auloge L, Pastural E, Lagelouse RD, Vilmer E, Cant AJ, Weissenbach J, Le Paslier D, Fischer A, Basile GS. Genetic and physical mapping of the Chediak-Higashi syndrome on chromosome 1q42-43. American Journal of Human Genetics. 1996;**59**:625-632. PMID: 8751864

[112] Blume RS, Wolff SM. The Chediak-Higashi syndrome: Studies in four patients and a review of the literature. Medicine. 1972;**51**:247-280. PMID: 5064229

[113] Sato A. Chediak and Higashi's disease: Probable identity of "a new leucocytal anomaly (Chediak)" and "congenital gigantism of peroxidase granules (Higashi)." The Tohoku Journal of Experimental Medicine. 1955;**61**:201-210. PMID: 14396888

[114] Cohen Jr MM, Hall BD, Smith DW, Graham CB, Lampert KJ. A new syndrome with hypotonia, obesity, mental deficiency and facial, oral, ocular and limb anomalies. The Journal of Pediatrics. 1973;**83**:280-284. PMID: 4717588

[115] Norio R, Raitta C, Lindahl E. Further delineation of the Cohen syndrome; report on chorioretinal dystrophy, leukopenia and consanguinity. Clinical Genetics. 1984;**25**:1-14. DOI: 10.1111/j.1399-0004.1984.tb00456.x

[116] Hennies HC, Rauch A, Seifert W, Schumi C, Moser E, Al-Taji E, Tariverdian G, Chrzanowska KH, Krajewska-Walasek M, Rajab A, Giugliani R, Neumann TE, Eckl KM, Karbasiyan M, Reis A, Horn D. Allelic heterogeneity in the COH1 gene explains clinical variability in Cohen syndrome. American Journal of Human Genetics. 2004;**75**:138-145. DOI: 10.1086/422219 DOI: 10.1086%2F422219#pmc_ext

[117] Hattori M, Fujiyama A, Taylor TD, Watanabe H, Yada T, Park HS, et al. The DNA sequence of human chromosome 21. Nature. 2000;**405**:311-319. DOI: 10.1038/35012518

[118] Gardiner K, Slavov D, Bechtel L, Davisson M. Annotation of human chromosome 21 for relevance to down syndrome: Gene structure and expression analysis. Genomics. 2002;**79**:833-843. DOI: 10.1006/geno.2002.6782

[119] Alfi OS, Chang R, Azen SP. Evidence for genetic control of nondisjunction in man. American Journal of Human Genetics. 1980;**32**:477-483. PMID: 6446853

[120] Sayee R, Thomas IM. Consanguinity, non-disjunction, parental age and Down's syndrome. Journal of the Indian Medical Association. 1998;**96**:335-337. PMID: 10218319

[121] Ghosh S, Hong CS, Feingold E, Ghosh P, Ghosh P, Bhaumik P, Dey SK. Epidemiology of Down syndrome: New insight into the multidimensional interactions among genetic and environmental risk factors in the oocyte. American Journal of Epidemiology. 2011;**174**:1009-1016. DOI: 10.1093/aje/kwr240

[122] Pyeritz RE, McKusick VA. The Marfan syndrome. The New England Journal of Medicine. 1979;**300**:772-777. DOI: 10.1056/NEJM197904053001406

[123] de Vries BB, Pals G, Odink R, Hamel BC. Homozygosity for a FBN1 missense mutation: Clinical and molecular evidence for recessive Marfan syndrome. European Journal of Human Genetics. 2007;**15**:930-935. DOI: 10.1038/sj.ejhg.5201865

[124] El Mouzan M, Al-Mofarreh M, Assiri A, Hamid Y, Saeed A. Consanguinity and inflammatory bowel diseases: Is there a relation? Journal of Pediatric Gastroenterology and Nutrition. 2013;**56**:182-185. DOI: 10.1097/MPG. 0b013e31826d9987

[125] Al-Mayouf SM, Albuhairan I, Muzaffer M, AlMehaidib A. Familial aggregation of Crohn's disease and necrotizing sarcoid-like granulomatous disease. European Journal of Rheumatology. 2015;**2**:122-124. DOI: 10.5152/eurjrheum. 2015.0102; DOI: 10.5152%2Feurjrheum.2015.0102#pmc_ext

[126] Youssefian L, Vahidnezhad H, Saeidian AH, Ahmadizadeh K, Has C, Uitto J. Kindler syndrome, an orphan disease of cell/matrix adhesion in the skin—molecular genetics and therapeutic opportunities. Expert Opinion on Orphan Drugs. 2016;**4**:845-854. DOI: 10.1080/21678707.2016.1207519

Chapter 4

Periodontitis and Chronic Obstructive Pulmonary Disease

Agathi Spiropoulou, Olga Lagiou,
Dimosthenis Lykouras, Kiriakos Karkoulias and
Kostas Spiropoulos

Additional information is available at the end of the chapter

http://dx.doi.org/10.5772/intechopen.69957

Abstract

Chronic periodontitis and chronic obstructive pulmonary disease (COPD) are chronic inflammatory diseases in which neutrophilic inflammation plays a major role. There are a few studies showing that these two entities share various predisposing factors and pathogenetic mechanisms; however, a direct connection between them has not yet been achieved. Epidemiology data may also show a connection between the two conditions. Neutrophilic inflammation in periodontitis and COPD is orchestrated by CD8+ lymphocytes and macrophages, leading to the aggregation of neutrophils and causing an imbalance to the proteases and antiproteases equilibrium. Finally, further research is needed to clarify the common pathogenesis of the two diseases to optimize their therapeutic management.

Keywords: chronic inflammation, neutrophils, oral hygiene

1. Introduction

Periodontitis is a chronic inflammatory disease of the oral cavity, affecting the structures that support the teeth. Almost half of the adult population has a great inflammation of the gums that causes loss of optimal contact between the teeth and periodontal tissues [1]. About 11% of adults develop clinical periodontitis. The dental plaque is caused by the development of anaerobic bacteria that cause accumulation and activation of neutrophils, which is orchestrated by various mediators and enzymes that destroy the connective tissue [2, 3]. Untreated periodontitis ultimately leads to loss of support of the teeth, and atrophy of the alveolar process, causing loss of the teeth.

Chronic obstructive pulmonary disease (COPD) is an inflammatory disorder of the airways, largely caused by smoking, and it is characterized by progressive and partially reversible airflow limitation [4]. The airflow obstruction and consequently the disease are confirmed by the presence of a postbronchodilator FEV1/FVC < 0.70 [5]. The disease constitutes one of the leading causes of morbidity and mortality in the industrialized world, affecting approximately 210 million people worldwide. In 2004, COPD was the fourth most common cause of death and it is expected to be the third cause of mortality by 2030 [6, 7].

COPD is a combination of chronic bronchitis and emphysema, and as a result, it constitutes a heterogeneous disease. The most common symptoms in patients suffering from COPD are dyspnea, cough, and production of sputum, which are chronic and progressive [8].

The lesions present in COPD and periodontitis are linked to various immunologic mechanisms, in which T-lymphocytes, macrophages, and neutrophils have a major role. Our chapter attempts to analyze the similarities in pathophysiology of COPD and chronic periodontitis and to elucidate the common pathogenetic mechanisms.

2. The role of chronic inflammation

COPD and chronic periodontitis are characterized by chronic neutrophilic inflammation, which mainly stems from the activity of enzymes released from granules of neutrophils. It is known that the development of COPD depends on the variable exposure to harmful factors, such as cigarette smoking, as well as on the susceptibility of the individual [9]. It is estimated that only a percentage of smokers (5–20%) develop COPD. Moreover, some patients develop mild disease, others moderate, and others serious disease. Among COPD patients, 80–90% have been current or ex-smokers. Air pollution and occupational exposure have also been responsible for some COPD cases at a lower rate.

On the other hand, in periodontitis, there is an interaction between environmental and genetic factors, which eventually leads to the development of the disease. In both COPD and periodontitis, the pathophysiological mechanisms include the accumulation and activation of neutrophils. Factors secreted by neutrophil granules cause damage to the connective tissue [10].

It is believed that COPD is a condition of chronic systemic inflammation, characterized by elevated C-reactive protein (CRP), interleukin-8 (IL-8), and tumor necrosis factor-α (TNF-α), whose levels determine the severity of disease, which is in line with the degree of muscle atrophy and dysfunction. These cytokines are also related to the development of coronary artery disease and diabetes [11]. Morbidity and mortality also depend on social and economic factors [12].

Inflammatory responses taking place in periodontitis are usually caused by the presence of anaerobic microbes. Thus, the levels of pro-inflammatory cytokines, such as CRP and TNF-α, are remarkably elevated. In both COPD and periodontitis, there is an increased incidence of heart attack, osteoporosis, diabetes mellitus and rheumatoid arthritis as a result of chronic inflammation [13].

3. Epidemiology of COPD and periodontitis

A variety of stimuli can induce the development of COPD, including heritable genes in conjunction with environmental risk factors. Air pollutants, cold temperature, lack of compliance with respiratory medication, and other noninfectious causes, as well as infections, are the usual triggers of acute exacerbations of COPD. Infections, which are the most frequent cause of exacerbations, could be of either bacterial or viral etiology [14]. It is known that almost half of the infections are caused by bacteria, while viruses are responsible for almost the rest of the infections. Moreover, coinfection with bacteria and viruses is identified in patients with severe COPD.

Smoking is an important predisposing factor both in COPD and in periodontitis. Almost 80% of COPD patients are current or ex-smokers. COPD is also associated with age, impaired lung function, and gender. Initially, it was believed that the impact was greater in men, but more recent data exhibit equal or greater sensitivity of women smokers to develop COPD [15].

A working environment involving exposure to dust and harmful gases increases the risk of developing the disease. When smoking coexists, there is a sixfold risk. Exposure to inhaled gases from burning biomass increases the risk. There are not causative microbes causing COPD to develop. However, several viruses and bacteria are responsible for COPD disease exacerbations that lead to impaired lung function and quality of life deterioration [16].

Smoking is also a risk factor for the development of periodontitis, and the severity of the disease depends on the density of smoking habit [17]. Men and elderly people are more susceptible for COPD and periodontitis. Other predisposing factors include diabetes and poor socioeconomic conditions. Since 1990, there has been an increasing interest in the possible links between COPD and periodontitis. There is a correlation between poor oral hygiene and COPD [18].

In a study of military veterans, a diagnosis of COPD was made in subjects with an FEV1/FVC ratio < 70% and a history of smoking. The existence of periodontitis was documented by X-ray results which show the loss of the alveolar bone. It was observed that a loss of 20% of the alveolar bone leads to an increased risk for development of COPD by 60%. However, it should be noted that the reduction of FEV1 is related not only to the existence of COPD but also to other respiratory diseases [19].

Other notable studies attempt to correlate COPD severity with the existence of periodontitis using more comprehensive definitions for the existence of COPD. In a study of 600 people with COPD was shown that the risk of developing COPD was associated directly with the quality of oral hygiene [20]. More specifically, patients with COPD had a higher dental plaque index, and an insufficient support of the tooth from the surrounding tissues. Moreover, the same patients had an unsatisfactory behavior regarding their oral hygiene, as measured by the frequency of toothbrushing, the use of dental yarns, and the frequency of visits to the dentist [21]. In another study, a direct correlation between COPD severity and poor hygiene was found in general. Therefore, this observation implies that the possibility of poor oral hygiene and the unfavorable course of COPD may be linked to nonhealthy lifestyle and poor socioeconomic conditions [22].

It is known that the pathogenesis of COPD is directly associated with the pathological relationship of proteases/antiproteases in the lung. The same theory has been suggested in periodontitis. Past studies have shown that in patients suffering from mild COPD and periodontitis the levels of metalloproteinase-8 (MMP-8) are elevated in saliva and serum. MMP-8 is a product of the secretion of neutrophils. However, levels of MMP-8 in saliva showed no statistically significant difference in patients with mild COPD who had no periodontitis compared to those that did not suffer from COPD. Some other studies demonstrate a poor correlation between COPD and periodontitis [23].

To sum up, several meta-analyses have shown that periodontitis increases the risk of developing COPD; however, the exact mechanism is still not fully understood. Future studies should focus on the elucidation of such pathogenetic mechanisms.

4. Pathophysiology of COPD and periodontitis

COPD is characterized by limitation of airflow which is partially reversible. Progressive decline of FEV1, inadequate lung emptying on expiration, and static and dynamic hyperinflation are the results of remodeling of the small-airway compartment and loss of elastic recoil by emphysematous destruction of parenchyma [24]. Exposure to smoke leads to infiltration of the mucosa, submucosa, and glandular tissue by inflammation cells. Increased mucus content, epithelial-cell hyperplasia, and disturbed tissue repair with wall thickening in the small conducting airways are the main features of COPD [25].

Smoking can cause injury of airway epithelial cells, and as a result, endogenous signals are released and recognized by receptors such as Toll-like receptors 4 and 2 on epithelial cells. This recognition leads to a nonspecific inflammatory response which involves the release of early cytokines, macrophages, neutrophils, and dendritic cells and the transportation of these features to the site of inflammation [26]. Self-antigens released from damaged tissue as well as foreign antigens from incoming pathogens are presented to naïve T-cells by dendritic cells. The T-cells are activated into T-helper-1 cells, and these specific CD4 and CD8 cells as well as B-cells which produce antibodies are transferred to the lungs so as to neutralize the antigens [27].

Alveolar macrophages and other immune cells produce proteinases that destroy the basal membrane and also cause damage to the collagen and elastic fibers of the connective tissue, leading to the development of emphysema [28]. Moreover, they secrete IL-4 and IL-3 that cause edema and increased production of mucus, which are both associated with airway hyperresponsiveness. These responses take place at the respiratory lobule of second order that is located after the terminal bronchiole. It consists of 3–5 generations of respiratory bronchioles that contain alveoli. This is the structure that is responsible for the exchange of respiratory gases, and its destruction may cause impaired gas exchange and respiratory failure [29]. Moreover, apart from the lack of α-1 antitrypsin, other genetic factors involved in the pathogenesis of the disease include interleukins and cysteine proteinases and elastases, which orchestrate an immune response which can lead to the destruction of the pulmonary parenchyma. Mast cells play an important role as antigen-presenting cells in the lung as well, and they have been shown to be valuable both in COPD and in periodontitis.

Smoking is the main factor that initiates immune system reaction in chronic inflammatory diseases as the chronic obstructive pulmonary disease and periodontitis [30]. In response to smoking, neutrophils accumulate rapidly in the lung, because the macrophages and epithelial cells of the lung are activated. They secrete neutrophil-attracting factors such as IL-8, C5a, and LTB4. The stimulation of neutrophils causes oxidative damage to the lung due to oxygen radicals produced by activated neutrophils. Moreover, free oxygen radicals cause oxidative injury to the lung [31]. Oxygen radicals play a role in premature cellular death, but also act on the epithelial and mesenchymal cells. The destruction of the cellular matrix causes a destruction of the supporting connective tissue. Some of these polypeptides as laminin and fibronectin have chemotactic effect and attract neutrophils, playing a key role in the sequence of events of the destruction of lung parenchyma due to smoking. Neutrophils contain proteinases stored in their granules, which are released and destroy the parenchyma. There are metalloproteinase-9 (MMP-9) and serine proteinases, which are released and destroy elastin. Elastin is the characteristic component of elastic fibers, which determine the elastic properties of the lung parenchyma. The destruction of the elastic fibers causes an increased lung compliance and reduction of elasticity, which are characteristic changes in pulmonary emphysema [32]. Elastin segments act as chemotactic agents for macrophages. The aggregated macrophages secrete metalloproteinases in turn and participate in the destruction of lung parenchyma. Macrophages secrete chemokines, which maintain the chronic inflammation that characterizes COPD (**Figure 1**) [33].

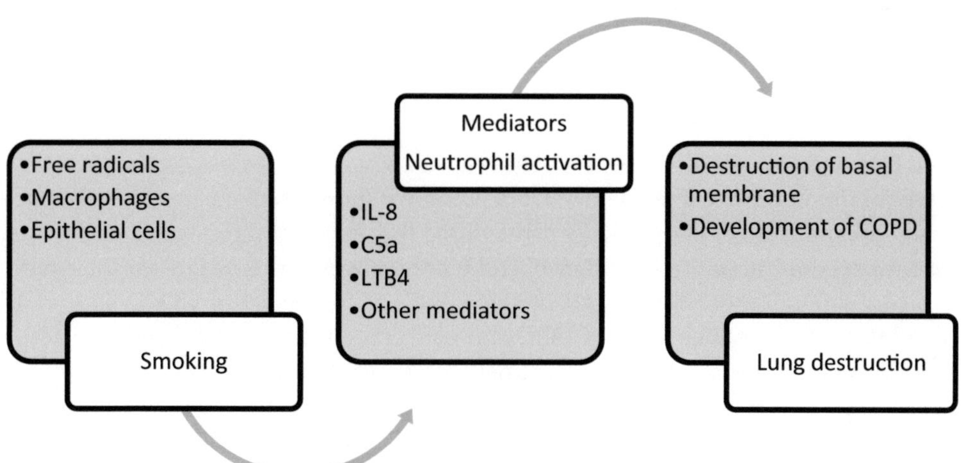

Figure 1. Pathogenetic mechanisms of lung destruction in COPD.

Apart from neutrophils and macrophages, there are also increased numbers of CD4+ T lymphocytes and CD8+ T lymphocytes in bronchioles and alveoli of COPD patients. Epithelial cells of smokers with COPD show an increased expression of CXC40 factor, which is a structural element of the agent of T-cell, CXRCR3 [34]. Although the precise role of T cells is not fully understood, it seems that they produce metalloproteinases, which have profound destructive effects on pulmonary parenchyma. The cytotoxic T-cells are also likely to affect epithelial cells, leading to premature cellular death. Other cells, such as dendritic cells and eosinophils, have also been reported to be increased in COPD. But their exact role is still unknown.

Cigarette smoking, as previously explained, is the main factor to initiate chronic inflammation. However, a few other factors cause inflammation to perpetuate, even years after smoking cessation. Indeed, in histological lung preparations derived from pneumonectomy, inflammation cells, such as macrophages, T-cells, neutrophils, and eosinophils are observed, even 9 years after the end of smoking habit [35]. The exact mechanism of persistent inflammation is not known, but it seems that the impaired mobility of the cilia of epithelial cells of the respiratory mucosa predisposes to the colonization of airways with bacteria, which in turn predisposes to viral infections, especially adenovirus infections, which trigger the inflammatory processes. Despite the controversial pathogenesis, numerous inflammatory cells participate in COPD pathogenesis and cause inflammation that proceeds even when the original trigger of cigarette smoke is absent.

These pathogenetic mechanisms have not yet been confirmed in the case of periodontitis. It is known that neutrophils are the inflammatory cells that predominate in cases of gingivitis [36] and their role in the pathogenesis of chronic periodontitis has been investigated. But, it is not yet fully understood whether the neutrophils have the same characteristics and the same role in both periodontitis and COPD. Further research is needed in the field. However, it is known that in both COPD and periodontitis, activated neutrophils secrete inflammatory mediators, such as proteinases and oxygen radicals, which are involved in tissue damage and in chronic inflammation. This is an important feature of both conditions. Moreover, increased free radicals are produced when cells are exogenously stimulated by the means of *Fusobacterium nucleatum*, a bacterium that frequently causes periodontitis [37].

It should be noted that adverse effects are also caused when local levels of antioxidant factors in interstitial fluid gum are disrupted. At this point, we should remark that if the hypothesis of diffuse inflammation is adopted, we can assume that successful treatment of one disease (periodontitis) could improve the other (COPD) and conversely. It is known that there is a positive correlation between poor oral hygiene and the frequency of COPD exacerbations [38]. In a recent study, patients with COPD and concomitant periodontitis were tested. Half of them (20 patients) received proper treatment for periodontitis, while the rest 20 patients did not receive any treatment at all. They were all observed for 12 months, and it was reported that in the first group a lower frequency of COPD exacerbations was documented. Although this is a significant finding, the study had some methodological problems such as the fact that the selection of patients was not randomized and the sample size was small.

Nevertheless, the findings of this study should be carefully considered in order to carry out further investigation in the field.

5. Antibiotic treatment in chronic periodontitis and COPD

Exacerbations are short periods in the course of COPD characterized by increased cough, dyspnea, and production of sputum that can become purulent. They can lead to accelerated lung function impairment, worse quality of life, and increased mortality [39]. Except from the severity, the frequency of the exacerbations, also, plays an important role in the management of the exacerbations. Depending on the severity of the exacerbation, different therapeutic strategies could be used. Therefore, increased doses of bronchodilators are required for mild exacerbations, systemic corticosteroids, and antibiotics can be used for moderate exacerbations, whereas severe exacerbations often require admission to hospital [40]. However, the most frequent causes of exacerbations are bacterial or viral infections, which are responsible for 60–80% of all exacerbations. These infectious exacerbations are more severe than the non-infectious exacerbations.

There are some articles concerning the possible relationship between chronic inflammatory diseases and their comorbidities. Both chronic periodontitis and COPD are neutrophilic, inflammatory conditions characterized by loss of local connective tissue. It is possible that there is an association and perhaps a casual link between the two diseases. It has been reported that respiratory pathogens such as *Pseudomonas aeruginosa* might adhere better to oral epithelial cells obtained from patients colonized by respiratory pathogens than to cells harvested from noncolonized patients. Trypsin treatment of epithelial cells from noncolonized patients in vitro resulted in increased adhesion of respiratory pathogens [41]. This suggests that mucosal alteration promoted enhanced bacterial adhesion of these bacteria. This alteration is perhaps the loss of fibronectin (by exposure to proteases) from the epithelial cell surface, which may unmask mucosal surface receptors for respiratory pathogen adhesions.

Subjects with poor hygiene may have elevated levels of hydrolytic enzymes in their saliva. These enzymes may process mucins to reduce their ability to bind to and clear pathogens such as *Haemophilus influenzae*. Conversely, the enzymes may process the respiratory epithelium to modulate the adhesion of such pathogens to the mucosal surface. Mannino et al. [42] postulated that oral pathogens continuously stimulate the cells of the periodontium (epithelial cells) to release a wide variety of cytokines and other biologically active molecules such as IL-1a, IL-1b, IL-6, IL-8, and TNF-a. Oral bacteria in secretions may adhere to the mucosal surface and stimulate the epithelial cells of the respiratory epithelium to secrete cytokines. These stimulated cells may then release other cytokines that recruit inflammatory cells to the site. These inflammatory cells release hydrolytic enzymes resulting in damaged epithelium that may be more susceptible to colonization by respiratory pathogens. It is possible that the poor oral health might work in concert with other factors (smoking, environmental pollution, viral infections, and genetic factors) to promote the progression and exacerbation of pulmonary disease.

6. Conclusions

The associations demonstrated between periodontitis and COPD suggest a basis for testing the effects of treatment for one condition upon the severity of the other. Improving oral hygiene might reduce the risk of respiratory infection among subjects who are at risk.

Our article describes similarities in epidemiology and pathogenetic mechanisms of COPD and periodontitis and proposes that improvement of one condition is linked to the treatment of the other. Future research is needed to clarify the existing pathogenetic mechanisms and extend possible therapeutic options.

Authors' contributions

Agathi Spiropoulou and Dimosthenis Lykouras have worked on manuscript concept, literature review, and manuscript preparation. Olga Lagiou worked on literature review and manuscript preparation. Kiriakos Karkoulias worked on manuscript preparation. Kostas Spiropoulos worked on revision of manuscript for important intellectual content.

Abbreviations

COPD	Chronic obstructive pulmonary disease
CD	Cluster of differentiation
CRP	C-reactive protein
MMP	Metalloproteinase
IL	Interleukin
TNF	Tumor necrosis factor
(FEV1/FVC) ratio	The ratio of the forced expiratory volume in the first one second to the forced vital capacity of the lungs
LTB4	Leukotriene B4
C5a	Complement component 5a

Author details

Agathi Spiropoulou, Olga Lagiou, Dimosthenis Lykouras, Kiriakos Karkoulias and Kostas Spiropoulos*

*Address all correspondence to: spircos@upatras.gr

Department of Pulmonary Medicine, University Hospital of Patras, Rio, Patras, Greece

References

[1] Morris AJ, Steele J, White DA. The oral cleanliness and periodontal health of UK adults in 1998. British Dental Journal. 2001;**191**:186-192

[2] Kinane DF, Preshaw PM, Loos BG, Working Group 2 of Seventh European Workshop on Periodontology. Host-response: Understanding the cellular and molecular mechanisms of host-microbial interactions—Consensus of the Seventh European Workshop on Periodontology. Journal of Clinical Periodontology. 2011;**38**(Suppl 11):44-48

[3] Listgarten MA. Pathogenesis of periodontitis. Journal of Clinical Periodontology. 1986;**13**:418-430

[4] Sampsonas E, Lykouras D, Drakatos P, Moschopoulou A, Spiropoulos K, Karkoulias K. Endothelin-1 polymorphisms involved in impaired exercise tolerance in COPD patients. A pilot study. European Review for Medical and Pharmacological Sciences. 2011;**15**(2):123-128

[5] Rabe KF, Hurd S, Anzueto A, et al. Global strategy for the diagnosis, management, and prevention of chronic obstructive pulmonary disease. American Journal of Respiratory and Critical Care Medicine. 2007;**176**(6):532-555

[6] GOLD. Global Strategy for the Diagnosis, Management and Prevention of COPD. Global Initiative for Chronic Obstructive Lung Disease (GOLD) [Online]. 2014. Available from: http://www.goldcopd.org/uploads/users/files/GOLD_Report_2014_Jun11.pdf

[7] Lopez AD, Mathers CD, Ezzati M, Jamison DT, Murray CJ. Global and regional burden of disease and risk factors, 2001: Systematic analysis of population health data. Lancet. 2011;**367**:1747-1757

[8] Tzortzaki E, Siafakas N. Paolo Palange, Anita K. Simonds. COPD and emphysema. In: ERS Handbook: Respiratory Medicine. 2nd ed. European Respiratory Society. UK; 2013. pp. 287-292. ISBN: 978-1-84984-040-8

[9] Stockley RA. Neutrophils and the pathogenesis of COPD. Chest. 2002;**121**(Suppl 5): 151S-155S

[10] Saetta M. Airway inflammation in chronic obstructive pulmonary disease. American Journal of Respiratory and Critical Care Medicine. 1999;**160**:S17-S20

[11] Barnes PJ, Celli BR. Systemic manifestations and comorbidities of COPD. European Respiratory Journal. 2009;**33**:1165-1185

[12] Sherrill DL, Lebowitz MD, Burrows B. Epidemiology of chronic obstructive pulmonary disease. Clinics in Chest Medicine. 1990;**11**:375-387

[13] Lee HJ, Garcia RI, Janket SJ, Jones JA, Mascarenhas AK, Scott TE, et al. The association between cumulative periodontal disease and stroke history in older adults. Journal of Periodontology. 2006;**77**:1744-1754

[14] Wedzicha J, Seemungal T. COPD exacerbations: Defining their cause and prevention. Lancet. 2007;**370**:786-796

[15] Connett JE, Murray RP, Buist AS, Wise RA, Bailey WC, Lindgren PG, et al. Changes in smoking status affect women more than men: Results of the Lung Health Study. American Journal of Epidemiology. 2003;**157**:973-979

[16] Mannino DM. COPD: Epidemiology, prevalence, morbidity and mortality, and disease heterogeneity. Chest. 2002;**121**(Suppl 5):121S-126S

[17] Pihlstrom BL. Periodontal risk assessment, diagnosis and treatment planning. Periodontal 2000. 2001;**25**:37-58

[18] Scannapieco FA, Papandonatos GD, Dunford RG. Associations between oral conditions and respiratory disease in a national sample survey population. Annals of Periodontology. 1998;**3**:251-256

[19] Deo V, Bhongade M, Ansari S, Chavan RS. Periodontitis as a potential risk factor for chronic obstructive pulmonary disease: A retrospective study. Indian Journal of Dental Research. 2009;**20**:466-470

[20] Zhou X, Wang Z, Song Y, Zhang J, Wang C. Periodontal health and quality of life in patients with chronic obstructive pulmonary disease. Respiratory Medicine. 2011;**105**:67-73

[21] Wang Z, Zhou X, Zhang J, Zhang L, Song Y, Hu FB, et al. Periodontal health, oral health behaviours, and chronic obstructive pulmonary disease. Journal of Clinical Periodontology. 2009;**36**:750-755

[22] Liu Z, Zhang W, Zhang J, Zhou X, Zhang L, Song Y, et al. Oral hygiene, periodontal health and chronic obstructive pulmonary disease exacerbations. Journal of Clinical Periodontology. 2012;**39**:45-52

[23] Yildirim E, Kormi I, Basoğlu ÖK, Gürgün A, Kaval B, Sorsa T, et al. Periodontal health and serum, saliva matrix metalloproteinases in patients with mild chronic obstructive pulmonary disease. Journal of Periodontal Research. 2013;**48**:269-275

[24] O'Donnell DE. Hyperinflation, dyspnea, and exercise intolerance in chronic obstructive pulmonary disease. Proceedings of the American Thoracic Society. 2006;**3**:180-184

[25] Hogg JC, Timens W. The pathology of chronic obstructive pulmonary disease. Annual Review of Pathology. 2009;**4**:435-459

[26] Barnes PJ, Shapiro SD, Pauwels RA. Chronic obstructive pulmonary disease: Molecular and cellular mechanisms. European Respiratory Journal. 2003;**22**:672-688

[27] Rahman I, Adcock IM. Oxidative stress and redox regulation of lung inflammation in COPD. European Respiratory Journal. 2006;**28**:219-242

[28] Shapiro SD. The macrophage in chronic obstructive pulmonary disease. American Journal of Respiratory and Critical Care Medicine. 1999;**160**:S29-S32

[29] Kheradmand F, Shan M, Xu C, Corry DB. Autoimmunity in chronic obstructive pulmonary disease: Clinical and experimental evidence. Expert Review of Clinical Immunology. 2012;**8**:285-292

[30] Ali J, Pramod K, Tahir MA, Ansari SH. Autoimmune responses in periodontal diseases. Autoimmunity Reviews. 2011;**10**:426-431

[31] Krinsky NI. Mechanism of action of biological antioxidants. Proceedings of the Society for Experimental Biology and Medicine. 1992;**200**:248-254

[32] Thurlbeck W. Pathology of chronic airflow obstruction. In: Cherniack NS, editor. Chronic Obstructive Pulmonary Diseases. Philadelphia: WB Saunders; 1991. pp. 3-20

[33] Silverman EK, Chapman HA, Dreazen JM, Weiss ST, Rosner B, Campbell EJ, et al. Genetic epidemiology of severe, early-onset chronic obstructive pulmonary disease: Risk to relatives for airflow obstruction and chronic bronchitis. American Journal of Respiratory and Critical Care Medicine. 1998;**157**:1770-1778

[34] Rennard SI. Repair. In: Calverley PMA, MacNee W, Pride NB, Rennard SI, editors. Chronic Obstructive Pulmonary Disease. London: Arnold; 2003. pp. 139-150

[35] Saetta M, Di Stefano A, Turato G, Facchini FM, Corbino L, Mapp CE, et al. CD8+ T-lymphocytes in peripheral airways of smokers with chronic obstructive pulmonary disease. American Journal of Respiratory and Critical Care Medicine. 1998;**157**:822-826

[36] Matthews JB, Wright HJ, Roberts A, Cooper PR, Chapple IL. Hyperactivity and reactivity of peripheral blood neutrophils in chronic periodontitis. Clinical & Experimental Immunology. 2007;**147**:255-264

[37] Nussbaum G, Shapira L. How has neutrophil research improved our understanding of periodontal pathogenesis? Journal of Clinical Periodontology. 2011;**38**(Suppl 11):49-59

[38] Kucukcoskun M, Baser U, Oztekin G, Kiyan E, Yalcin F. Initial periodontal treatment for prevention of chronic obstructive pulmonary disease exacerbations. Journal of Periodontology. 2012;**84**:863-870

[39] Llor C, Moragas A, Hernandez S, Bayona C, Miravitlles M. Efficacy of antibiotic therapy for acute exacerbations of mild to moderate chronic obstructive pulmonary disease. American Journal of Respiratory and Critical Care Medicine. 2012;**186**:716-723

[40] Decramer M, Janssens W, Miravitlles M. Chronic obstructive pulmonary disease. Lancet. 2012;**379**:1341-1351

[41] Zandvoort A, van der Geld YM, Jonker MR, Noordhoek JA, Vos JT, et al. High ICAM-1 gene expression in pulmonary fibroblasts of COPD patients: A reflection of an enhanced immunological function. European Respiratory Journal. 2006;**28**:113-122

[42] Mannino DM, Doherty DE, Sonia Buist A. Global Initiative on Obstructive Lung Disease (GOLD) classification of lung disease and mortality: Findings from the Atherosclerosis Risk in Communities (ARIC) study. Respiratory Medicine. 2006;**100**:115-122

Chapter 5

Probiotics and Periodontal Diseases

Alicia Morales, Joel Bravo-Bown, Javier Bedoya and
Jorge Gamonal

Additional information is available at the end of the chapter

http://dx.doi.org/10.5772/intechopen.68814

Abstract

Probiotics are defined as live microorganisms that, when administered in adequate amounts, confer a health benefit on the host. Probiotics have been used to directly modify the resident oral microbiome and proposed to modulate immune responses. In dentistry, probiotics have been employed as useful adjuncts for the reduction of caries development, suppressing oral Candida infection and controlling halitosis. Plaque-induced gingivitis is a gingival inflammation caused by the adherent bacterial biofilm around teeth. Gingivitis and periodontitis are considered to be a continuum of the same inflammatory process, although many gingivitis lesions do not progress to periodontitis. Periodontitis is an inflammatory process that affects the attachment structures of teeth. It constitutes a second cause of tooth loss worldwide. Conventional treatment modalities of periodontal disease include non-surgical and/or surgical management, with an emphasis on mechanical debridement. However, mechanical debridement as a sole therapy is not always effective to improve clinical parameters. A growing number of studies support probiotic therapy to prevent or treat gingivitis and periodontitis. Oral administration of probiotics is an effective adjunct in reducing pathogenic bacteria and improving clinical signs of disease. Probiotics may serve as adjunct or replacement therapy substitute antibiotics in managing human periodontal infections in future.

Keywords: probiotics, periodontitis, gingivitis, periodontal diseases, dental scaling

1. Introduction

In order to speak about probiotics, we have to go back to the twentieth century when the Russian scientist Elie Metchnikoff postulated the theory about the influence of gastrointestinal micro biota (gut flora) over ageing. In 1908, this Nobel Prize winner attached the longevity of some Balkans towns to the frequent consumption of fermented dairy, containing Lactobacillus, which reduced the toxins produced by intestinal bacteria, promoting health and prolonging life [1].

The discovery of Lactic Acid Bacteria (LAB) in the middle of the nineteenth century confirmed the interest in microorganism and since then many people have concluded that dairy fermented by lactobacillales provide numerous benefits to our health [2].

For a long time, microorganisms have been responsible for the production of numerous foods and drinks and also have had an important impact on human health. The discovery of a symbiotic relationship between bacteria and humans awoke the curiosity of seeing the bacteria as potentially beneficial rather than pathogenic [2].

Lilly and Stillwell coined the term "probiotics" first definition in 1965 as: "Living microorganisms that confer a benefit to the host's health when given in adequate amounts" [3]. The term "prebiotic" was defined as "a non-digestible food ingredient that beneficially affects the host by selectively stimulating the growth and/or activity of one or a limited number of bacteria in the colon, and thus improves host health" by Gibson and Roberfroid [4].

Symbiotic is the relationship between probiotics and prebiotics, which benefits the host by increasing the survival and implantation of live microorganisms from dietary supplements in the gastrointestinal system [5]. This has not been deeply studied, but it could increase bacteria potential to develop their function in the colon because symbiotic products could increase the survival of probiotic in their intestinal transit phase. Also, a synergic effect has been described. Prebiotics contribute to the installation of a specific bacterial flora with beneficial effects on health because they stimulate the growth of specific strains [6].

Nowadays the term probiotic has evolved and is now described as "living microorganisms, mostly bacteria, non-pathogenic, used as nutritional supplement, which after being ingested in the right amount, improve the intestinal microbial balance and cause beneficial effects on the health of those who ingest them" [7]. They are considered safe for human health [8]. Since the 1980s scientific investigation about healthy properties of ingesting probiotics has increased considerably, which boosted their use and led to their appearance in clinical practice as treatment for diseases such as chronic diarrhea, immune regulation, allergies, inflammatory bowel disease, constipation, lactose intolerance and lipid intolerance [9]. Lately there is big concern regarding the use of probiotics to treat oral infections like dental cavities (caries) and periodontal diseases. However, available information about the effects of probiotics on periodontal health is still minimal [10].

Chronic oral infections in soft tissues cause inflammatory alterations releasing pro-inflammatory substances such as cytokines, which through the circulatory system, access any area of the body, increasing the risk of muscular, digestive and cardiovascular problems, premature birth, diabetes and sports injuries. Hence, the treatment of chronic oral diseases and the maintenance of oral health should be considered as an asset in the prevention of systemic problems for general health [11].

Periodontal diseases and dental cavities have high prevalence [12], and according to the World Health Organization, the majority of children have signs of gingivitis and among adults the initial stages of periodontal disease are highly prevalent [13]. Bacterial biofilm that forms in the hard and soft tissues of the oral cavity is considered the main etiological factor in most pathological conditions of the oral cavity. The accumulation of bacteria inside the biofilm, provided by a poor oral health, influences changes in the microbial community, leading to periodontal inflammation [14].

Several studies such as Gorbach and Goldin (1985) [15], Näse et al. (2001) [16], Grudianov et al. (2002) [17], Wei et al. [18], Von Bultzingslowen et al. [19], Hatakka et al. (2007) [20] have spoken about the relation between bacterial strains like *Lactobacillus rhamnosus, Bifidobacterium* spp, and *Lactobacillus plantarum,* which have a positive effect on tooth adhesion and their action against diseases such as dental cavities (caries) and yeast infection. In recent years, treatments of periodontal diseases have changed to an antibiotic or antimicrobial kind. Nonetheless, with the increased incidence of antibiotic resistance, probiotics may be a promising area of research in periodontal therapy [21]. Currently, there is a probiotic that can be used for oral hygiene, as it combats dental plaque, gingivitis and cariogenic bacteria through the patented combination of two strains of *Lactobacillus reuteri*. This is 100% natural due to its residence in the human gastrointestinal tract and production of an antibiotic substance of broad-spectrum called "reuterina", which administrated in the right amount, causes the desired antimicrobial effect to keep the intestinal microbiota intact [11].

Increasingly, antibiotics become complex elements to manage in medical therapies due to the increment of bacterial resistance to them. However, inversely proportional, clinical studies have shown the positive effects in human health associated with the use of probiotics. This is the reason why the World Health Organization supports the use of probiotics as microbial interference therapy. Consequently, the use of probiotics could be postulated as a useful alternative in the control of periodontal diseases, since it improves the conditions of the host, reducing periodontal pocket depth, inflammation, bleeding and halitosis.

2. Local mechanisms of probiotic action

Several mechanisms have been suggested to contribute to the probiotic action. Their effects at local level are mentioned as follows:

1. Production of lactic acid (a short chain fatty acid) can penetrate the bacterial membrane and acidify the cytoplasm by inhibiting the proliferation of *Porphyromonas gingivalis, Streptococcus mutans* [22] and *Prevotella intermedia* [23]. *Lactobacillus gasseri* is a homofermentative bacteria (metabolism via glycolysis) that is able to produce large quantities of lactic acid.

2. Production of hydrogen peroxide can inhibit the growth of pathogenic bacteria [24–26]. *Streptococcus sanguinis* reduces the levels of *Aggregatibacter actinomycetemcomitans* (in about 45 times) and *S. mutans.*

3. Protein modification on the site of attachment, removal of aglutinina gp 340, which is necessary for the attachment of *S. mutans* [16].

4. Production of biosurfactants that prevent bacterial adhesion. *Streptococcus mitis* produces a biosurfactant that prevents adhesion of *S. mutans* and some periodontopathogenic bacteria to the tooth surface.

5. Production of bacteriocins (cationic peptides synthesized on ribosomes with antimicrobial activity that have a narrow spectrum of action) [27–29].

   (a) Salivaricin A and B: Bacteriocins produced by *Streptococcus salivarius*. Salivaricin decreases the proliferation of *S. mutans* and *Streptococcus sobrinus* in carious lesions. Salivaricin B inhibits the growth of *Prevotella* spp. and *Micromonas micros* in halitosis.

   (b) Reuterin: Bacteriocin produced by *L. reuteri,* has antibacterial activity on bacterial Gram (+) and Gram (−), fungi (*Candida albicans*) and protozoa. Among them *S. mutans* and *P. intermedia*.

6. Production of inhibitory substances like bacteriocins: peptides synthesized on ribosomes with antimicrobial activity and broad spectrum of action.

7. Production of vitamins and other substances.

   (a) *Lactobacillus acidophilus* can participate in the production of niacin, folic acid and vitamin B6.

   (b) *Bifidobacterium dentium* increases the absorption of iron, zinc, calcium and magnesium.

   (c) *Streptococcus thermophilus* synthesizes polysaccharides such as hyaluronic acid and produces urease.

8. Changes in the cellular envelope: *Lactobacillus paracasei* HL32 inhibits *P. gingivalis* to induce a change in the cellular envelope [30].

9. Glucosiltransferasa enzyme inhibition. *L. rhamnosus* inhibits the glycosyl-transferase enzyme by reducing the synthesis of glucans in the formation of the biofilm.

10. Anti-oxidant effect.

   (a) *Bifidobacterium longum* has anti-oxidant effect by inhibiting the formation of linolenic acid in the form of hydrogen peroxide.

   (b) *Lactobacillus brevis* decreases the levels of nitric oxide synthetases (NOS).

11. Ingested probiotics can impact resident communities through trophic interactions, a direct alteration in fitness or an indirect alteration in fitness through altered production of host-derived molecules [31]. The major changes of gastrointestinal microbiome occur in stomach and small intestine. These are important not only quantitatively; they may also alter the relative abundance of major phyla [32–35].

3. Systemic mechanisms of probiotic action

The systemic mechanisms of probiotic action are associated with its effect on immune response. In past years, there have been an increasing number of studies linking gut health with several chronic diseases. In order to understand these mechanisms, it is necessary to review this literature.

3.1. Use of probiotics in medicine

Clinical studies have demonstrated the clinical potential of probiotic against many diseases. However, generalizations concerning the potential health benefits of probiotic should not be made because its effects are strain-specific [36]. Probiotics have been used in some conditions, such as:

3.1.1. Atopic dermatitis

Atopic dermatitis is a chronically relapsing skin disease that occurs most commonly during early infancy and childhood. It is associated with allergen sensitization, recurrent skin infections and abnormalities in skin barriers function [37]. Foolad et al. published a meta-analysis study aimed to find evidence about the effect of probiotics in children with atopic dermatitis [38]. They concluded that the use of probiotics, specifically *L. rhamnosus* GG [39], showed to be effective in mothers and infants in preventing the development and reducing severity of atopic dermatitis [38]. In adult patients, the use of *L. salivarius* LS01 [40] and a combination of *L. salivarius* LS01 with *Bifidobacterium breve* BR03 [41] were associated with significant improvement of clinical manifestations of atopic dermatitis.

3.1.2. Antibiotic-associated diarrhea

Diarrhea is a common side effect of antibiotic use. It can be classified as *Clostridium*-associated antibiotic diarrhea or non-*Clostridium difficile*-associated antibiotic diarrhea. The first one is benign. In contrast, the second one refers to a wide spectrum of diarrhea illnesses caused by the toxins produced by *C. difficile*, including cases of severe colitis with or without the presence of pseudomembranes [42]. A series of meta-analysis concluded that probiotics significantly reduce the risk of antibiotic-associated diarrhea in children [43] and adult patients [44]. It was associated with the use of *L. rhamnosus* GG, *B. lactis* and *S. thermophiles* [43]. *S. boulardii* was reported to be effective in *C. difficile* disease [45, 46].

3.1.3. Irritable bowel syndrome (IBS)

IBS is defined as an abdominal discomfort or pain associated with altered bowel habits for at least 3 days in the previous 3 months, with the absence of organic disease [42]. A meta-analysis demonstrated that, compared with placebo, the use *L. rhamnosus* GG was associated with a significantly higher rate of treatment responders in the overall population with abdominal pain-related functional gastrointestinal disorders and in the irritable bowel syndrome patients [47].

3.1.4. Inflammatory bowel disease (IBD)

IBD consists of two disorders: ulcerative colitis (UC) and Crohn's disease (CD). The gut mucosa suffers a chronic, uncontrolled inflammation. CD is characterized by focal transmural inflammatory lesions and ulcerations that can be present anywhere in the gastrointestinal tract. UC is more superficial and limited to colon.

A meta-analysis concluded that remission rates in patients with active UC were significantly higher in patients who were treated with probiotics, specifically, VSL#3 (a combination of probiotics containing *B. breve, B. longum, Bifidobacterium infantis, L. acidophilus, L. plantarum, L. paracasei, L. bulgaricus* and *S. thermophiles*) [48].

3.1.5. Helicobacter pylori

Probiotics do not eradicate *H. pylori*, but they can diminish the levels of this bacterium in the stomach. In association with antibiotic treatments, some probiotics increased eradication rates and/or decreased adverse effects due to the antibiotics [49].

3.1.6. Necrotizing enterocolitis

It is a severe condition occurring especially in preterm infants. A Cochrane review concluded in 2011 that enteral supplementation with probiotics prevents sever necrotizing enterocolitis in preterm infants [50].

3.1.7. Hypocholesterolemic treatment

The combinations of prebiotics and probiotics such as bifidobacteria and FOS, lactobacilli and lactitol, and bifidobacteria and galactooligosacharides were used in trials and have shown promising results in hypocholesterolemic effect [51].

3.1.8. Radiation enteritis

Pelvic malignancies are commonly treated with radiation therapy. Chronic gastrointestinal side effects occur in over 30% of patients [42]. A meta-analysis concluded that probiotic treatment with *Lactobacillus* spp could prevent chemotherapy and radiation enteritis-induced diarrhea in patients with pelvic malignancies [52].

3.2. Probiotic effect on immune responses

Probiotics help maintain gut immune homeostasis by modulating immune response, enhancing epithelial barrier function and inhibiting pathogen growth. Probiotic interaction with mucosal immune system is through the same pathways as commensal bacteria. Its effect appears to be more immune regulating than immune activating [37].

Probiotics modulate epithelial barrier function through interactions with Toll-like receptor (TLR)-2 [53]. The initiation of TLRs signalling regulates synthesis of pro-inflammatory cytokines, chemokines and antimicrobial peptides, recruitment of B cells and production of IgA [54]. Probiotics have been shown to suppress systemic inflammatory response, modulating epithelial signal transduction pathways and cytokine production [55]. For example, *Lactobacillus johnsonni* N6.2 up-regulated type-1 interferon and IFN regulators Stat1 and IRF7 in a TLR-9 dependent way, in rats [56].

Several strains of lactic acid bacteria induce *in vitro* release of pro-inflammatory cytokines TNF-α and IL-6, reflecting stimulation of nonspecific immunity [57]. *L. acidophilus* Lal enhances phagocytosis in humans [58]. *L. casei* Shirota can enhance natural killer cell activity *in vivo* and *in vitro* in humans [59]. However, there are some bacteria that can decrease pro-inflammatory molecules. For example, *L. brevis* CD2 decreases inflammatory markers in saliva from patients with periodontal disease, including prostaglandin E2 (PGE2) [60]. Also, it was reported that probiotics, specifically, *L. reuteri* ATCC PTA 5289 decreased in CGF levels of TNF-α and IL-1β in patients with chronic periodontitis [61]. *Streptococcus cristatus, S. salivarius, S. mitis* and *S. sanguinis* may decrease the release of IL-8 by the epithelial cells stimulated with *Fusobacterium nucleatum* and *A. actinomycetemcomitans* [62–64].

Some specific strains generate an effect on maturation of dendritic cells (DC). DC has a central role in directing the T cell response. They can change to T helper cell (Th) 1, Th2, Th17 and T regulatory cells (Treg) [65]. Certain bacterial strains induce the production of Th polarizing key cytokines by DCs, such as IL-10, IL-12 and IL-23 [66, 67]. Also, some *Lactobacillus* strains have been shown to stimulate Th1 cytokine production while others have increased Th2 responses or induced a mixed Th1/Th2 response [37]. An example of this is the use of a combination of *L. salivarius* LS01 and *Bifidobacterium breve* BR03 in treatment of atopic dermatitis. This probiotic mix generated a significant reduction in microbial translocation, immune activation, improved Th17/Treg cell and Th1/Th2 [41]. Intervention with *B. bifidum, L. acidophilus, L. casei* and *L. salivarius* effectively reduced signs of atopic dermatitis and serum cytokines interleukin (IL-5, IL-6, IFN-γ and serum IgE) [68]. *L. rhamnosus* GG could up-regulate IFN-γ and IL-10 in infants with cow's milk allergy or with IgE-associated dermatitis [69]. The use of *Lactobacillus delbruekii* and *Lactobacillus fermentum* significantly reduced IL-6 concentration and expression of TNF-α and NFκB in colon of patients with ulcerative colitis [70]. *L. brevis* CD2 decreased IFN-γ levels in saliva [60]. *L. reuteri* ATCC PTA 5289 decreased in CGF levels of IL-17 in patients with chronic periodontitis [61].

Anti-inflammatory effect of probiotics has been associated with Treg. For example, oral administration of *L. casei* alleviated colitis and increased the suppressive function of Treg of colon lamina propia. Consumption of *B. infantis* drives the generation of Treg cells, which attenuate nuclear factor kappa B (NFκB) activation induced by LPS of *Salmonella typhimurium* [71].

There is evidence of the effect of some probiotics on matrix metalloproteinases (MMP). They represent a family of human zinc-dependent endopeptidases [65]. *L. brevis* CD2 decreased MMP in saliva [60]. *L. reuteri* DSM 17938 + ATCC PTA 5289 decreased GCF MMP-8 and increased tissue inhibitors of matrix metalloproteinase (TIMP)-1 levels in patients with periodontitis [72].

Current studies also mentioned the role of probiotics in modulation of cell signal transduction pathways, specifically NFκB, which monitors the inflammatory response in the host [73]. *L. reuteri* inhibited inhibitory κB (IκB) degradation and IL-8 expression in TNF-α induced T84 cells and NFκB translocation to the nucleus in HeLa cells [74]. In the same way, *L. rhamnosus* GG diminished nucleus translocation of NFκB, restored decreased cytoplasmic IκB and limited IL-8 secretion in Caco-2 cell model [75]. These actions impede the stimulation of transcription of a series of pro-inflammatory genes such as the encode cytokines, chemokines and grow factors that modulate the proliferation of immune cells [76]. In bronchial epithelial cells cocultured with *S. salivarius* K12, an immunosuppression was observed, coincident with the inhibition of activation of the NF-κB pathway.

Certain strains of *Bifidobacteria, Lactobacilli, Escherichia coli, Propionibacterium, Bacillus* and *Saccharomyces* influence gene expression of TLRs, NFκB and interleukins. *In vitro,* the interaction of probiotics with antigen presenting cells results in downregulation of pro-inflammatory genes and upregulation of anti-inflammatory genes [36].

4. Probiotics and gingivitis

The adherent bacterial biofilm around the teeth produces a gingival inflammation called plaque-induced gingivitis [77]. It is the most common form of periodontal disease worldwide and plenty of data exist, from different countries and age groups, about the prevalence, extent and severity of gingivitis. Studies on population have shown that regardless of age, gender and race, gingivitis is always associated with the level of oral hygiene [78]. Large-scale population studies on children, adolescents, adults and elderly people have reported very high prevalence of gingivitis, ranging from 50 to 100% [79–82]. Gingivitis and periodontitis are regarded as a continuum of a same inflammatory process. However, it is necessary to point out that in many cases gingivitis does not progress to periodontitis [83, 84].

Once the teeth erupt, a bacterial biofilm immediately begins to form at their surfaces exposed to the oral cavity and in intimate contact with the gingival margin. The level of biofilm accumulation, the virulence of the biofilm bacteria and the humoral and cellular immune responses to the biofilm microbiome are the factors that determine the severity of the periodontal disease [85]. Normally gingivitis in young subjects remains chronic for an extended period of time and does not cause any damage to the periodontal ligament or bone. Nevertheless, an alteration of the balance between biofilm and host can originate a loss of periodontal attachment. Chronic and aggressive periodontitis start as gingivitis. However, the biological processes involved in the progression from gingivitis to periodontitis have been difficult to determine [86]. It is probable that the following elements are implicated in the disease progression to periodontitis: microbial dysbiosis, overgrowth of pathogenic bacteria, herpes virus reactivation, immune-system disruption and acquired and/or genetic susceptibility factors [87–89].

Mechanical removal of supragingival plaque is the most effective tool to prevent gingivitis [90] but most individuals do not adequately control plaque accumulation and gingivitis continues to be prevalent. To overcome this hindrance, antimicrobial products in the form of dentifrices or mouthwashes have been tested for their adjunctive efficacy in reducing plaque and gingivitis.

Probiotic technology represents a breakthrough approach to maintain oral health by utilizing natural beneficial bacteria commonly found in healthy mouths to provide a natural defence against the bacteria thought to be harmful to teeth and gums [15]. Within dentistry, the previous studies with *lactobacilli* strains such as *L. rhamnosus, L. casei, L. reuteri*, or a *Lactobacilli* mix have revealed mixed results on oral microorganisms.

Krasse et al. conducted one of the first clinical trial randomized double-blind placebo controlled. The principal aim of the study was to assess if the probiotic *L. reuteri* could be effective in the management of gingivitis and then to evaluate the influence of the probiotic on plaque and the lactobacilli population in the saliva. Fifty-nine patients with moderate to severe gingivitis were included and given either/or specific *L. reuteri* formulations (LR-1 or LR-2) at a dose of 2 × 108 CFU/day, or a corresponding placebo. At baseline (day 0), they collected saliva to determine the lactobacilli and measured gingival index and plaque on two surfaces. They taught patients to brush and to floss their teeth carefully and the treatment began. The patients returned on day 14 for final assessment of gingivitis and saliva and plaque were collected. Twenty patients were randomly given LR-1, 21 took LR-2 and 18 received inactive substances. The gingival index decreased evenly in all three groups ($p < 0.0001$). LR-1 only (not LR-2) improved more than placebo ($p < 0.0001$). Plaque index fell evenly in LR-1 ($p < 0.05$) and in LR-2 ($p < 0.01$) between day 0 and day 14 but without significant change in the inactive substance. On day 14, 65% of the patients in the LR-1 group were colonized with *L. reuteri* and 95% in the LR-2. *L. reuteri* reduce both gingivitis and plaque in patients with moderate to severe gingivitis [91].

Twetman et al. conducted a clinical trial randomized double-blind placebo controlled in patients with gingivitis (n = 42). The subjects were randomly assigned to one of three comparable arms: Group A/P (n = 15) was given one active and one test substance gum daily, Group A/A (n = 14) received two active chewing gums and Group P/P (n = 13) two placebo gums. They used chewing gum (2 times a day for 10 min in the morning and evening) with *L. reuteri* (ATCC 55730 and ATCC PTA 5289, 1×10^8 CFU). They taught the patients to chew the gums 10 min for 2 weeks and conducted bleeding on probing and GCF sampling at baseline and after 1, 2 and 4 weeks. The levels of IL-1β, TNFα IL-6, IL-8 and IL-10 were measured using luminex technology and multiplex immunoassay kits. Bleeding on probing improved and GCF volume decreased in all groups during the chewing period. Still, the results were statistically different ($p < 0.05$) only in Groups A/P and A/A. TNFα and IL-8 levels decreased significantly ($p < 0.05$) in Group A/A compared with baseline after 1 and 2 weeks, respectively. They also observed a non-significant tendency to decrease in IL-1β during the chewing period. The levels of IL-6 and IL-10 remained unchanged in all groups after 1 and 3 weeks. The elemental basis of the probiotic approach to confront inflammation in the oral cavity could be the decrease of pro-inflammatory cytokines in GCF [92].

Staab et al. conducted a parallel-designed non-blinded study. Fifty volunteer students took part in this study. The test group took a probiotic drink (*L. casei*, 100 billion per 100 ml everyday); the control group did not drink any product. After 8 weeks, individual mechanical plaque control was delayed for 96 h. Papilla bleeding index, interproximal plaque and Turesky plaque index were measured at baseline, after 8 weeks and again 96 h later. At the coincidence points, we collected GCF for evaluation of polymorphonuclear elastase, myeloperoxidase (MPO) and MMP-3. There was no difference in the interproximal plaque index and papillary bleeding between the groups. In the test group, the elastase activity and the amount of MMP-3 were significantly lower after the intake of the probiotic drink ($p < 0.001$ and 0.016). A significant increase of MPO activity was noted in the control group; both groups had differences at the end of the survey ($p = 0.014$). According to the data, it is suggested that the probiotic milk drink has a beneficial effect on the gingival inflammation [93].

Ierardo et al. conducted a clinical trial in patients with gingivitis: Test group (n = 21) consumed chewing gum (3 times per day for 60 days) containing probiotic *L. brevis*. Control group was used for the laboratory variables (n = 16). Measurements were taken at baseline, 30 and 60 days. It was concluded that *L. brevis* has anti-inflammatory effects showing clinical improvement. In addition, it allows to reduce the levels of immunoglobulin (Ig)-A [94].

Iniesta et al. conducted a clinical trial randomized double-blind in patients with gingivitis: Test Group (n = 20) obtained lozenges with *L. reuteri* (DSM-17938 and ATCC PTA 5289, 2×10^8 CFU) for two periods of 12 weeks (with an intermediate period of 4 weeks without measures of hygiene). Microbiological and clinical differences and the pattern of colonization of *L. reuteri* were determined again. In conclusion, no significant changes occurred between and within the groups in the clinical variables. Total anaerobic counts in saliva after 4 weeks ($p = 0.021$) and counts of *P. intermedia* after 8 weeks ($p = 0.030$) decreased in the test group. In subgingival samples, *P. gingivalis* counts reduced significantly from baseline to 4 weeks ($p = 0.008$). With PCR, the presence of *L. reuteri* ATCC-PTA-5289 was higher than *L. reuteri* DSM-17938. The administration of *L. reuteri* in tablets reduced the number of selected periodontal pathogens in the subgingival microbiota, with no associated clinical impact [95].

Hallstrom et al. conducted a clinical trial randomized double-blind controlled in patients with gingivitis: Group test (n = 18) accepted lozenges of *L. reuteri* (ATCC 55730 and PTA TM9061, 1×10^8 CFU), two times a day for 3 weeks (with a period of 2 weeks of experimental gingivitis). During the intervention periods, all the patients presented local plaque accumulation together with manifest gingivitis at the test sites. Both groups had an increase in the volume of GCF but it was statistically significant only in the placebo group ($p < 0.05$). The concentrations of IL1-β and IL-18 ($p < 0.05$) increased significantly, while IL-8 and macrophage inflammatory protein (MIP)1-β decreased ($p < 0.05$). No differences were found between test and inactive substance. Similarly, the microbial composition was not different between the groups. The plaque accumulation, inflammatory reaction or composition of the biofilm did not seem to be significantly affected by the daily intake of probiotic lozenges during experimental gingivitis [96].

Karuppaia et al. conducted a randomized double-blind clinical trial in patients with gingivitis (aged 14–17 years): Test group (n = 108) used curd (clump of milk) 4 weeks. The control group (n = 108) excluded curd in their diet for 30 days. Clinical differences were found, the probiotic was efficacious in reducing the plaque index and gingival index [97].

Purunaik et al. conducted a clinical trial randomized double-blind placebo controlled in patients (aged 15–16 years) (n = 90) with gingivitis: Group A (n = 30) used chlorhexidine 0.2%, Group B (n = 30) mouthwash of probiotic (*L. acidophilus, L. rhamnosus, B. longum* and *Saccharomyces boulardii*) (dose: 1.25 million mix, 2 times a day for 14 days), and Group C (n = 30) placebo (20 mL per day for 60 s.). It was found that both the chlorhexidine and the probiotic group can significantly reduce the plaque index (best chlorhexidine) and the gingival index (best probiotic) [98].

Lee et al. conducted a clinical trial randomized double-blind placebo controlled in patients (n = 34) with gingivitis: Group Test (n = 17) used lozenges of *L. brevis* (CD2, 1×10^9 CFU), three times per day × 2 weeks and Control group (n = 17) took placebo for the same period of time. It was found that probiotic reduced the bleeding on probing. There were no differences with respect to the gingival index. The levels of NO (nitric oxid) increased in proportional form in the placebo group. The levels of MMP-8 and PGE-2 did not change [99].

Nadkerny et al. conducted a clinical trial randomized double-blind placebo controlled in three groups of patients (n = 45) with gingivitis: Group A (Test) used a mouthwash of probiotic (*L. acidophilus, L. rhamnosus, Lactibacillus sporogenes, B. longum* and *S. boulardii*; n = 15), Group B (positive control) with chlorhexidine 0.2% (n = 15), and Group C (placebo: saline solution; n = 15) for 4 weeks. The mouthwash of probiotic and chlorhexidine was efficacious in reducing the plaque index and gingival index [100].

5. Probiotics and periodontitis

Periodontitis is an inflammatory process caused by an infection, and it implicates the interaction of biofilm and immuno-inflammatory response of host [101]. Its consequence is the destruction of attachment structures of teeth, or periodontium. There are three signs of disease: clinical attachment loss, alveolar bone resorption and presence of periodontal pocket [102].

Periodontitis constitutes the second cause of tooth loss worldwide [103–105]. Moreover, studies [106, 107] performed in South and Central America have shown that the prevalence of severe disease is high (>30%) in these populations.

Periodontitis is caused by complex subgingival microbial communities, which are in a dysbiotic state [108]. However, a few bacteria in the subgingival biofilm have been associated with disease. Strong evidence concluded that *P. gingivalis, A. actinomycetemcomitans* and *T. forsythia* are periodontal pathogens [65]. Although the tooth-associated biofilm plays a role in the development of periodontitis, it is primarily the host inflammatory response that inflicts the irreversible damage on the periodontium [108]. T helper 1 and Th17 lymphocyte have been described in the pathogenesis of disease [65].

The aim of periodontal treatment is mechanical debridement of root surface. When periodontal pathogens are effectively reduced after therapy and higher proportions of host-compatible microorganisms is established, improvements in clinical parameters are achieved [109]. However, mechanical debridement as a sole therapy is not always effective to improve clinical parameters [110]. Therefore, systemic antibiotics were introduced as an adjunct to mechanical treatment [111]. This treatment modality eliminates the entire microbiota, irrespective of its pathogenicity. Also, it could generate antibiotic resistance and recolonization of treated sites with pathogenic bacteria is frequent [112, 113]. Hence, there is a need of new treatment paradigms in periodontal disease management.

Several clinical trials were conducted in order to study the effect of administration of probiotics in initial treatment of periodontitis [114–117]. The bacteria most frequently used as probiotic are *L. reuteri* (DSM 17938 + ATCC PTA 5289) [72, 118–120], *Lactibacillus salivarius* WB21 [121, 122], *L. reuteri* (ATCC 55730 + ATCC PTA 5289) [123], *L. reuteri* (ATCC PTA 5289) [61], *Streptoccus oralis* KJ3 + *Streptococcus uberis* KJ2 + *Streptoccus rattus* JH145 [124] and *L. rhamnosus* SP1 [125].

Vivekananda et al. conducted a randomized, placebo-controlled, double blind, split-mouth designed clinical study to evaluate the effect of *L. reuteri* (DSM 17938 + ATCC PTA 5289) lozenges with and without scaling and root planning (SRP) on clinical and microbiological parameters of chronic periodontitis patients. The study period was 42 days. The lozenges were used two times a day for 21 days, from day 21 to day 42. Thirty systemically healthy subjects were recruited. On day 42, plaque index, gingival index and bleeding on probing decreased for all treatments. However, the level of this reduction was higher in SRP + probiotic, and lower, in placebo (p <0.05). Probiotic, with or without SRP, reduced significantly *P. gingivalis, A. actinomycetemcomitans* and *P. intermedia* [118].

Teughels et al. conducted a randomized, parallel, controlled and double blinded clinical, whose aim was to evaluate the effect of *L. reuteri* (DSM 17938 + ATCC PTA 5289, 1×10^8 CFU)-containing lozenges as an adjunct to full mouth disinfection protocol (FMD). Thirty systemically healthy patients were recruited (n = 15 in each group). Clinical measurements and microbiological samples were collected at baseline and 3, 6, 9 and 12 months after initial therapy with FMD. The lozenges were used two times a day for 12 weeks. At the end of intervention, i.e., 12 weeks after FMD, all clinical parameters were significantly reduced in both groups. In probiotic group, there was more pocket depth reduction and attachment gain ($p <$ 0.05). Also, there was more *P. gingivalis* reduction ($p < 0.05$) [119].

Tekce et al. and Ince et al. conducted a randomized, parallel, controlled and double blinded clinical trial in order to evaluate the effect of lozenges containing *L. reuteri* (DSM 17938 + ATCC PTA 5289, 1×10^8 CFU) as an adjuvant to full mouth scaling and root planning treatment for chronic periodontitis. The lozenges were used two times a day for 3 weeks. Forty systemically healthy subjects were recruited (n = 20 in test group). Clinical measurements, microbiological and GCF samples were obtained at baseline and on days 21, 90, 180 and 360. After treatment, plaque index, gingival index, bleeding on probing and probing pocket depth were lower in test group at all times points (p <0.05) [120]. Attachment gain was significantly higher in the test group on days 90, 180 and 360 (p <0.05) [72]. Total viable cell counts and the proportions of obligate anaerobes in subgingival plaque were lower in test group at all time points (p <0.05), with the exception of day 360 [120]. Also, decreased GCF MMP-8 and increased TIMP-1 levels were found to be significant up to day 180 in test group (p <0.05) [72].

Shimauchi et al. and Mayanagi et al. conducted a randomized placebo-controlled clinical trial, whose objective was to evaluate the effect of *L. salivarius* (WB21, 6.7×10^8 CFU)-containing tablet or a placebo in treatment of mild and moderate periodontitis. The dose was three tablets taken orally every day during 8 weeks. Periodontal treatment was not performed. Sixty-six systemically healthy volunteers were recruited (n = 34 in test group). Periodontal clinical parameters, whole saliva samples and supra and subgingival plaque samples were obtained at baseline, 4 weeks, and at the end of the interventional period (8 weeks). Current smokers in the test group showed a significantly greater improvement of plaque index and probing pocket depth when compared with placebo group. Salivary lactoferrin level was also significantly decreased in the test group smokers [121]. The numerical sum of five selected periodontopathic bacteria and *T. forsythia* in subgingival plaque decreased significantly in test group (p <0.05) at 4 weeks of treatment [122].

Vicario et al. conducted a randomized placebo-controlled, parallel design, double-blind clinical trial. The aim was to evaluate the effect of *L. reuteri* (ATCC 55730 + ATCC PTA 5289, 2×10^8 CFU)-containing lozenges in treatment of chronic periodontitis. Twenty systemically healthy subjects were recruited. Periodontal treatment was not performed. Subjects were advised to use a lozenge every day for 30 days. Clinical measurements were performed at baseline and at the end of interventional period. Only test group demonstrated a significant reduction in plaque index, bleeding on probing and pocket depth at the end of interventional period ($p < 0.05$) [123].

Szkaradkiewicz et al. conducted a clinical trial aimed to evaluate the pro-inflammatory cytokine response in patients with chronic periodontitis administered with probiotic *L. reuteri* (ATCC PTA 5289, 1×10^8 CFU)-containing lozenges. Control group did not receive lozenges. All patients were treated with SRP. They recruited 38 systemically healthy subjects (n = 24 in test group). The dose was two lozenges per day (authors did not mention the duration of intervention). Test group experimented a significant improvement of clinical measurements and a decrease in CGF levels of TNF-α, IL-1β and IL-17 (p <0.05) [61].

Laleman et al. conducted a double-blind, placebo-controlled, randomized clinical trial with two parallel arms in chronic periodontitis. The aim was to evaluate the adjunctive effect of probiotic (*Streptoccus oralis* KJ3 + *Streptococcus uberis* KJ2 + *Streptoccus rattus* JH145, 1×10^8 CFU)-containing lozenges after FMD. The dose was two lozenges per day during 3 months. Forty-eight subjects were recruited. Clinical parameters and microbiological samples were collected at baseline, 4, 8, 12 and 24 weeks follow-up visit. In test group, plaque index was significantly lower at the 24-week evaluation (p <0.05) Also, salivary *P. intermedia* counts were significantly lower at the 12-week visit in probiotic group (p <0.05) [124].

Morales et al. conducted a double-blind placebo controlled parallel-arm randomized clinical trial whose objective was to evaluate the clinical effect of *L. rhamnosus* (SP1, 2×10^7 CFU)-containing sachet as an adjunct to non-surgical therapy (SRP) of chronic periodontitis. Twenty-eight systemically healthy subject were recruited (n = 14 in test group). The dose was one sachet of probiotic or placebo taken orally every day during 3 months. Treatment involved SRP per quadrant performed with 1-week intervals in four to six sessions. A periodontal supportive therapy was performed every 3 months. Clinical parameters were measured at baseline, 3, 6, 9 and 12 months follow-up visit. Both groups showed improvements in clinical parameters at all time points evaluated. However, there were no differences between groups in any visit [125, 126].

There are some systematic reviews whose aim was to explore the available clinical evidence on the efficacy of probiotic therapy in initial treatment of chronic periodontitis. There was a significant reduction in probing pocket depth, bleeding on probing, plaque index and attachment gain in probiotic group [116]. In the studies where *L. reuteri* was selected as probiotic, the reduction of probing pocket depth was 1.31–1.74 mm in probiotic group and 0.49–1.39 mm in placebo group. Also, the attachment gain was 0.99–1.39 mm in probiotic group and 0.29–0.76 mm in placebo group [117]. Finally, the authors concluded that oral administration of probiotics is a safe and effective adjunct to scaling and root planning in the treatment of chronic periodontitis. Their adjunctive use is likely to improve diseases indices and reduce the need for antibiotics [116].

The use of probiotics in supportive periodontal therapy (SPT) was reported in a clinical trial conducted by Iwasaki et al. The aim of this randomised, double-blind, placebo controlled clinical trial was to evaluate the effect of heat-killed *L. plantarum* L-137 on the outcome of SPT. Thirty-nine SPT subjects (n = 20 in test group) who completed active treatment for chronic periodontitis followed by SPT every 4 weeks were recruited. Subjects consumed a hard gelatine capsule of 50 mg of probiotic or placebo per day during 12 weeks. The SPT programmes and clinical examinations were performed at baseline 4, 8, and 12 weeks after start intervention. Bleeding on probing and sites with pocket probing depth ≥4 mm were significantly reduced in both groups. In test group, there was a significantly greater probing pocket depth (PPD) reduction in teeth with sites with PPD ≥ 4 mm at week 12 (p <0.05). This result indicates that daily intake of probiotic may be useful in SPT [127].

6. Conclusions

Oral diseases are a recognized public health problem worldwide [128, 129]. Dental caries, periodontitis and oral cancer, among other oral diseases, currently occupy the health agenda, seeking to establish policies that, when integrated with other health intervention programs, will impact the oral health of our population. Along with the economic impact on governments and individuals [130], a higher cost is added in terms of pain, discomfort, social and functional limitations, and time lost and absenteeism in schools and workplaces [131, 132].

The goals of periodontal therapy are to reduce probing pocket depth, to gain attachment level and to reduce bleeding on probing suppuration. A new microbial community is needed in order to achieve the clinical results [109]. Therefore, with the aim of potentiating the effects of periodontal treatment, other protocols, such as the association of mechanical debridement with systemic antibiotics, have been used successfully in the treatment of periodontal diseases. The problems of antibiotics are in association with the elimination of the entire microflora, irrespective of their pathogenicity, and the emergence of antibiotic resistance; the shift towards a less pathogenic microbiota is only temporary with a frequent recolonization of treated sites with pathogenic bacteria; and the temporary use of antibiotics locally or systemically, does not really improve the long-term effect of periodontal therapy.

Considering the beneficial effects of probiotics, this therapy could serve as a useful adjunct or alternative to periodontal treatment. The use of probiotics in oral care applications is gaining momentum [118]. There is increasing evidence that the use of existing probiotic strains can deliver oral health benefits. Therefore, proposing a treatment involving the non-surgical treatment plus probiotic intake may result in better regulation of bacterial plaque and thus contribute to a successful periodontal treatment, and they can also exert effects on modulating immunological parameters.

Acknowledgements

This study was supported by a grant provided by the Scientific and Technologic Investigation Resource, Santiago, Chile (Fondecyt Project N° 1130570) and CONICYT-PCHA/Magíster

Nacional/2013-22130172. Thanks to Mr. Juan Fernandez from the Language and Translation services of the Faculty of Dentistry, University of Chile for kindly correcting the English spelling and grammar of this paper. The authors declare that there are no conflicts of interest in this study.

Author details

Alicia Morales[1], Joel Bravo-Bown[2], Javier Bedoya[3] and Jorge Gamonal[1*]

*Address all correspondence to: jgamonal@odontologia.uchile.cl

1 Laboratory of Periodontal Biology, Department of Conservative Dentistry, Faculty of Dentistry, University of Chile, Santiago, Chile

2 Faculty of Medicine and Dentistry, University of Antofagasta, Antofagasta, Chile

3 Faculty of Dentistry, University of Antioquia, Medellin, Colombia

References

[1] Metchnikoff E. The prolongation of life. Journal of Dairy Science. 1907;**36**:356

[2] Grandy G, Medina M, Soria R, Teran CG, Araya M. Probiotics in the treatment of acute rotavirus diarrhoea. A randomized, double-blind, controlled trial using two different probiotic preparations in Bolivian children. BMC Infectious Diseases. 2010 **10**:253. DOI: 10.1186/1471-2334-10-253

[3] Lilly DM, Stillwell RH. Probiotics: Growth-promoting factors produced by microorganisms. Science. 1965;**147**:747-748

[4] Gibson GR, Roberfroid MB. Dietary modulation of the human colonic microbiota: Introducing the concept of prebiotics. Journal of Nutrition. 1995;**125**:1401-1412

[5] Scientific concepts of functional foods in Europe: Consensus document. British Journal of Nutrition. 1999;**81 Suppl 1**:S1-27

[6] Roberfroid MB. Prebiotics and probiotics: are they functional foods. The American Journal of Clinical Nutrition. 2000;**71**:1682S-1687S;discussion 1688S–1690S

[7] Isolauri E, Kirjavainen PV, Salminen S. Probiotics: A role in the treatment of intestinal infection and inflammation? Gut. 2002;**50 Suppl 3**:III54-59

[8] Didari T, Solki S, Mozaffari S, Nikfar S, Abdollahi M. A systematic review of the safety of probiotics. Expert Opinion on Drug Safety. 2014;**13**:227-239. DOI: 10.1517/14740338.2014.872627

[9] Manzano C, Estupiñan D, Poveda E. Clinical effects of probiotcis: What does the evidencia says? Revista Chilena de Nutrición. 2012;**39**:98-110.

[10] Muñoz K, Alarcon M. Effect of probiotics in periodontal conditions. Revista Clínica de Periodoncia. 2010;**3**:136-139

[11] Zalba Elizari JI, Flichy-Fernández AJ. Empleo de probióticos en odontología. Nutr Hosp. 2013;**28**:49-50

[12] Frencken JE. Global epidemiology of dental caries and severe periodontitis—A comprehensive review. Journal of Clinical Periodontology. 2017;**44 Suppl 18**:S94–S105. DOI: 10.1111/jcpe.12677

[13] WHO. What is the burden of oral disease? <http://www.who.int/oral_health/disease_burden/global/en/>

[14] Newman HN. Plaque and chronic inflammatory periodontal disease. A question of ecology. Journal of Clinical Periodontology. 1990;**17**:533-541

[15] Gorbach S.L. The discovery of Lactibacillus GG. Nutr Today. 1996;**31**:2S–4S

[16] Näse L., Hatakka K., Savilahti E., Saxelin M., Pönkä A., Poussa T., et al. Effect of long-term consumption of a probiotic bacterium, Lactobacillus rhamnosus GG, in milk on dental caries and caries risk in children. Caries Res. 2001;**35**:412-420

[17] Grudianov A.I., Dmitrieva N.A., Fomenko E.V. Use of probiotic Bifidumbacterin and Acilact in tablets un therapy of periodontal inflammations. Stomatologiia Mosk. 2002; **81**:39-43

[18] Wei H, et al. Stability and activity of specific antibodies against *Streptococcus mutans* and *Streptococcus sobrinus* in bovine milk fermented with Lactobacillus rhamnosus strain GG or treated at ultra-high temperature. Oral microbiology and immunology. 2002;**17**:9-15

[19] Von Bultzingslowen I, Adlerberth I, Wold AE, Dahlen G, Jontell M. Oral and intestinal microflora in 5-fluorouracil treated rats, translocation to cervical and mesenteric lymph nodes and effects of probiotic bacteria. Oral Microbiology and Immunology 2003;**18**:278-284

[20] Hatakka K, et al. Probiotics reduce the prevalence of oral candida in the elderly—A randomized controlled trial. Journal of Dental Research. 2007:**86**;125-130. DOI: 10.1177/154405910708600204 [2007]

[21] Koduganti RR, Sandeep N, Guduguntla S, Chandana Gorthi VS. Probiotics and prebiotics in periodontal therapy. Indian Journal of Dental Research. 2011;**22**:324-330, DOI: 10.4103/0970-9290.84312

[22] Sookkhee S, Chulasiri M, Prachyabrued W. Lactic acid bacteria from healthy oral cavity of Thai volunteers: Inhibition of oral pathogens. Indian Journal of Applied Microbiology. 2001;**90**:172-179

[23] Koll-Klais P, et al. Oral lactobacilli in chronic periodontitis and periodontal health: Species composition and antimicrobial activity. Oral Microbiology and Immunology. 2005;**20**:354-361. DOI: 10.1111/j.1399-302X.2005.00239.x

[24] Mashimo PA, Yamamoto Y, Nakamura M, Reynolds HS, Genco RJ. Lactic acid production by oral *Streptococcus mitis* inhibits the growth of oral Capnocytophaga. Journal of Periodontology Online. 1985;**56**:548-552

[25] Makras L De, Vuyst L. The in vitro inhibition of Gram-negative pathogenic bacteria by Bifidobacteria is caused by the production of organic acids. International Dairy Journal. 2006;**9**:1049-1057

[26] Falagas M, Betsi GI, Athanasiou S. Probiotics for the treatment of women with bacterial vaginosis. Clinical Microbiology and Infection 2007;**13**:657-664

[27] Balakrishnan M, Simmonds RS, Tagg JR. Dental caries is a preventable infectious disease. Australian Dental Journal. 2000;**45**:235-245

[28] Burton JP, Chilcott CN, Tagg JR. The rationale and potential for the reduction of oral malodour using *Streptococcus salivarius* probiotics. Oral Diseases. 2005;**11**:29-31

[29] Burton JP, Chilcott CN, Moore CJ, Speiser G, Tagg JR. A preliminary study of the effect of probiotic *Streptococcus salivarius* K12 on oral malodour parameters. Journal of Applied Microbiology. 2006;**100**: 754-764

[30] Pangsomboon K, Kaewnopparat S, Pitakpornpreecha T, Srichana T. Antibacterial activity of a bacteriocin from Lactobacillus paracasei HL32 against Porphyromonas gingivalis. Archives of Oral Biology. 2006;**51**: 784-793

[31] Derrien M, van Hylckama Vlieg JE. Fate, activity, and impact of ingested bacteria within the human gut microbiota. Trends in Microbiology. 2015;**23**:354-366. DOI: 10.1016/j.tim.2015.03.002

[32] Schiller C, et al. Intestinal fluid volumes and transit of dosage forms as assessed by magnetic resonance imaging. Alimentary Pharmacology and Therapeutics. 2005;**22**:971-979. DOI: 10.1111/j.1365-2036.2005.02683.x

[33] Bik EM, et al. Molecular analysis of the bacterial microbiota in the human stomach. Proceedings of the National Academy of Sciences of the United States. 2006;**103**:732-737. DOI: 10.1073/pnas.0506655103

[34] Zoetendal EG, et al. The human small intestinal microbiota is driven by rapid uptake and conversion of simple carbohydrates. The ISME Journal. 2012;**6**:1415-1426. DOI: 10.1038/ismej.2011.212

[35] Claesson MJ, et al. Composition, variability, and temporal stability of the intestinal microbiota of the elderly. Proceedings of the National Academy of Sciences of the United States. 2011;**108(Suppl 1)**:4586-4591. DOI: 10.1073/pnas.1000097107

[36] Plaza-Diaz J, Gomez-Llorente C, Fontana L, Gil A. Modulation of immunity and inflammatory gene expression in the gut, in inflammatory diseases of the gut and in the liver by probiotics. World Journal of Gastroenterology. 2014;**20**:15632-15649. DOI: 10.3748/wjg.v20.i42.15632

[37] Fuchs-Tarlovsky V, Marquez-Barba MF, Sriram K. Probiotics in dermatologic practice. Nutrition. 2016;**32**:289-295. DOI: 10.1016/j.nut.2015.09.001

[38] Foolad N, Brezinski EA, Chase EP, Armstrong AW. Effect of nutrient supplementation on atopic dermatitis in children: A systematic review of probiotics, prebiotics, formula, and fatty acids. JAMA Dermatology. 2013;**149**:350-355

[39] Foolad N, Armstrong AW. Prebiotics and probiotics: The prevention and reduction in severity of atopic dermatitis in children. Beneficial Microbes. 2014;**5**:151-160. DOI: 10.3920/BM2013.0034

[40] Drago L, et al. Effects of *Lactobacillus salivarius* LS01 [DSM 22775] treatment on adult atopic dermatitis: A randomized placebo-controlled study. International Journal of Immunopathology and Pharmacology. 2011;**24**:1037-1048. DOI: 10.1177/039463201102400421

[41] Iemoli E, et al. Probiotics reduce gut microbial translocation and improve adult atopic dermatitis. Journal of Clinical Gastroenterology. 2012;**46 Suppl**:S33-40. DOI: 10.1097/MCG.0b013e31826a8468

[42] Mizock BA. Probiotics. Disease-a-Month. 2015;**61**:259-290. DOI: 10.1016/j.disamonth.2015.03.011

[43] Sazawal S, et al. Efficacy of probiotics in prevention of acute diarrhoea: A meta-analysis of masked, randomised, placebo-controlled trials. The Lancet Infectious Diseases, 2006;**6**:374-382. DOI: 10.1016/S1473-3099[06]70495-9

[44] Hempel S, et al. Probiotics for the prevention and treatment of antibiotic-associated diarrhea: A systematic review and meta-analysis. JAMA. 2012;**307**:1959-1969. DOI: 10.1001/jama.2012.3507

[45] McFarland LV. Meta-analysis of probiotics for the prevention of antibiotic associated diarrhea and the treatment of *Clostridium difficile* disease. The American Journal of Gastroenterology. 2006;**101**:812-822. DOI: 10.1111/j.1572-0241.2006.00465.x

[46] Tung JM, Dolovich LR, Lee CH. Prevention of *Clostridium difficile* infection with *Saccharomyces boulardii*: A systematic review. Canadian Journal of Gastroenterology and Hepatology. 2009;**23**:817-821

[47] Horvath A, Dziechciarz P, Szajewska H. Meta-analysis: *Lactobacillus rhamnosus* GG for abdominal pain-related functional gastrointestinal disorders in childhood. Alimentary Pharmacology and Therapeutics. 2011;**33:**1302-1310. DOI: 10.1111/j.1365-2036.2011.04665.x

[48] Shen J, Zuo ZX, Mao AP. Effect of probiotics on inducing remission and maintaining therapy in ulcerative colitis, Crohn's disease, and pouchitis: Meta-analysis of randomized controlled trials. Inflammatory Bowel Disease. 2014;**20**:21-35. DOI: 10.1097/01.MIB.0000437495.30052.be

[49] Szajewska H, Horvath A, Piwowarczyk A. Meta-analysis: The effects of *Saccharomyces boulardii* supplementation on *Helicobacter pylori* eradication rates and side effects

during treatment. Alimentary Pharmacology & Therapeutics. 2010;**32**:1069-1079. DOI: 10.1111/j.1365-2036.2010.04457.x

[50] Alfaleh K, Anabrees J, Bassler D, Al-Kharfi T. Probiotics for prevention of necrotizing enterocolitis in preterm infants. Cochrane Database Systematic Reviews. 2011;CD005496. DOI: 10.1002/14651858.CD005496.pub3

[51] Ishimwe N, Daliri EB, Lee BH, Fang F, Du G. The perspective on cholesterol-lowering mechanisms of probiotics. Molecular Nutrition & Food Research. 2015;**59**:94-105. DOI: 10.1002/mnfr.201400548

[52] Gibson RJ, et al. Systematic review of agents for the management of gastrointestinal mucositis in cancer patients. Support Care Cancer. 2013;**21**:313-326. DOI: 10.1007/s00520-012-1644-z

[53] Kalliomaki MA, Walker WA. Physiologic and pathologic interactions of bacteria with gastrointestinal epithelium. Gastroenterology Clinics of North America. 2005;**34**:383-399. vii. DOI: 10.1016/j.gtc.2005.05.007

[54] Wan LYM, Chen ZJ, Shah NP, El-Nezami H. Modulation of intestinal epithelial defense responses by probiotic bacteria. Critical Reviews in Food Science and Nutrition. 2016;**56**:2628-2641

[55] Neish AS. Bacterial inhibition of eukaryotic pro-inflammatory pathways. Immunologic Research. 2004;**9**:175-186. DOI: 10.1385/IR:29:1-3:175

[56] Kingma SD, et al. *Lactobacillus johnsonii* N6.2 stimulates the innate immune response through Toll-like receptor 9 in Caco-2 cells and increases intestinal crypt Paneth cell number in biobreeding diabetes-prone rats. Journal of Nutrition. 2011;**141**:1023-1028. DOI: 10.3945/jn.110.135517

[57] Miettinen M, Vuopio-Varkila J, Varkila K. Production of human tumor necrosis factor alpha, interleukin-6, and interleukin-10 is induced by lactic acid bacteria. Infection and Immunity. 1996;**64**:5403-5405

[58] Schiffrin EJ, Rochat F, Link-Amster H, Aeschlimann JM, Donnet-Hughes A. Immunomodulation of human blood cells following the ingestion of lactic acid bacteria. Journal of Dairy Science. 1995;**78**:491-497

[59] Takeda K, et al. Interleukin-12 is involved in the enhancement of human natural killer cell activity by *Lactobacillus casei* Shirota. Clinical & Experimental Immunology. 2006;**146**:109-115

[60] Riccia DN, et al. Anti-inflammatory effects of *Lactobacillus brevis* [CD2] on periodontal disease. Oral Diseases. 2007;**13**:376-385. DOI: 10.1111/j.1601-0825.2006.01291.x

[61] Szkaradkiewicz AK, Stopa J, Karpinski TM. Effect of oral administration involving a probiotic strain of Lactobacillus reuteri on pro-inflammatory cytokine response in patients with chronic periodontitis. Archivum Immunologiae et Therapia Experimentalis. 2014;**62**:495-500

[62] Cosseau C, et al. The commensal *Streptococcus salivarius* K12 downregulates the innate immune responses of human epithelial cells and promotes host-microbe homeostasis. Infection and Immunity. 2008;**76**:4163-4175. DOI: 10.1128/IAI.00188-08

[63] Zhang G, Chen R, Rudney JD. *Streptococcus cristatus* attenuates *Fusobacterium nucleatum*-induced interleukin-8 expression in oral epithelial cells. Journal of Periodontal Research. 2008;**43**:408-416

[64] Sliepen I, et al. Interference with *Aggregatibacter actinomycetemcomitans*: Colonization of epithelial cells under hydrodynamic conditions. Oral Microbiology and Immunology. 2009;**24**:390-395. DOI: 10.1111/j.1399-302X.2009.00531.x

[65] Silva N, et al. Host response mechanisms in periodontal diseases. Journal of Applied Oral Science. 2015;**23**:329-355. DOI: 10.1590/1678-775720140259

[66] Hart AL, et al. Modulation of human dendritic cell phenotype and function by probiotic bacteria. Gut. 2004;**53**:1602-1609. DOI: 10.1136/gut.2003.037325

[67] Barberi C, et al. T cell polarizing properties of probiotic bacteria. Immunology Letters. 2015;**168**:337-342. DOI: 10.1016/j.imlet.2015.11.005

[68] Yesilova Y, Calka O, Akdeniz N, Berktas M. Effect of probiotics on the treatment of children with atopic dermatitis. Annals of Dermatology. 2012;**24**:189-193. DOI: 10.5021/ad.2012.24.2.189

[69] Pohjavuori E, et al. Lactobacillus GG effect in increasing IFN-gamma production in infants with cow's milk allergy. Journal of Allergy and Clinical Immunology. 2004;**114**:131-136. DOI: 10.1016/j.jaci.2004.03.036

[70] Hegazy SK, El-Bedewy MM. Effect of probiotics on pro-inflammatory cytokines and NF-kappaB activation in ulcerative colitis. World Journal of Gastroenterology. 2010;**16**:4145-4151

[71] O'Mahony C, et al. Commensal-induced regulatory T cells mediate protection against pathogen-stimulated NF-kappaB activation. PLoS Pathogens. 2008;**4**:e1000112. DOI: 10.1371/journal.ppat.1000112

[72] Ince G, et al. Clinical and biochemical evaluation of lozenges containing *Lactobacillus reuteri* as an adjunct to non-surgical periodontal therapy in chronic periodontitis. Journal of Periodontology. 2015;**86**:746-754. DOI: 10.1902/jop.2015.140612

[73] Sherman PM, Ossa JC, Johnson-Henry K. Unraveling mechanisms of action of probiotics. Nutrition in Clinical Practice. 2009;**24**:10-14. DOI: 10.1177/0884533608329231

[74] Ma DS, Forsythe P, Bienenstock J. Live Lactobacillus reuteri is essential for the inhibitory effect on tumor necrosis factor alpha-induced interleukin-8 expression. Infection and Immunity. 2004;**72**:5308-5314

[75] Zhang L, Li N, Caicedo R, Neu J. Alive and dead *Lactobacillus rhamnosus* GG decrease tumor necrosis factor-alpha-induced interleukin-8 production in Caco-2 cells. Journal of Nutrition. 2005;**135**:1752-1756

[76] Kim JG, Lee SJ, Kagnoff MF. Nod1 is an essential signal transducer in intestinal epithelial cells infected with bacteria that avoid recognition by toll-like receptors. Infection and Immunity. 2004;**72**:1487-1495

[77] Mariotti A. Dental plaque-induced gingival diseases. Journal of Periodontology Online. 1999;**4**:7-19

[78] Haytac MC, Ozcelik O, Mariotti A. Periodontal disease in men. Periodontology. 2013;**61:** 252-265

[79] Albandar JM, Kingman A. Gingival recession, gingival bleeding, and dental calculus in adults 30 years of age and older in the United States, 1988-1994. Journal of Periodontology Online. 1999;**70**:30-43

[80] Albandar JM, Rams TE. Global epidemiology of periodontal diseases: An overview. Periodontology 2000. 2002;**29:**7-10

[81] Brown LJ, Brunelle JA, Kingman A. Periodontal status in the United States, 1988-1991: Prevalence, extent, and demographic variation. Journal of Dental Research. 1996;**75**:672-683

[82] Zhang J. Severity and prevalence of plaque-induced gingivitis in the Chinese population. Compendium of Continuing Education in Dentistry. 2010;**31**:624-629

[83] Kinane DF, Attstrom R, Group B. Advances in the pathogenesis of periodontitis. Journal of Clinical Periodontology 2005;**32:**130-131

[84] Smith M, Seymour GJ, Cullinan MP. Histopathological features of chronic and aggressive periodontitis. Journal of Periodontology Online. 2000;**53**:45-54. DOI: 10.1111/j.1600-0757.2010.00354.x

[85] Botero JE, Rösing CK, Duque A, Jaramillo A, Contreras A. Periodontal disease in children and adolescents of Latin America. Journal of Periodontology Online. 2015;**67**:34-57. DOI: 10.1111/prd.12072

[86] Armitage GC, Cullinan MP. Comparison of the clinical features of chronic and aggressive periodontitis. Journal of Periodontology Online. 2010;**53**:12-27. DOI: 10.1111/j.1600-0757.2010.00353.x

[87] Contreras A, Slots J. Mammalian viruses in human periodontitis. Molecular Oral Microbiology. 1996;**11**:381-386

[88] Offenbacher S. Periodontal disease at the biofilm-gingival interface. Journal of Periodontology 2007;**78**:1911-1925

[89] Darveau RP. Periodontitis: A polymicrobial disruption of host homeostasis. Nature Reviews Microbiology. 2010;**8**:481-490. DOI: 10.1038/nrmicro2337

[90] Loe H, Theilade E, Jensen SB. Experimental gingivitis in man. Journal of Periodontology Online. 1965;**36**:177-187. DOI: 10.1902/jop.1965.36.3.177

[91] Krasse P, et al. Decreased gum bleeding and reduced gingivitis by the probiotic *Lactobacillus reuteri*. Swedish Dental Journal. 2006;**30**:55-60

[92] Twetman S. Short-term effect of chewing gums containing probiotic *Lactobacillus reuteri* on the levels of inflammatory mediators in gingival crevicular fluid. Acta Odontologica Scandinavica. 2009;**67**:19-24

[93] Staab B, Eick S, Knofler G, Jentsch H. The influence of a probiotic milk drink on the development of gingivitis: A pilot study. Journal of Clinical Periodontology. 2009;**36**:850-856. DOI: 10.1111/j.1600-051X.2009.01459.x

[94] Ierardo G. The arginine-deiminase enzymatic system on gingivitis: Preliminary pediatric study. Annali di Stomatologia Roma. 2010;**1**:8-13

[95] Iniesta M. Probiotic effects of orally administered *Lactobacillus reuteri*-containing tablets on the subgingival and salivary microbiota in patients with gingivitis. Journal of Clinical Periodontology. 2012;**39**:736-744. DOI: 10.1111/j.1600-051X.2012.01914.x

[96] Hallström H. Effect of probiotic lozenges on inflammatory reactions and oral biofilm during experimental gingivitis. Acta Odontologica Scandinavica. 2012;**71**:828-833

[97] Karuppaiah RM, et al. Evaluation of the efficacy of probiotics in plaque reduction and gingival health maintenance among school children—Control Trial. Journal of International Oral Health. 2013;**5**:33-37

[98] Purunaik S, Thippeswamy HM, Chavan SS. To evaluate the effect of probiotic mouth rinse on plaque and gingivitis among year old school children of Mysore, India—Randomized controlled trial. Global Journal of Medical Research. 2014;**14**:15-16

[99] Lee J, Kim SJ, Ko S, Ouwehand AC, Ma DS. Modulation of the host response by probiotic *Lactobacillus brevis* CD2 in experimental gingivitis. Oral Diseases. 2015;**21**:705-712

[100] Nadkerny PV, Ravishankar PL, Pramod V, Agarwal LA, Bhandari S. A comparative evaluation of the efficacy of probiotic and chlorhexidine mouthrinses on clinical inflammatory parameters of gingivitis: A randomized controlled clinical study. Journal of Indian Society of Periodontology. 2015;**19:**633-639

[101] Kornman KS. Mapping the pathogenesis of periodontitis: A new look. Journal of Periodontology Online. 2008;**79**:1560-1568. DOI: 10.1902/jop.2008.080213

[102] van der Velden U. Purpose and problems of periodontal disease classification. Periodontology 2000. 2005;**39**:13-21. DOI: 10.1111/j.1600-0757.2005.00127.x

[103] Mai X, et al. Associations between smoking and tooth loss according to the reason for tooth loss: The Buffalo OsteoPerio study. The Journal of the American Dental Association. 2013;**144**:252-265

[104] Niessen LC, Weyant RJ. Causes of tooth loss in a veteran population. Journal of Public Health Dentistry. 1989;**49**:19-23

[105] Baelum V, Lopez R. Periodontal disease epidemiology—Learned and unlearned? Periodontology 2000. 2013;**62**:37-58. DOI: 10.1111/j.1600-0757.2012.00449.x

[106] Gjermo P, Rosing CK, Susin C, Oppermann R. Periodontal diseases in Central and South America. Periodontology 2000. 2002;**29**:70-78. DOI: 10.1034/j.1600-0757.2002.290104.x

[107] Susin C, Dalla Vecchia CF, Oppermann RV, Haugejorden O, Albandar JM. Periodontal attachment loss in an urban population of Brazilian adults: Effect of demographic, behavioral, and environmental risk indicators. Journal of Periodontology Online. 2004;**75**:1033-1041. DOI: 10.1902/jop.2004.75.7.1033

[108] Hajishengallis G, Darveau RP, Curtis MA. The keystone-pathogen hypothesis. Nature Reviews Microbiology. 2012;**10**:717-725. DOI: 10.1038/nrmicro2873

[109] Teles RP, Haffajee AD, Socransky SS. Microbiological goals of periodontal therapy. Periodontology 2000. 2006;**42**:180-218. DOI: 10.1111/j.1600-0757.2006.00192.x

[110] Haffajee AD, Patel M, Socransky SS. Microbiological changes associated with four different periodontal therapies for the treatment of chronic periodontitis. Molecular Oral Microbiology. 2008;**23**:148-157. DOI: 10.1111/j.1399-302X.2007.00403.x

[111] Feres M, Figueiredo LC, Soares GM, Faveri M. Systemic antibiotics in the treatment of periodontitis. Periodontology 2000. 2015;**67**:131-186. DOI: 10.1111/prd.12075

[112] Rams TE, Degener JE, van Winkelhoff AJ. Antibiotic resistance in human chronic periodontitis microbiota. Journal of Periodontology Online. 2014;**85**:160-169. DOI: 10.1902/jop.2013.130142

[113] Haffajee AD, Teles RP, Socransky SS. The effect of periodontal therapy on the composition of the subgingival microbiota. Periodontology 2000. 2006;**42**:219-258. DOI: 10.1111/j.1600-0757.2006.00191.x

[114] Yanine N, et al. Effects of probiotics in periodontal diseases: A systematic review. Clinical Oral Investigations. 2013;**17**:1627-1634. DOI: 10.1007/s00784-013-0990-7

[115] Gruner D, Paris S, Schwendicke F. Probiotics for managing caries and periodontitis: Systematic review and meta-analysis. Journal of Dentistry. 2016;**48**:16-25. DOI: 10.1016/j.jdent.2016.03.002

[116] Matsubara VH, Bandara HM, Ishikawa KH, Mayer MP, Samaranayake LP. The role of probiotic bacteria in managing periodontal disease: A systematic review. Expert Review of Anti-infective Therapy. 2016;**14**:643-655. DOI: 10.1080/14787210.2016.1194198

[117] Martin-Cabezas R, Davideau JL, Tenenbaum H, Huck O. Clinical efficacy of probiotics as an adjunctive therapy to non-surgical periodontal treatment of chronic periodontitis: A systematic review and meta-analysis. Journal of Clinical Periodontology. 2016;**43**:520-530. DOI: 10.1111/jcpe.12545

[118] Vivekananda MR, Vandana KL, Bhat KG. Effect of the probiotic Lactobacilli reuteri [Prodentis] in the management of periodontal disease: A preliminary randomized clinical trial. Journal of Oral Microbiology. 2010;**2**:1-9. DOI: 10.3402/jom.v2i0.5344

[119] Teughels W, et al. Clinical and microbiological effects of *Lactobacillus reuteri* probiotics in the treatment of chronic periodontitis: A randomized placebo-controlled study. Journal of Clinical Periodontology. 2013;**40**:1025-1035. DOI: 10.1111/jcpe.12155

[120] Tekce M, et al. Clinical and microbiological effects of probiotic lozenges in the treatment of chronic periodontitis: A 1-year follow-up study. Journal of Clinical Periodontology. 2015;**42**:363-372. DOI: 10.1111/jcpe.12387

[121] Shimauchi H, et al. Improvement of periodontal condition by probiotics with *Lactobacillus salivarius* WB21: A randomized, double-blind, placebo-controlled study. Journal of Clinical Periodontology. 2008;**35**:897-905. DOI: 10.1111/j.1600-051X.2008.01306.x

[122] Mayanagi G, et al. Probiotic effects of orally administered *Lactobacillus salivarius* WB21-containing tablets on periodontopathic bacteria: A double-blinded, placebo-controlled, randomized clinical trial. Journal of Clinical Periodontology. 2009;**36**:506-513. DOI: 10.1111/j.1600-051X.2009.01392.x

[123] Vicario M, Santos A, Violant D, Nart J, Giner L. Clinical changes in periodontal subjects with the probiotic *Lactobacillus reuteri* Prodentis: A preliminary randomized clinical trial. Acta Odontologica Scandinavica. 2013;**71**:813-819. DOI: 10.3109/00016357.2012.734404

[124] Laleman I, et al. The effect of a streptococci containing probiotic in periodontal therapy: A randomized controlled trial. Journal of Clinical Periodontology. 2015;**42**:1032-1041. DOI: 10.1111/jcpe.12464

[125] Morales A, et al. Clinical effects of *Lactobacillus rhamnosus* in non-surgical treatment of chronic periodontitis: A randomized placebo-controlled trial with 1-year follow-up. Journal of Periodontology Online. 2016;**87**:944-952. DOI: 10.1902/jop.2016.150665

[126] Morales A, et al. Efecto clínico del uso de probiótico en el tratamiento de la periodontitis crónica: ensayo clínico. Revista Clínica de Periodoncia, Implantología y Rehabilitación Oral. 2016;**9**:146-152

[127] Iwasaki K. et al. Daily intake of heat-killed *Lactobacillus plantarum* L-137 decreases the probing depth in patients undergoing supportive periodontal therapy. Oral Health & Preventive Dentistry. 2016;**14**:207-214. DOI: 10.3290/j.ohpd.a36099

[128] Beaglehole R, Benzian H, Crail J, Mackay J. The Oral Health Atlas: Mapping a Neglected Global Health Issue. FDI World Dental Education Ltd & Myriad Editions. Switzerland; 2009

[129] Petersen PE, Bourgeois D, Ogawa H, Estupinan-Day S, Ndiaye C. The global burden of oral diseases and risks to oral health. Bulletin of the World Health Organization. 2005;**83**:661-669. DOI: /S0042-96862005000900011

[130] Patel R. The State of Oral Health in Europe. 2012. <http://www.oralhealthplatform.eu/wp-content/uploads/2015/09/Report-the-State-of-Oral-Health-in-Europe.pdf>

[131] Casamassimo PS, Thikkurissy S, Edelstein BL, Maiorini E. Beyond the dmft: The human and economic cost of early childhood caries. The Journal of the American Dental Association. 2009;**140**:650-657

[132] Rockville MD. Oral Health in America: A Report of the Surgeon General—Executive Summary. U.S. Department of Health and Human Services, National Institute of Dental and Craniofacial Research, National Institute of Health, USA; 2000

Section 2

Functional Rehabilitation of the Dental Status

Chapter 6

Cleft Lip and Palate Management from Birth to Adulthood: An Overview

Maen Hussni Zreaqat, Rozita Hassan and
Abdulfattah Hanoun

Additional information is available at the end of the chapter

http://dx.doi.org/10.5772/intechopen.68448

Abstract

Cleft lip and palate (CLP) is the most common congenital deformity of the orofacial. Clefts are thought to be of multifactorial etiology due to genetic and environmental factors. Different dental abnormalities are usually seen in cleft patients, including midface deficiency, collapsed dental arches, malformation of teeth, hypodontia, and supernumerary teeth. Moreover, feeding and speech are major functional dilemmas for those patients. The goal of treatment is to restore esthetics and functional impairments associated with clefts. The nature and the extent of medical and dental problems among CLP patients dictate the need toward multidisciplinary approach where different medical and dental specialists are involved in the treatment. The purpose of this section is to codify and synthesize a literature about management of cleft lip and palate deformity from birth until adulthood so that general concepts, principles, and axioms can be formulated. In this regard, feeding plates, nasoalveolar molding (NAM), lip and palate repair, palatal expansion, alveolar bone grafting, rhinoplasty, orthodontic treatment, and orthognathic surgery will be discussed. Furthermore, the question of proper timing for each therapeutic procedure is scrutinized in this chapter. Suggested clinical tips and changes of treatment modalities are summarized and illustrated as well.

Keywords: cleft lip and palate, multidisciplinary management, lip repair, palate repair, orthognathic surgery

1. Introduction

Cleft lip and palate (CLP) is the most common orofacial malformation affecting one in every 700–1000 newborns worldwide [1]. The anomaly is characterized by the lack continuity of tissues forming the lip, alveolus, and soft and hard palate. The severity ranges from a small notch in the lip to a complete fissure extending into the roof of the mouth and nose. Due to their disturbing appearance in many cases, these deformities have attracted much attention in terms of treatment and research. The large impact of the cleft lip and palate on appearance and function renders them a major public health problem worldwide [2]. Data from human and animal studies have suggested that the etiology of cleft lip and palate results from gene-environment interaction where genes have a major influence. Current research is emphasizing on detection of location and nature of mutations in genes associated with cleft lip and palate.

In comparison with unaffected children, individuals with unilateral cleft lip and palate (UCLP) present with striking asymmetries of the soft tissues as well as the nasomaxillary and lower facial structures. The facial profile is significantly affected by the cleft anomaly; the profile is generally concave due to the maxillary retrognathia. Several studies had reported that unilateral cleft lip and palate children have increased nose width, reduced mouth width, nose asymmetry, increased nose width/mouth width ratio, reduced upper lip length [3], and reduced lip elasticity [4]. For the dentoalveolar relationships, crossbite and open bite are common findings among unilateral cleft lip and palate patients [5].

Bishara et al. suggested that differences in dentoalveolar morphology between cleft and noncleft subjects could be related to many factors. These include the morphogenetic pattern of the cleft anomaly, long-term management, and adaptive changes due to the mechanical presence of the cleft or lack of continuity of tissues [6].

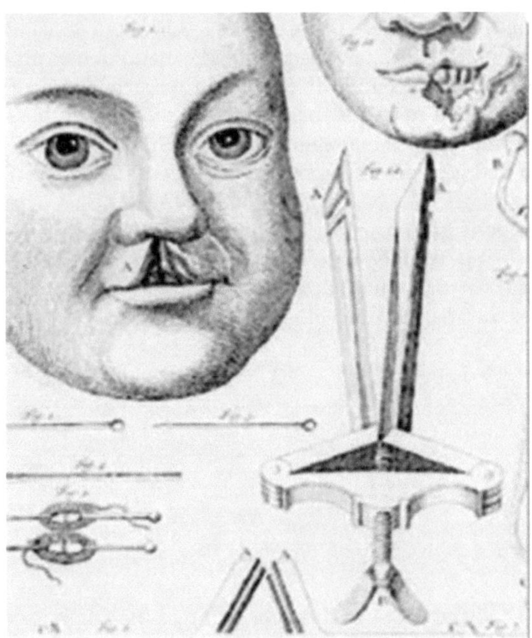

Figure 1. Surgical instruments for cleft surgery (Heister's surgical textbook, 1731).

The management of children with cleft lip and palate is a real challenge. Intervention of cleft patients starts as early as intrauterine and continues into late adulthood. Related families are involved as well. Those patients are presented with various problems, and thus, effective therapeutic outcomes can be only through a multidisciplinary approach. The cleft team consists of different specialists work closely together, so that maximum care can be delivered in the optimum way. There is a consensus that understanding of the requirements and specialist skills of the other team members is necessary so that all members within the team can work coordinately which leads to improving outcomes.

The first proven description of treatment of a cleft lip and palate appeared in ancient China in the fourth century after Christ. Heister in 1731 described a clinical picture of cleft lip and palate management (**Figure 1**). It was Hagedorn who laid the basics of geometrical anatomical and surgical lip repair in 1884. He developed the surgical technique of repair using a geometric cutting procedure, the flap exchange, which in principle is in practice up to now. Thus, he founded basics of oriented surgical procedures that were described later by clinicians in the twentieth century [7].

2. Incidence of cleft lip and palate

Incidence of cleft lip and palate had been the subjects of many studies. There are significant differences in the incidence of cleft lip and palate, with the highest rates in Asian populations and Native Americans, intermediate rates in Caucasians, and lowest rates in African American. According to the European registration of congenital and twins (EUROCAT), incidence rates of cleft lip and palate for various regions in Europe between the year 1980 and 1988 were 1.45–1.57/1000 living birth [8]. Unilateral cleft lip and palate (UCLP) occurred in 40% of all cleft groups with male/female ratio (2:1) and was more common on the left side [9]. On the other hand, isolated cleft palate occurs more in females and is usually associated with syndromes [10].

3. Classification of cleft lip and palate

Different systems were introduced to classify cleft lip and palate.

3.1. Veau classification (1931)

Veau (1931) classified oral clefts based on the anatomy of the oral cavity into four groups:

1. Cleft of soft palate.
2. Cleft of soft and hard palate from incisive foramen up to the secondary palate.

3. Complete unilateral cleft from the uvula to incisive foramen, going on one side through the alveolus at the side of the future lateral incisor tooth.
4. Complete bilateral cleft from the incisive foramen to the alveolus, the premaxilla remains suspended from the nasal septum.

3.2. Classification by International Confederation for Plastic and Reconstructive Surgery (1966)

International Confederation for Plastic and Reconstructive Surgery had classified oral cleft into three groups:

1. Clefts of anterior primary palate, where the lip and alveolus are affected.
2. Clefts of anterior and posterior palate, where the alveolus and the hard palate are affected.
3. Clefts of the posterior palate, where the hard and soft palate are affected.

3.3. Kernahan and Stark classification (1958)

This classification is based on embryology and classifies oral clefts into two main groups:

1. Cleft of primary palate: extends from alveolus up to the incisive foramen.
2. Cleft of secondary palate: extends from soft and hard palate up to incisive foramen. Both groups could be complete or incomplete, unilateral or bilateral (Kernahan and Stark, 1958).

Kernahan and Stark classification was widely accepted because it is simple and embryologically sound [11].

3.4. Kernahan stripped "Y" classification

This classification is represented as a stripped "Y" with numbered blocks. Different numbers represent a specific affected area in the cleft deformity (**Figure 2**).

- Blocks 1 and 4 indicate the lip.
- Blocks 2 and 5 indicate the alveolus.
- Blocks 3 and 6 indicate hard palate to the incisive foramen.
- Blocks 7 and 8 indicate hard palate to incisive foramen.
- Block 9 indicates the soft palate.

The shaded boxes represent the site of cleft deformity.

http://dx.doi.org/10.5772/intechopen.68448

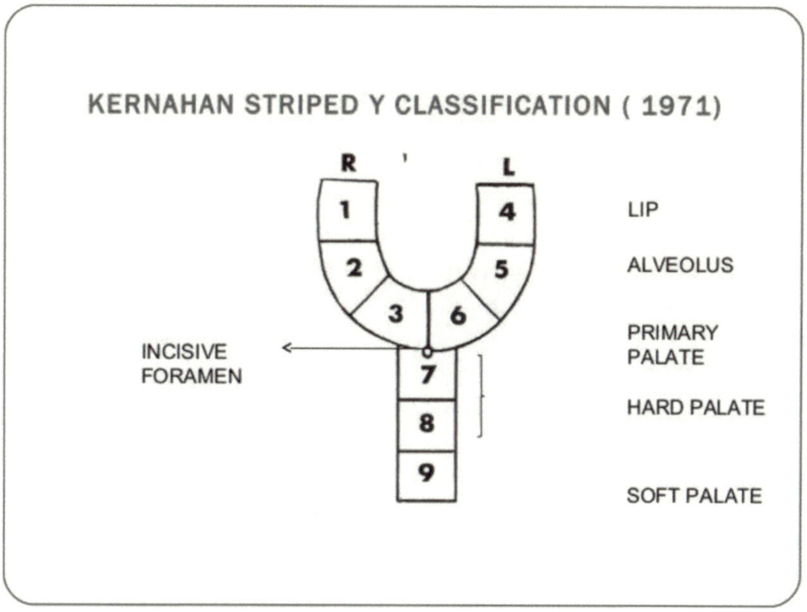

Figure 2. Kernahan's stripped "Y" classification.

3.5. Iowa classification

Iowa classification had classified cleft lip and palate into five groups (**Figure 3**). This descriptive classification was a variation of Veau classification and is more commonly used.

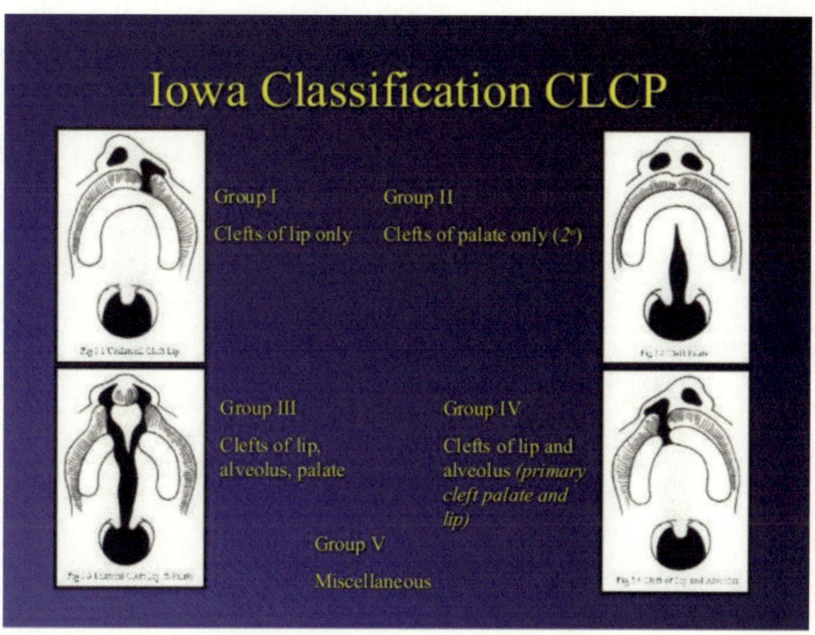

Figure 3. Iowa classification of cleft lip and palate.

4. Embryology background

Knowledge of the normal embryological development of the lip and palate is essential for understanding and management of cleft lip and palate. The face is formed by the fusion of a number of embryonic processes that form around the primitive oral cavity (stomodeum). By the 4th week of intrauterine life, five branchial arches develop at the site of future neck. The nasomaxillary complex is formed through the development of the first branchial arch (the mandibular arch). The upper boundary of the stomodeum (primitive oral cavity) originates as a large frontal prominence. The primary mouth is divided from the foregut by the bucco-pharyngeal membrane. The dorsal end of developing mandibular arch gives off a bud called maxillary process with the formation of the nasal pit. One medial and two lateral nasal processes are formed as the frontonasal process gets divided [12] (**Figure 4**).

4.1. Development of the primary palate (upper lip and premaxilla)

The maxillary process undergoes rapid growth between the 5th and the 6th weeks of intrauterine life. By the 7th week, the maxillary, the medial, and lateral nasal processes are integrated to form the intermaxillary segment with its labial component forming the philtrum of the upper lip while its triangular palatal component forming the maxillary incisors and extend backwards to the incisive foramen. As a result, the upper lip and the maxilla are formed. Cleft lip may develop due to inadequate proliferation of the maxillary and medial nasal processes.

4.2. Development of the secondary palate

The rest of the palatal shelves forms hard and soft palates, which are formed from secondary palate. By the 6th week of the intrauterine life, palatal shelves are formed from the medial surface of the maxillary process. These will grow medially and downwards, lateral to the tongue being elevated in the 7th week, and more marked in the anterior region and leading to growth of the mandible.

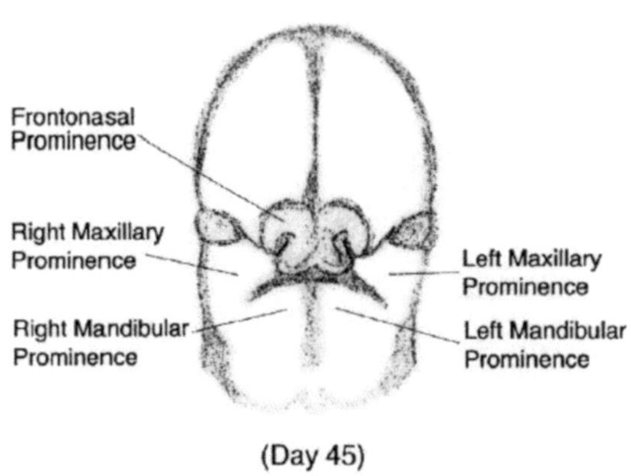

Figure 4. Facial embryo at day 45.

The tongue plays a vital role in the initial prevention of the palatal shelves union. Thus, the shelves grow vertically down. By the 8th week of intrauterine life, palatal shelves approximate touching each other. As a result, the related epithelium degenerates and mesenchyme from both shelves join in the midline. Final closure by fusion is completed by the 10th week and usually occurs a little bit later in males than females. Failure of fusion of the maxillary shelves with each other and with the frontonasal processes results in cleft palate.

5. Etiology of cleft lip and palate

Recent studies have shown that the etiology of cleft lip and palate is multifactorial. The underlying genetic factors are enhanced by environmental factors [13].

5.1. Genetic factors

The genetic factors for the etiology of nonsyndromic cleft lip with or without cleft palate and for nonsyndromic cleft palate only were first indicated in the population studies of Fogh-Anderson. Animal studies of cleft deformity were directed toward the importance of the secondary palate formation. These studies have pointed out the importance of extracellular matrix proteins and soluble factors in normal palate formation. Transforming growth factor-α (TGF-α), epidermal growth factor, fibroblast growth factor, and TGF-β3 are of clinical significance in this process. Moreover, transforming growth factor-α (TGF-α) has been suggested as a target gene in the etiology of nonsyndromic cleft deformity. In animal studies, high levels of TGFA were detected in the epithelial tissue of the medial edge of the palatal shelves at the time of shelf fusion. The biologic support for the role of TGFA gene in cleft etiology was addressed due to the reported association of TGFA alleles with human cleft lip and palate [14].

Glu mutation of the PVRL 1 gene proved to be a genetic factor for nonsyndromic clefts of the primary and the secondary palates, but simultaneous occurrence of PVRL1 and CLPTM 1 gene mutations in cleft patients does not correlate with the type of cleft (left, right, bilateral) or the gender of the patients [15, 16].

5.2. Environmental factors

A positive association between maternal cigarette smoking and cleft lip and palate has been observed in number of studies [17]. A case-control study of the association between cleft lip and palate and maternal exposure to tobacco smoke during the first trimester of pregnancy in United Kingdom proved that there is a statistically significant positive association between active smoking during pregnancy and the risk of developing cleft lip and palate [18]. B group vitamin deficiency (including folic acid) during pregnancy has been shown to be a teratogen in the etiology of cleft lip and palate formation in humans [19].

Krost and Schubert evaluated the seasonal influence on the occurrence of cleft lip and palate and proved a significant maximum risk in spring and minimum in winter for the conception date. They claimed that there are seasonal factors implicated in the etiology of cleft lip and palate.

These include deficiency of vitamins and fluctuations in mother's diet, intensive UV light exposure, the use of fertilizers and pesticides in agriculture, and infectious disease cycles [20].

6. Cleft management

Management of children with cleft lip and palate should go through a multidisciplinary team who will provide the optimal treatment (Bill, 2006). The managing team should provide comprehensive diagnosis, planning, and treatment. The cleft team usually includes orthodontist, maxillofacial surgeon, plastic surgeon, prosthodontist, speech therapist, audiologist (ENT specialist), psychologist, and pediatrician [21]. Goals of treatment of the child with a cleft lip and palate should include the repairing the birth defect (lip, palate, and nose), achieving normal speech, language, hearing, functional occlusion, and good dental health. It should also optimize the psychosocial and developmental outcomes [22]. However, protocols for the management of CLP patients vary from center to center. According to the Eurocleft project between 1996 and 2000, there were 194 different surgical approaches followed for treatment of unilateral cleft alone [23]. Management is discussed according to specific time periods as shown below.

6.1. Pre-natal diagnosis

Ultrasound examination may detect clefts of the lip and alveolus unlike cleft palate, which is difficult to diagnose through routine screening (**Figure 5**). Additional examinations and tests can confirm the presence of deformity. These include cephalic presentation of the child, low body mass index of the mother, and examination preferably around the 20th gestational week [24]. Moreover, information about family history should be addressed so that provisions for postnatal measures in adequately equipped hospitals can be made in with improvement in ultrasound technology.

In case of cleft identification, genetic counseling the family including amniocentesis should be performed. For this purpose, a complete pregnancy progress and family history should be addressed. Exposure to any teratogenic factors, the presence of family members with cleft or other birth defects, developmental problems, and genetic syndromes are all important parameter to explore during counseling. In cases where clefts are diagnosed prenatally, the cleft team will be involved in the management so that the family can learn about the nature of the deformity and its care and treatment strategies. Psychological and emotional support of the family is very essential procedure at this time due to the very negative effect once the diagnosis was confirmed.

6.2. Birth time

The most immediate problem caused by orofacial clefting is likely to be difficulty with feeding. The anatomical characteristics of cleft lip and palate greatly hinder infants' ability to feed. Poor intraoral suction may produce choking, emission of milk through the nose, and

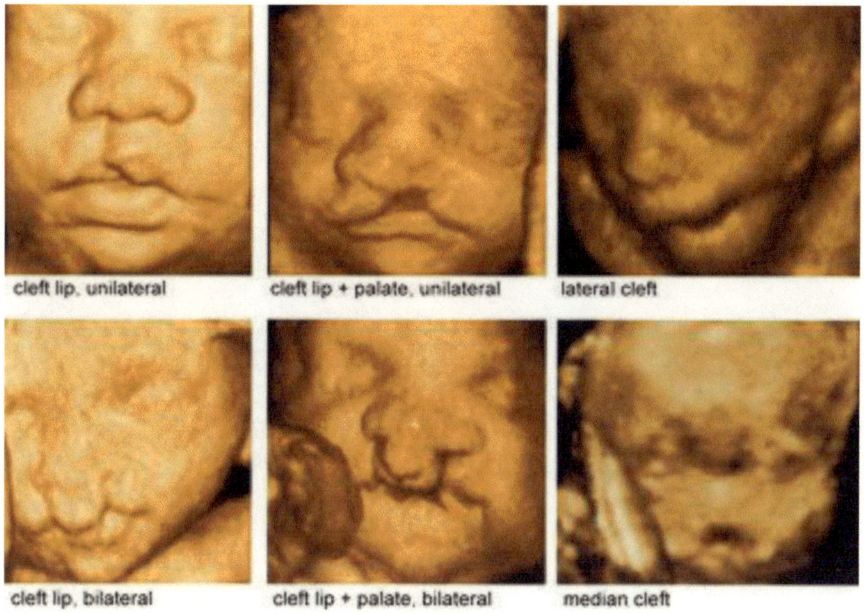

Figure 5. Three-dimensional neonatal view—various cleft deformities.

excessive air intake. The feeding process can also be extremely stressful for the parents of such infants who often struggle to find effective feeding method [25]. Early referral to the infant-feeding specialist or nurses associated with cleft teams can facilitate to solve this problem. Those children need special teat and bottles that allow milk to be delivered to the back of throat where it can be swallowed (**Figure 6**). In addition, we may use special dental plates (palatal prosthesis) to seal the cleft side. Such prosthesis could be effective in increasing the volume of fluid intake, decreasing time of feeding, and promoting adequate growth and gain in infants with cleft lip and palate [26]. Some babies may not have the energy to suck from a teat, and here a cup and spoon method may be helpful (**Figure 7**).

Presurgical orthopedics and nasoalveolar molding have become part of the treatment protocol in many cleft centers to improve the treatment outcome. Presurgical orthopedics approximates the maxillary alveolar segments and results in reduction of the tension on the repaired lip. The Latham appliance is an active presurgical orthopedic device used for cleft defects (**Figure 8**). Its long-term effects are debated. The basic idea behind appliance is to decrease the anatomical dilemma in cleft deformity so that better surgical outcome can be obtained. The device has proved its success in expanding and aligning the maxillary segments; retruding protruded premaxilla; aligning bilateral alveolar ridges; reducing tension on surgical closures; and reducing rates of fistula development. However, its long-term effect on maxillary development or occlusion has not been proven [27].

On the other hand, presurgical nasoalveolar molding (PNAM) can reduce soft tissues and cartilaginous cleft deformity to facilitate surgical soft tissue repair with minimum tension

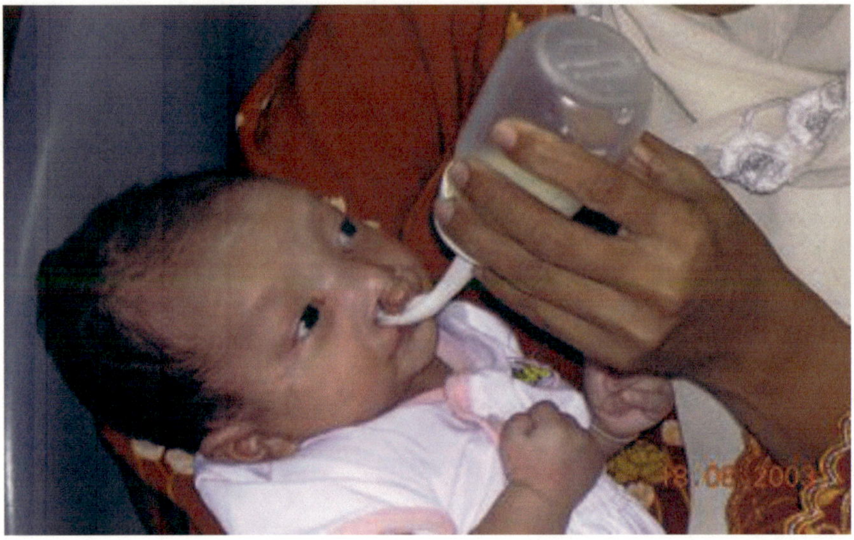

Figure 6. Special feeding bottle for cleft patients.

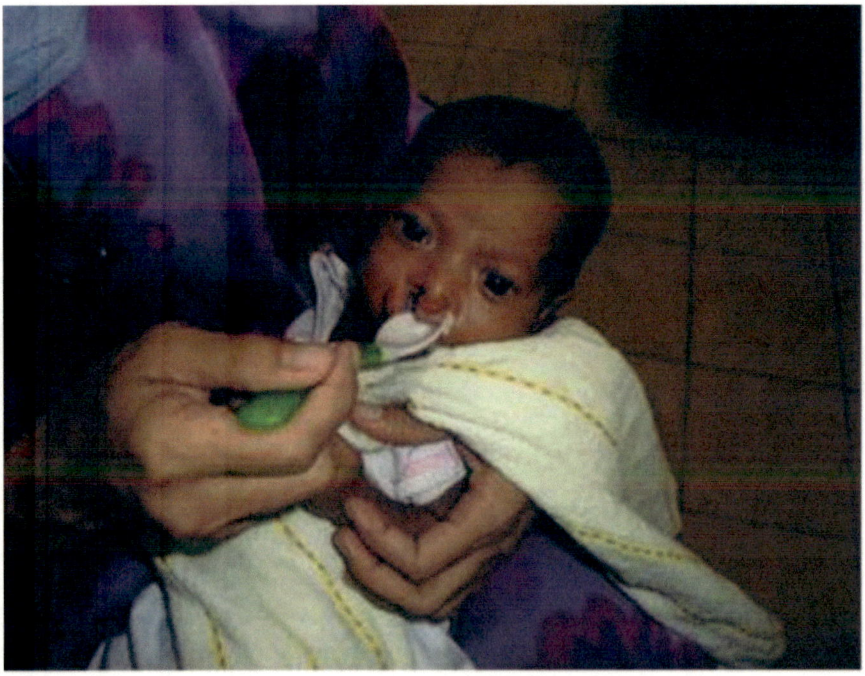

Figure 7. Spoon feeding for cleft patients.

to minimize scar formation [28]. It stimulates and redirects growth of the alveolar segments, which will lead to ideal arch formation. Moreover, it aids in normal speech development through better positioning of the tongue. Other benefits include improvement of appearance

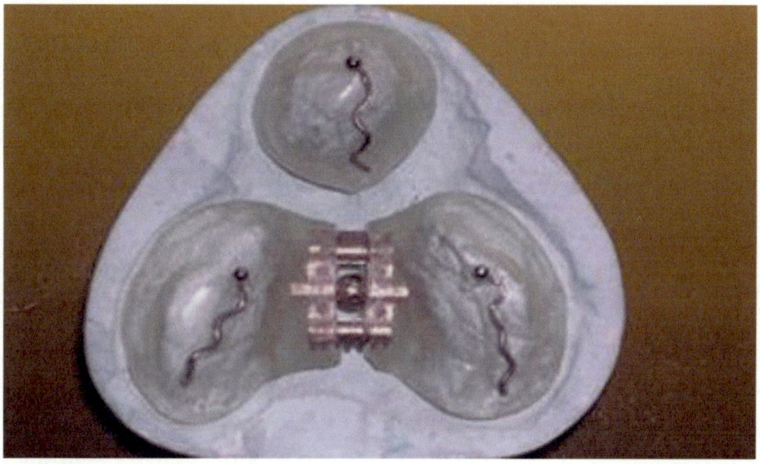

Figure 8. Pre-surgical orthopedic plate—Latham appliance.

psychosocial wellbeing, better feeding, and bone contour [29]. PNAM appliance consists of a removable alveolar molding plate made of orthodontic acrylic from a dental cast of the infant's maxilla. The nasal stent is bent at the end of a 0.032-inch stainless steel wire that is embedded into the anterior portion of the alveolar molding plate (**Figure 9**). The nasal stent

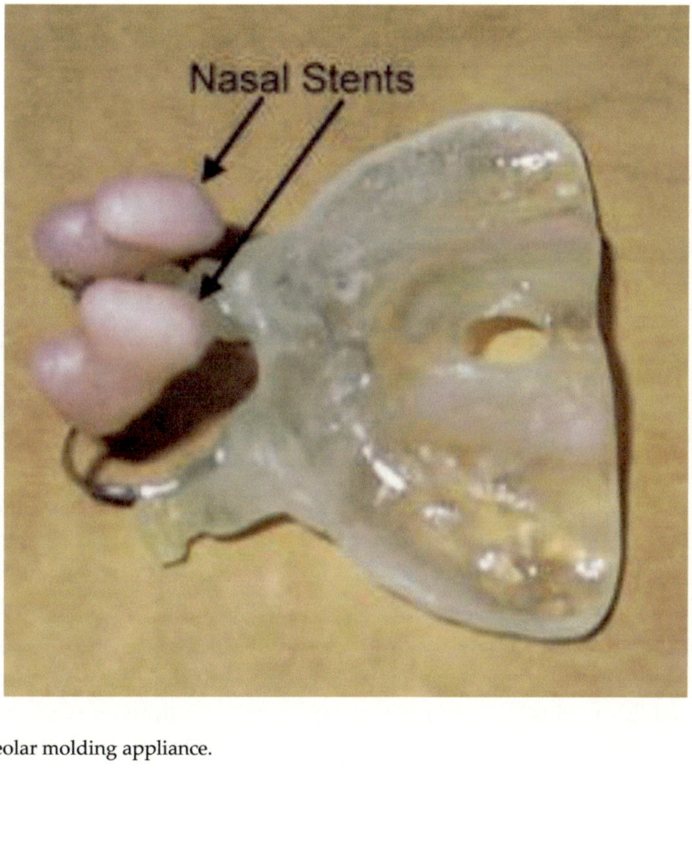

Figure 9. Active alveolar molding appliance.

and the intraoral molding plate are adjusted weekly or biweekly to gradually correct the nasal and alveolar deformities, giving rise to the name nasoalveolar molding. PNAM can be applied to the entire range of cleft deformities including complete clefts without an intact nasal floor [30].

6.3. Lip repair

There is a wide variation in the timing and techniques of primary lip repair depending upon the preference and protocol of the surgeon and cleft team involved. These include LeMesurier—1949, Tennison—1952, Randall—1959, Pfeifer—1970, Millard—1976, Del cheilorhinoplasty technique (Delaire—1978), "alar-leapfrog" technique (Pigott—1985) and many others. In broad terms, lip repair is performed at 3 months of age and palate repair at 12 months of age (Millard technique). Other schools perform surgery earlier (soft palate repair at 3 months of age and lip and hard palate repair at 6 months of age) as in the case of Malek protocol [31]. Cleft surgery has a major target in dissecting and approximating the muscles of the lip and alar base in their correct anatomical position. Debates continue to point out the suitable dissection procedure (subperipostal dissection or supraperiosteal dissection) [32].

Neonatal repair is still being evaluated. Some schools suggest doing the surgery as early as possible. According to them, the early surgery improves the facial appearance and reduces parent's apprehension. Moreover, earlier surgeries would help in the development of normal articulation [33]. On the other hand, some schools oppose earlier surgical intervention as this will restrict future growth leading to maxillary collapse and occlusal crossbites. Moreover, delayed surgery means that surgeons will have more tissues to deal with giving better outcome.

6.4. Palate repair

Cleft palate repair is a challenging procedure to learn because of the delicate tissue handling required and the small confines of the infant oral cavity. Hard and soft palate repair is performed at the age range of 9–18 months. The idea behind this relatively early intervention is giving priority to development of normal articulation, which can be extremely difficult to eradicate after the age of 5 years [34]. Different surgical protocols are followed to repair the palate; these include: Von Langbeck repair, vomer flap repair, and Z-plasty repair. In general, scar retraction due to exposed bone in palatoplasty is the leading cause of constricted maxilla. Modern techniques have focused on minimizing the effects of scarring by reducing the exposure of the bone area.

It is self-evident that a physical defect that affects the structures of the mouth and face has the potential to influence articulatory development [35]. Cleft palate often causes problems with speech and hearing. It has been primarily considered as a disorder of the vocal tract. Parents are encouraged to stimulate and converse with infants normally expecting the development of good speech. Speech and language therapist should carry out early assessment with special expertise in clefts. Assessment at 18 months gives a good indication and is repeated, for example, at 3 years. In most cases, the majority of children following cleft palate repair have normal intelligibility. On the other hand, many babies with cleft lip and palate have recurrent otitis media and develop glue ear. A possible etiology for this is that palatal muscles (levator palati and tensor palati) are involved in cleft deformity leading to eustachian tube dysfunction. Cleft subjects need extensive screening in ENT department [36].

6.5. Primary dentition (2–6 years)

Velopharyngeal insufficiency (VPI) is a common finding in cleft patients. VPI is the incomplete closure of the velopharyngeal sphincter resulting in hypernasal resonance, which can compromise speech intelligibility. Most sounds are divided to be oral (produced in the oral cavity) and nasal (m & n only). Speech nasality happens when the oral cavity is not completely sealed from the nasal cavity. As a result, air escapes through the nose. Even after palate repair, cleft patients can still sound nasal due to the inability of the soft palate to seal and separate these two cavities. The reason for that is weakness in muscles of the soft palate. Moreover, the soft palate is short, which hinders its contact with pharyngeal wall [37]. Speech assessment might be commenced as early as 18 months of age taking into consideration the needs of the patient [38]. Assessment of speech must continue through childhood along with cleft team to detect any developing problems that may arise with growth. ENT surgeon will be involved throughout all monitoring phase. Lip revision and closure of any residual palatal fistula before schooling might be considered to support speech development [39].

Orthodontic treatment in this stage is limited to the correction of certain posterior crossbite and anterior crossbite of mild-to-moderate degree. Posterior crossbites are of both skeletal and dental origin. A crossbite of a dental origin and accompanied with occlusal shift can be managed by selective grinding; anterior crossbite of mild-to-moderate degree can be managed by the use of elastic protraction forces delivered through a facial mask [40]. However, if this crossbite is related to severe maxillary hypoplasia, the patient is best managed with surgical procedures that are done at later stages. During this age, it is important to develop good dental care habits, instituting fluoride supplements in nonfluoridated areas [41].

6.6. Mixed dentition (6–12 years)

The negative effects of surgical repair become clear during this phase including maxillary collapse and arch discrepancies. Moreover, defects in alveolar bone, tooth number, formation, and position can be detected. Surgeons start to consider alveolar bone graft to correct the maxillary defects at this stage (**Figure 10**). Grafting is best performed with autogenously cancellous bone. Alveolar bone grafting will provide maxillary-alveolar ridge continuity for tooth eruption and alignment. It also provides nasal base support and provides bone through which the permanent canines and laterals can erupt into the dental arch. In bilateral cases, alveolar bone grafting stabilizes the premaxillary segment with bone support [42]. Alveolar bone grafting is performed using a gingival flap of mucoperiosteum, turned back "book" flaps and cancellous bone harvested from the iliac crest. The covering flap of gingival mucoperiosteum is used to cover the graft in the alveolus, nostril floor, and anterior maxilla. The ideal age for bone grafting is 9–11 years to give chance for the lateral incisor or the canine to erupt through the graft and stabilize it. Supernumerary teeth in the surgical site should be extracted 8–12 weeks before surgery. This will allow the surgeon to have intact

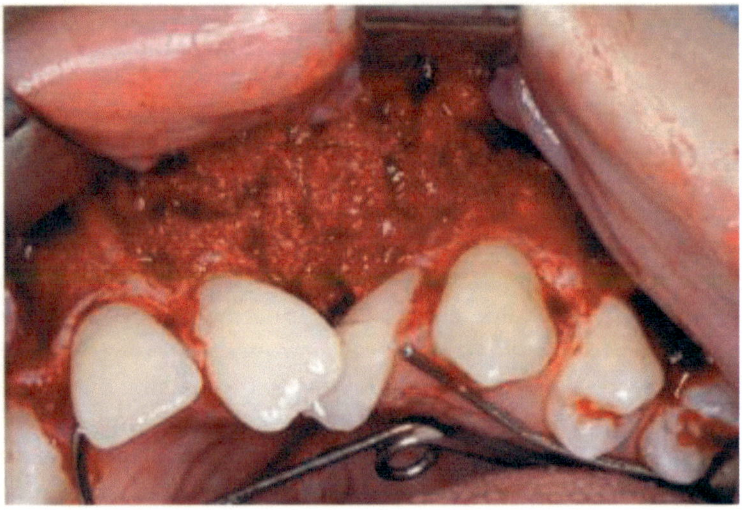

Figure 10. Alveolar bone graft.

gingival tissues for proper coverage of the alveolar bone graft. At the time of complete eruption of permanent dentition (approximately 12 or 13 years of age), orthodontic treatment is commenced.

The timing of bone grafting will be decided on the basis of the dental development of individual patients [43]. In patients with well-formed lateral incisors that are in the line of the dental arch, bone grafting can be done quite early, around 7 or 8 years. However, most patients with complete unilateral cleft lip and palate have a missing, ectopic, or deformed lateral incisor, so it is preferable that bone grafting is postponed until they are 10 or 11 years of age (**Figure 11**). This allows the root development of the cleft-side canine to progress more and may help in better canine eruption [44].

An interceptive orthodontic treatment is undertaken in the mixed dentition to reposition the dentition adjacent to the cleft preparing the cleft side for the secondary alveolar bone graft,

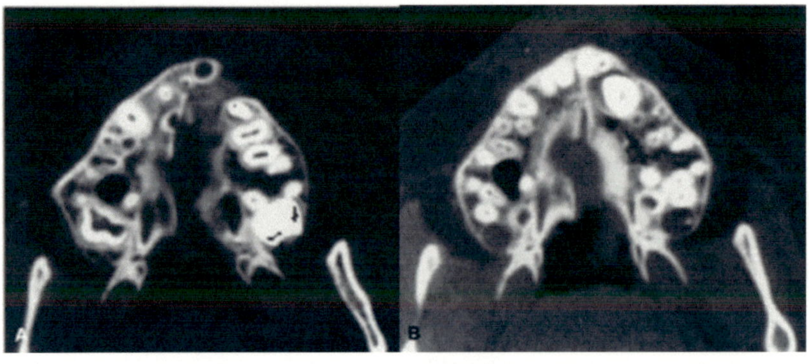

Figure 11. CBCT of alveolar bone graft in UCLP patient (A: before and B: after).

but such procedure must be postponed until the development of the incisor roots to avoid any resorptive effect on teeth. If maxillary segments and dentition on either side of the cleft are well aligned, it is not necessary to do presurgical orthodontics [45]. Thus, orthodontic treatment is not generally commenced until age 9 or 10 years when, if necessary, the maxillary segments are expanded to correct the transverse relationship using palatal expansion appliances, these include upper removable appliance, quad helix (**Figure 12**), rapid maxillary expansion, bonded "fan" appliance (**Figure 13**), and others [46, 47].

6.7. Permanent dentition

Definitive orthodontic treatment must be commenced at this time. The goals of treatment are similar to those for noncleft patients, but certain conditions must be taken into consideration during the treatment planning. These include maintenance of the integrity of the dentition and supporting structures especially for teeth adjacent to the cleft side, correction of impacted and transposed teeth, and management of congenitally missing teeth [48].

If the cleft side lateral incisor is missing, management will be based on either replacing the missing tooth with prosthesis or closing the space. In those patients with missing lateral incisor in whom the maxillary canine has migrated mesially and is erupting into the grafted alveolar ridge, replacement of the missing lateral incisor by the canine and movement of all posterior teeth forward will be the treatment of choice. In cases where the alveolar bone graft is not ideal, bone morphology can be improved by moving the canine forward into graft side [49].

Extractions may be required to create space for arch alignment with the second premolars being first choice in the maxilla. This is related to formation of scar tissue during the course of primary palatal repair, which pulls the premolars palatally. However, relapse is common after orthodontic correction. Invariably, fixed appliances are required to achieve a satisfactory degree of precision in tooth alignment with sound values of tip and torque movements [50]. Once the permanent dentition has been established, planning for orthognathic surgery must take place in a tempt to correct mid-face retrusion. Factors such as maxillary retrognathia, the magnitude and effect of any future growth, and patient wishes should be taken into consideration. Surgical correction is indicated only when growth is complete. Surgical revision of the nose (rhinoplasty) will be the last surgical step. This is because movement of the underlying bone will affect the contour of the nose [51].

Hypodontia, microdontia, and conical crowns are common findings in cleft lip and palate (**Figure 14**). In broad terms, treatment strategies reflect the pattern of tooth absence, the amount of residual spacing, existing malocclusions, and patient's attitude [52, 53]. The congenital missing of teeth may result in minimal spacing; still, it may not be an esthetic concern to patients and can be accepted. Space closure and modification of the canine to resemble a lateral incisor is a common treatment option where maxillary lateral incisors are missing. However, where several teeth are congenitally absent, the orthodontic redistribution of space to allow restoration with prostheses is frequently the treatment of choice. The esthetic and functional outcomes of such an approach should be confirmed with a trial diagnostic set-up.

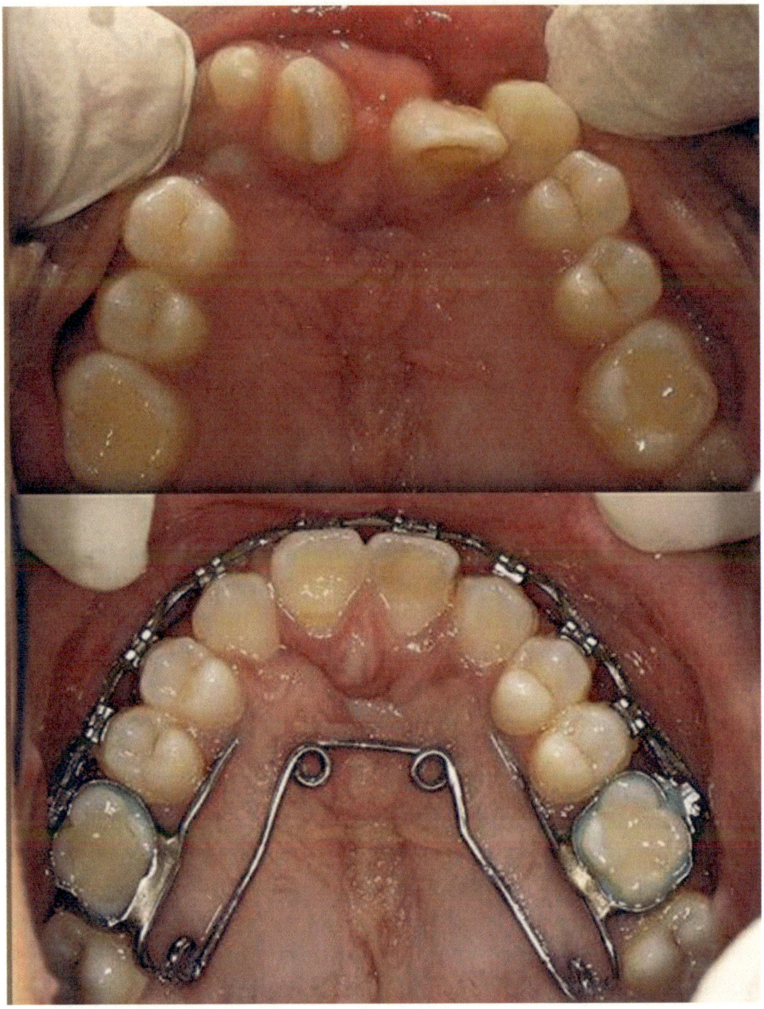

Figure 12. Quad helix expansion in UCLP.

Replacement of missing teeth with prosthesis includes removable partial dentures, conventional and adhesive bridges, and implant supported prostheses. Clearly, both the timing and manner of their application must reflect the needs and limitations imposed by a young, growing individual [54].

6.8. Orthognathic surgery

The midfacial hypoplasia or maxillary constriction is a common secondary deformity in cleft deformity involving primary palate. This hypoplasia and constriction are related to growth impairment and scar formation in hard palate during the palate repair. Despite of orthodontic treatment, up to 25% of patients with cleft lip and palate needs surgical interventions to achieve balanced and harmonious facial appearance.

http://dx.doi.org/10.5772/intechopen.68448

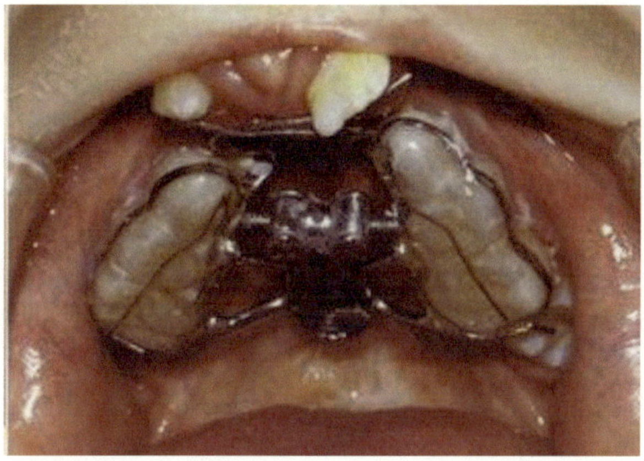

Figure 13. Bonded "fan" expansion appliance.

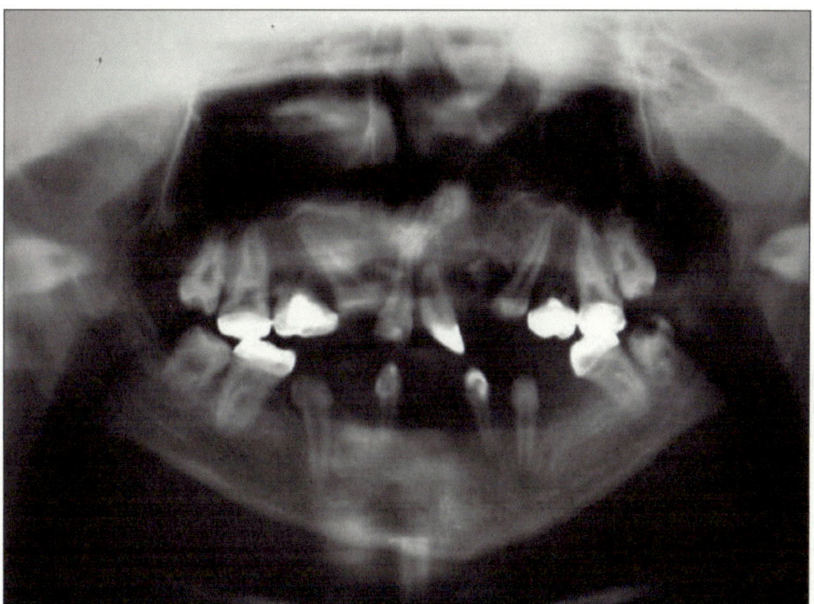

Figure 14. Hypodontia in cleft lip and palate.

At approximately the age of 17–18, a final assessment of facial pattern is carried out clinically. Detailed cephalometric assessment and growth analyses are carried out to plan for orthognathic surgery. No orthognathic surgery is carried out until growth is complete. Surgeons perform the corrective surgery in the maxillary bone or both jaws according to the severity of the underlying skeletal discrepancy. The advantage of this surgical-orthodontic approach is that the clinicians can provide the patient with occlusal relations close to ideal and markedly improved function and esthetics.

6.9. Psychological effects

Children with craniofacial anomalies are at greater risk of developing behavioral, emotional, or social competence problems [55]. Some children with oral clefts have decreased social competence as shown by fewer friends and poor social interaction. Slifer et al. have found that 30–50% of children with cleft lip and/or palate between the ages of 6 and 16 are rated by their parents to be 1.0 or more standard deviations below the mean compared to noncleft peers on measures of social adjustment and competence (sharing their friends in social activities, degree, and quality of social interaction). Unfortunately, this tendency continued through adolescence and into adulthood [56].

All the above features will have psychological effects on cleft patients as well as their families; these effects become more significant when patients get younger. Two stages where those children have a real challenge to deal with; are when they go to school (5–6) years i.e. the difficulty of being different. The second when they start to look after their appearance, i.e. the pre-puberty and adolescence time. Children with visible clefts are often very self-conscious about their appearance, speech, and schooling.

6.10. Learning disorders and behavioral problems

Children with cleft lip and palate are at an increased risk for learning disorders. There is a consensus that language skills of cleft palate patients tend to be delayed even if the cleft was a small one [57]. Broder et al. have examined the prevalence of learning disability, level of school achievement, and prevalence of grade retention by type of cleft and gender at two craniofacial centers. The results showed that 46% of subjects with cleft had learning disability and 47% had deficient educational progress. Moreover, 27% had repeated a grade in the school. The results also showed that males with only cleft palate and females with cleft lip and palate were at higher risk among all cleft subjects [58].

Acknowledgments

To my wife Huda Zurigat whose never-failing sympathy and encouragement, without your support, this chapter would not have been finished on time.

Author details

Maen Hussni Zreaqat[1]*, Rozita Hassan[1] and Abdulfattah Hanoun[2]

*Address all correspondence to: maenzreqat@yahoo.com

1 Universiti Sanins Malaysia, Kota Bharu, Malaysia

2 Orthodontic Department, Universiti Sains Malaysia, Penang, Malaysia

References

[1] Murray J. Gene/environment causes of cleft lip and/or palate. Clinical Genetics. 2002;**61**(4):248-256. DOI: 10.1016/j.coms.2016.01.004

[2] Bender P. Genetics of cleft lip and palate. Journal of Pediatric Nursing. 2000;**15**(4):242-249. DOI: 10.1016/j.coms.2016.01.2300

[3] Duffy S, Noar J, Evans R, Sanders R. Three-dimensional analysis of the child cleft face. Cleft Palate Craniofacial Journal. 2000;**37**(2):137-144. DOI: 10.1016/j.coms.2016.01.004

[4] Susami T, Kamiyama H, Uji M, Motohashi N, Kuroda T. Quantitative evaluation of the shape and the elasticity of repaired cleft lip. Cleft Palate Craniofacial Journal. 1993;**30**(3):309-312. DOI: 10.1016/j.fsc.2016.06.015

[5] Mars M, Asher-McDade C, Brattstrom V, Dahl E, McWilliam J, Molsted K, Plint D, Prahl-Andersen B, Semb G, Shaw W. A six-center international study of treatment outcome in patients with clefts of the lip and palate: Part 3. Dental arch relationships. Cleft Palate Craniofacial Journal. 1992;**29**(5):405-408. DOI: 10.1016/j.fsc.2016.06.052

[6] Bishara SE, de Arrendondo RS, Vales HP, Jakobsen JR. Dentofacial relationships in persons with unoperated clefts: Comparisons between three cleft types. American Journal of Orthodontics. 1985;**87**(6):481-507. DOI: 10.1097/SCS.0000000000002889

[7] Bill J, Proff P, Bayerlein T, Weingaertner J, Fanghanel J, Reuther J. Treatment of patients with cleft lip, alveolus and palate – A short outline of history and current interdisciplinary treatment approaches. Journal of Cranio-maxillofacial Surgery. 2006; **34**(2):17-21. DOI: 10.1016/j.ijporl.2016.12.030

[8] Derijcke A, Eerens A, Carels C. The incidence of oral clefts: A review. British Journal of Oral and Maxillofacial Surgery. 1996;**34**(6):488-494. DOI: 10.1097/MCD.0000000000000172

[9] Daskalogiannakis J, Kuntz K, Chudley A, Ross B. Unilateral cleft lip with or without cleft palate and handedness: Is there an association?. Cleft Palate Craniofacial Journal. 1998;**35**(1):46-51. DOI: 10.1097/SCS.0000000000003506

[10] Shprintzen R, Higgins M, Antshel K, Fremont W, Roizen N, Kates W. Velo-cardio-facial syndrome. Current Opinion in Pediatrics. 2005;**17**(6):725-30. DOI: 10.1111/1460-6984.12307

[11] Sandham A. Classification of clefting deformity. Early Human Development. 1985;**12**(1): 81-85 DOI: 10.1007/s00268-017-3896-8

[12] Thornton J, Nimer S, Howard P. The incidence, classification, etiology, and embryology of oral clefts. Seminars in Orthodontics. 1996;**2**(3):162-168. DOI: 10.1016/j.actbio.2017.01.053

[13] Wong F, Hagg U. An update on the aetiology of orofacial clefts. Hong Kong Medical Journal. 2004;**10**(5):331-336. DOI: 10.1597/14-296

[14] Machida J, Yoshiura K, Funkhauser C, Natsume N, Kawai T, Murray J. Transforming growth factor-a (TGFA): Genomic structure, boundary sequences, and mutation analysis in nonsyndromic cleft lip/palate and cleft palate only. Genomics. 1999;**61**:237-242. DOI: 10.1597/16-156

[15] Turhani D, Item C, Watzinger E, Sinko K, Watzinger F, Lauer G, Ewers R. Mutation analysis of CLPTM 1 and PVRL 1 genes in patients with non-syndromic clefts of lip, alveolus and palate. Journal of Cranio-maxillofacial Surgery. 2005;**33**(5):301-306. DOI: 10.1093/hmg/ddx012

[16] Arosarena O. Cleft lip and palate. Otolaryngologic Clinics of North America. 2007; **40**(1):27-60. DOI: 10.1597/16-008

[17] Seller MJ, Bnait KS. Effects of tobacco smoke inhalation on the developing mouse embryo and fetus. Reproductive Toxicology. 1995;**9**(5):449-459. DOI: 10.1097/SCS.0000000000003324

[18] Little J, Cardy A, Arslan M, Gilmour M, Mossey A. Smoking and orofacial clefts: A United Kingdom-based case-control study. Cleft Palate Craniofacial Journal. 2004;**41**(4):381-386. DOI: 10.1038/srep38872

[19] Schubert J, Schmidt R, Syska E. B group vitamins and cleft lip and cleft palate. International Journal of Oral and Maxillofacial Surgery. 2002;**31**(4):410-413. DOI: 10.3889/oamjms

[20] Krost B, Schubert J. Influence of season on prevalence of cleft lip and palate. International Journal of Oral and Maxillofacial Surgery. 2006;**35**(3):215-218. DOI: 10.3892/mmr.2017.6107

[21] Schnitt D, Agir H, David D. From birth to maturity: A group of patients who have completed their protocol management. Part I. Unilateral cleft lip and palate. Plastic and Reconstructive Surgery. 2004;**113**(3):805-817. DOI: 10.1186/s12887

[22] Sommerlad B, Mehendale F, Birch M, Sell D, Hattee C, Harland K. Palate re-repair revisited. Cleft Palate Craniofacial Journal. 2002;**39**(3):295-307. DOI: 10.1080/08870446.2016.1275630

[23] Shaw W, Semb G, Nelson P, Brattstrom V, Molsted K, Prahl-Andersen B, Gundlach K. The eurocleft project 1996–2000: Overview. Journal of Maxillofacial Surgery. 2001;**29**(3):131-140. DOI: 10.1111/jop.12548

[24] Heinrich A, Proff P, Michel T, Ruhland F, Kirbschus A, Gedrange T. Prenatal diagnostics of cleft deformities and its significance for parent and infant care. Journal of Craniomaxillofacial Surgery. 2006;**34**(2):14-16. DOI: 10.1155/2016/3054578

[25] Endriga C, Speltz L, Mark L, Jones K. Do psychosocial variables predict the physical growth of infants with orofacial clefts? Infant Behavior & Development. 1998;**21**(4):700-712. DOI: 10.1002/ajmg.a.37740

[26] Turner C, Zagirova A, Frolova E, Courts F, Williams W. Oral health status of Russian children with unilateral cleft lip and palate. Cleft Palate Craniofacial Journal. 1998;**35**(6):489-494. DOI: 10.1002/bdra.23512

[27] Cruz C. Presurgical orthopedics appliance: The latham technique. Oral and Maxillofacial Surgery Clinics of North America. 2016;**28**(2):161-168. DOI: 10.1016/j.coms.2016.01.004

[28] Attiguppe P, Karuna Y, Yavagal C, Naik S, Deepak M, Maganti R, Krishna G. Presurgical nasoalveolar molding: A boon to facilitate the surgical repair in infants with cleft lip and palate. Contemporary Clinical Dentistry. 2016;**7**(4):569-573. DOI: 10.1001/jamaoto.2016.3175

[29] Liang Z, Yao J, Chen PK, Zheng C, Yang J. Effect of presurgical nasoalveolar molding on nasal symmetry in unilateral complete cleft lip/palate patients after primary cheiloplasty without concomitant nasal cartilage dissection: Early childhood evaluation. Cleft Palate Craniofacial Journal. 2017;**13**(7):75-81. DOI: 10.1597/14-296

[30] Grayson B, Garfinkle S. Early cleft management: The case for nasoalveolar molding. American Journal of Orthodontics and Dentofacial Orthopedics. 2014;**145**:134-142. DOI: 10.1016/j.oooo.2016.08.007

[31] da Silva FO, de Castro MM, de Andrade A, de Souza Freitas A, Bishara S. Upper dental arch morphology of adult unoperated complete bilateral cleft lip and palate. American Journal of Orthodontics and Dentofacial Orthopedics. 1998;**114**(2):154-161. DOI: 10.7196/SAMJ.2016.v106i10.11314

[32] Mitchell L. An Introduction to Orthodontics. 2nd ed. Oxford University Press, New York; 2012. pp. 177-189. DOI:10.1111/jan.12994

[33] Taub P, Piccolo P. Cleft lip repair: Through the looking glass. Journal of Craniofacial Surgery. 2016;**27**(8):2031-2035. DOI: 10.1097/SCS.0000000000002889

[34] Woo A. Evidence-based medicine: Cleft palate. Plastic and Reconstructive Surgery. 2017;**139**(1):191e-203e. DOI: 10.1097/PRS.0000000000002854

[35] Larsson A, Schölin J, Mark H, Jönsson R, Persson C. Speech production in 3-year-old internationally adopted children with unilateral cleft lip and palate. International Journal of Language and Communication Disorders. 2017;**14**(5):52-59. DOI: 10.1111/1460-6984.1230

[36] Prathanee B, Pumnum T, Seepuaham C, Jaiyong P. Five-year speech and language outcomes in children with cleft lip-palate. Craniomaxillofacial Surgery. 2016;**44**(10):1553-1560. DOI: 10.1016/j.jcms.2016.08.004

[37] Lam D, Starr R, Perkins A, Lewis W, Eblen E, Dunlap J, Sie K. A comparison of nasendoscopy and multiview videofluoroscopy in assessing velopharyngeal insufficiency. Otolaryngology Head and Neck Surgery. 2006;**134**(3):394-402. DOI: 10.1016/j.coms.2016.01.003

[38] Nyberg J, Havstam C. Speech in 10-year-olds born with cleft lip and palate: What do peers say?. Cleft Palate Craniofacial Journal. 2016;**53**(5):516-526. DOI: 10.1597/15-140

[39] Paliobei V, Psifidis A, Anagnostopoulos D. Hearing and speech assessment of cleft palate patients after palatal closure. Long-term results. International Journal of Pediatric Otorhinolaryngology. 2005;**69**(10):1373-1381. DOI: 10.1097/SCS.0b013e3181b6c82d

[40] Subtelny D. Oral respiration: Facial maldevelopment and corrective dentofacial orthopedics. The Angle Orthodontist. 1980;**50**:147-164. DOI: 10.1097/SCS.0b013e3181b6c69f

[41] Rivkin C, Keith O, Crawford P, Hathorn S. Dental care for the patient with a cleft lip and palate. Part 2: The mixed dentition stage through to adolescence and young adulthood. British Dental Journal. 2000;**188**(3):131-134. DOI: 10.1097/SCS.0b013e3181b5d4c0

[42] Takahashi T, Fukuda M, Yamaguchi T, Kochi S, Inai T, Watanabe M, Echigo S. Use of an osseointegrated implant for dental rehabilitation after cleft repair by periosteoplasty: A case report. Cleft Palate Craniofacial Journal. 1997;**34**(3):268-271. DOI: 10.1097/SCS.0b013e3181b5d08e

[43] Gürsoy S, Hukki J, Hurmerinta K. Five-year follow-up of maxillary distraction osteogenesis on the dentofacial structures of children with cleft lip and palate. Journal of Oral and Maxillofacial Surgery. 2010;**68**(4):744-750. DOI: 10.1016/j.joms.2009.07.036

[44] Newlands C. Secondary alveolar bone grafting in cleft lip and palate patients. British Journal of Oral and Maxillofacial Surgery. 2000;**38**(5):488-491. DOI: 10.1097/SCS.0b013e3181b3

[45] Solis A, Figueroa A, Cohen M, Polley J, Evans A. Maxillary dental development in complete unilateral alveolar clefts. Cleft Palate Craniofacial Journal. 1998;**35**:320-328. DOI: 10.1597/14-136

[46] Figueiredo D, Cardinal L, Bartolomeo F, Palomo M, Horta C, Andrade I, Oliveira DD. Effects of rapid maxillary expansion in cleft patients resulting from the use of two different expanders. Dental Press Journal of Orthodontics. 2016;**21**(6):82-90. DOI: 10.1590/2177-6709.2016-001.aop

[47] Garib DG, Garcia LC, Pereira V, Lauris RC, Yen S. A rapid maxillary expander with differential opening. Journal of Clinical Orthodontics. 2014;**48**(7):430-435 DOI: 10.3109/2000656X.2015

[48] Vig K, Mercado M. Overview of orthodontic care for children with cleft lip and palate, 1915-2015. American Journal of Orthodontics and Dentofacial Orthopedics. 2015;**148**(4):543-556. DOI: 10.1016/j.ajodo.2015.07.021

[49] Tome W, Yashiro K, Kogo M, Yamashiro T. Cephalometric outcomes of maxillary expansion and protraction in patients with unilateral cleft lip and palate after two types of palatoplasty. Cleft Palate Craniofacial Journal. 2016;**53**(6):690-694. DOI: 10.1097/01.prs.0000472269.61556.61

[50] Hammond J. The Belle Maudsley memorial lecture 1986. Treatment of maxillary retrusion in a case of cleft lip and palate. Dental Update. 1987;**14**(5):193-196, 198, 200. DOI: 10.1007/s12663-013-0490-y

[51] Bhuskute A, Tollefson T. Cleft lip repair, nasoalveolar molding, and primary cleft rhinoplasty review. Facial Plastic Surgery Clinics of North America. 2016;**24**(4):453-466. DOI: 10.1016/j.fsc.2016.06.015

[52] Berniczei-Roykó Á, Tappe JH, Krinner A, Gredes T, Végh A, Gábor K, Linkowska-Świdzińska K, Botzenhart UU. Radiographic study of the prevalence and distribution of hypodontia associated with unilateral and bilateral cleft lip and palate in a Hungarian population. Medical Science Monitor. 2016;**21**(22):3868-3885. DOI: 10.4103/2231-0746.161060

[53] Al-Kharboush G, Al-Balkhi K, Al-Moammar K. The prevalence of specific dental anomalies in a group of Saudi cleft lip and palate patients. Saudi Dental Journal. 2015;**27**(2):75-80. DOI: 10.1016/j.sdentj.2014.11.007

[54] Jepson M, Noh S, Carter E, Gillgrass J, Meechan G, Hobson S, Nunn H. The interdisciplinary management of hypodontia: Restorative dentistry. British Dental Journal. 2003;**194**(6):299-304. DOI: 10.1093/jamia/ocv125

[55] Pruzinsky T. Social and psychological effects of major craniofacial deformity. Cleft Palate Craniofacial Journal. 1992;**29**(6):578-584. discussion 570. DOI: 10.1093/jamia/ocv125

[56] Slifer K, Diver T, Amari A, Cohn F, Hilley L, Beck M, McDonnell S, Kane A. Assessment of facial emotion encoding and decoding skills in children with and without oral clefts. Journal of Craniomaxillofacial Surgery. 2003;**31**(5):304-315. DOI: 10.1002/ajmg.a.37342

[57] Millard T, Richman C. Different cleft conditions, facial appearance, and speech: Relationship to psychological variables. Cleft Palate Craniofacial Journal. 2001;**38**(1):68-75. DOI: 10.1002/ajmg.a.35767

[58] Broder H, Richman C, Matheson B. Learning disability, school achievement, and grade retention among children with cleft: A two-center study. Cleft Palate Craniofacial Journal. 1998;**35**(2):127-131. DOI: 10.4103/1817-1745.131491

Chapter 7

Treatment of Class II Malocclusion (Hypodivergent Face) with MEAW Therapy

Paulo Augusto de Sousa Beltrão

Additional information is available at the end of the chapter

http://dx.doi.org/10.5772/intechopen.69331

Abstract

Patients with class II deep bite malocclusion and hypodivergent skeletal typology represent complex and prolonged cases of treatment due to their muscular characteristics. The etiology of the class II deep bite is multifactorial: environmental and/or genetic factors represent an important part in the establishment of class II deep bite. However, there is a close connection between three class II factors and the adaptation of mandible and occlusal function. These factors are lack of vertical dimension, inclination of the upper occlusal plane, lack of occlusal support, and pressure of TMJ. According to Tanaka and Sato, there is a relationship between the inclination of the maxillary posterior occlusal plane and the mandibular position, consistent with the etiology of different dento-skeletal structures. The occlusal plane is more tilted in patients with class II and more flat in patients with class III than in individuals with class I occlusions. **Patients and methods**: Two male teenagers were treated with MEAW therapy, and both treatments lasted 24 months. **Results**: The MEAW therapy appropriately corrected the class II deep bite over a period of 24 months, achieving a good occlusal, functional, and esthetic result. **Conclusions**: The MEAW therapy proved to be effective in the treatment of class II deep bite malocclusion, in growing patients.

Keywords: class II deep bite, steep occlusal plane, hypodivergent, MEAW

1. Introduction

During the process development of skeletal class II, there are three important factors (insufficient height of bite, strong inclination of the occlusal plane, lack of occlusal support), which are closely related with the adaptation of the mandible and the occlusal function [1–3].

The maxillary dentition of patients with class II malocclusion has low vertical dimension in the posterior area, and the upper posterior occlusal plane is steep. The occlusal interferences in the molar area prevent the mandible to adapt to a forward position, instead the mandible adapts posteriorly, aggravating the distoclusion. Actually, 70% of the class II malocclusion does not imply the protrusion of the maxilla but is known to be caused by retrusion of the mandible (McNamara [4]).

Morphological characteristics of the class II deep overbite are the following: the mandible is small and retruded, insufficient vertical dimension and occlusal support, steepening of the occlusal plane in the upper posterior area, occlusal interferences in the molar area, and labial tipping of the upper anterior teeth. The skeletal characteristics of class II deep bite malocclusion are closely related to the lack of vertical dimension and the steepness of the occlusal plane. Some authors proved that the vertical disproportion was in many cases at the origin of anterior-posterior dysplasias.

Therefore, a treatment approach based on the control of the occlusal plane and vertical dimension is essential to the success of the treatment. The treatment objectives for class II deep bite are the following: to increase the vertical dimension, to rebuild and flatten the upper posterior occlusal plane, to coordinate upper and lower dental arch width, to move the mandible forward, to improve overbite (deep bite), to obtain normal intercuspidation, and to improve the profile.

The treatment of low-angle class II malocclusions must prevent occlusal interferences and extrude the upper molars to increase their vertical height and flatten the occlusal plane. As a result, the mandible readapts to the physiological position, and occlusal function is attained. The steps of the class II deep overbite malocclusion are leveling, elimination of occlusal interferences, establishing mandibular position, reconstruction of the occlusal plane, and achieving a physiological occlusion.

2. The multiloop edgewise arch wire (MEAW)

In 1967, Young H. Kim created the multiloop edgewise arch wire (MEAW) to treat open bite malocclusions, which he achieved with great efficiency. Subsequently, Prof. Sadao Sato (Kanagawa Dental College, Japan) [5] developed the MEAW philosophy of treatment and applied it to all types of malocclusions. MEAW can be constructed with stainless steel 0.016 × 0.022 (bracket 0.018 inch slot) or 0.017 × 0.025 ss (bracket 0.022 inch slot).

The arches have ideal dental arch shape with five loops on each side of the arch. The loops between the teeth act as a force breaker and allow smooth and continuous forces to be distributed through the teeth, as well as individual control of vertical, horizontal, and torque forces on the teeth. The use of MEAW arches with activation must be done together with the use of intraoral elastics (appropriate to the malocclusion), in order to obtain a successful reconstruction of the posterior occlusal plane (**Figure 1**).

http://dx.doi.org/10.5772/intechopen.69331

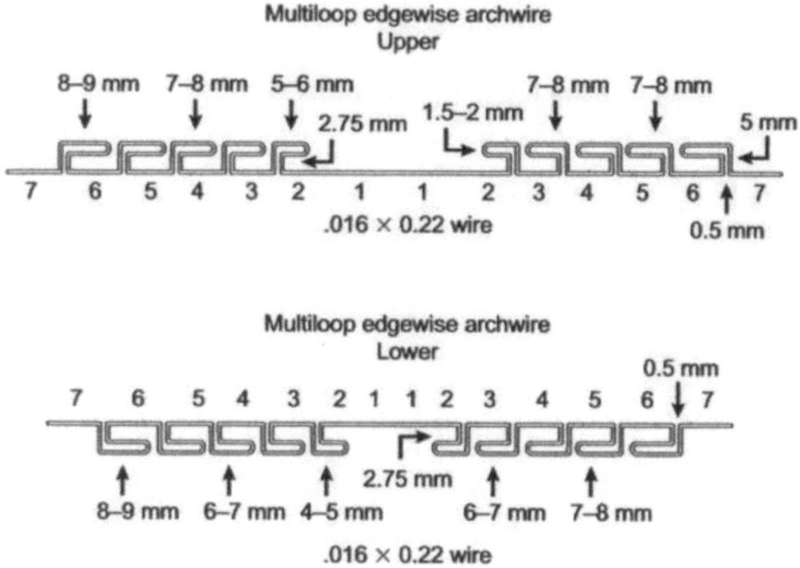

Figure 1. Upper and lower multiloop edgewise arch wire (MEAWs).

3. Cephalometric analysis

3.1. Analysis of Kim

Kim [6, 7] developed his cephalometric analysis in order to identify the types of vertical and anterior-posterior growth and their connection with the inclination of the occlusal plane:

- Overbite depth indicator (ODI)
- Anterior-posterior dysplasia indicator (APDI)
- Combination factor (CF)

3.2. Overbite depth indicator (ODI)

The ODI is the sum of two angles: the A–B plane with the mandibular plane (MP) and the palatal plane with the Frankfort horizontal (FH) plane. The angle is negative when the palatal plane inclines superiorly in relation to the FH plane and is read as a positive angle when the palatal plane inclines inferiorly in relation to the FH plane.

There is a norm of 74.5 degrees with a standard deviation of 6.07. A value lower than 74.5 (±6.07 degrees) shows a skeletal open bite tendency. A highest value of 74.5 (±6.07 degrees) shows a deep bite skeletal pattern tendency. In these patients with skeletal deep bite tendency, tooth extractions should be avoided, in order not to lose occlusal support, because loss of occlusal support increases the risk of relapse (**Figure 2**).

3.3. Anteroposterior dysplasia indicator (APDI)

The APDI consists of three angles: the angle of the facial plane (Frankfurt horizontal (FH)/ facial plane (FP)), added or decreased to the angle Downs, and added or decreased to the angle of the palatine plane in relation to the plane HF. The APDI can also be calculated by the value of the angle formed by the palatine plane (PP) (line linking points A and B).

APDI = (FH-FP) + (AB-FP) + (FH-PP). The average APDI value is 81.4°. A value higher than 81.4° shows a trend skeletal class III; on the contrary a smaller value shows the tendency for skeletal class II and molar class II relationship. APDI unlike ODI (which is slight altered by the treatment) shows the potential of the treatment of the clinical case, because the APDI can be significantly changed by growth and treatment. Kim (Kim and Vietas, 1978) [5] considered

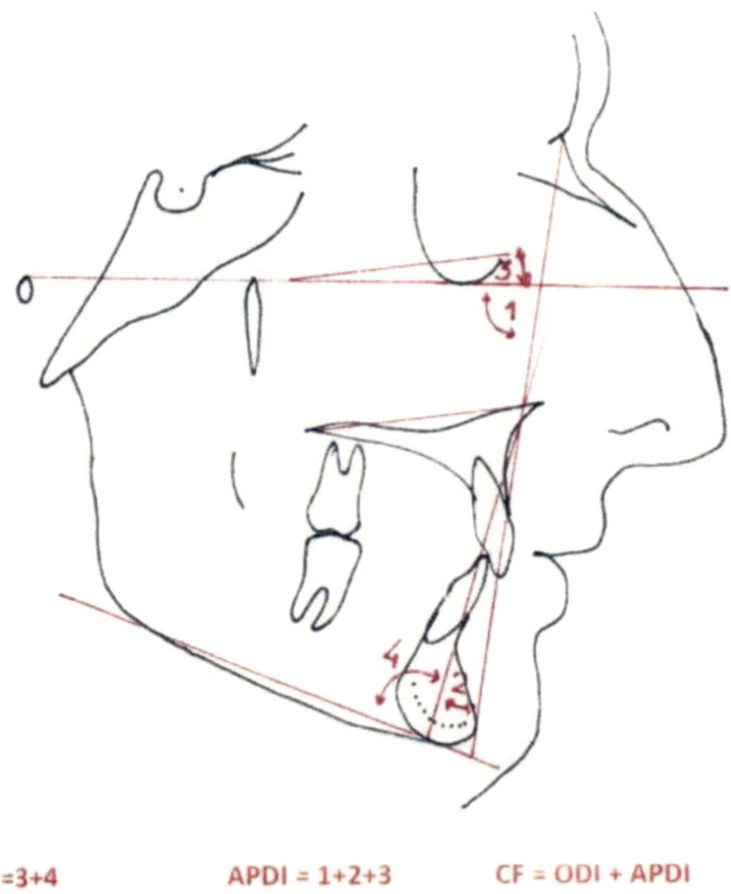

Figure 2. Kim cephalometric analysis.

http://dx.doi.org/10.5772/intechopen.69331

that at the end of the treatment the APDI should be close to the norm (81.4°) in order to have a clinical case with stability and the risk of relapse decreased.

3.4. Combination factor (CF)

The combination factor (CF) [8] is a combination of ODI and APDI.

A value of CF above 155° shows a trend for a skeletal pattern of low angle. A value of CF below 155° exhibits the trend for high angle, and the necessity for tooth extraction is increased.

The CF provides guidance if the clinical case should be treated with or without extractions.

4. The importance of cranial base and the development scheme of skeletal class II deep bite malocclusion

The base of the skull is formed by the ethmoid, sphenoid, and occipital bones, joined by spheno-occipital and sphenoethmoidal synchondrosis. The sutures fuse with age, sphenoethmoidal at 7–8 years and spheno-occipital at 18–20 years, but allow small movements. Hooper in 1986 referred to spheno-occipital synchondrosis as the most important at the base of the skull where the flexion/extension movements occurred. The various malocclusions show different cranial base angles. Thus, in class I occlusions, the angle of the base of the skull (Na-S-Ar) approaches to 124.2°, in class II the angle is more obtuse approaching to 130°, and in class III, the base of the skull presents flexion, being the angle approximately 120°. The movement of flexion/extension occurred in the spheno-occipital suture is transmitted by the Vomer to maxillary. According to the movement occurred in the spheno-occipital suture, also the direction of growth of the maxillary will be different. When sphenoid flexion occurs, the maxillary growth is more vertical, growing more in height and less in length, resulting in posterior dental discrepancy; this is what happens in class III skeletal frame. On the contrary, when extension at the base of the skull occurs, the force transmitted by the Vomer to maxillary will push it protrusively, and maxillary will grow more in length and less in height. This protrusive rotation of maxillary is responsible for the inclination of the incisors and spaces between them (typical in class II/1 malocclusion).

The results of a poor maxillary vertical dimension are:

- Low vertical dimension
- Decrease of occlusal support
- Steep posterior occlusal plane

When the posterior occlusal plane (POP) is steep, the mandible adapts posteriorly with molar distoclusion; on the contrary, when the POP is flat, the mandible adapts in an anterior position producing molar mesioclusion. In 1975, Petrovic [9] reported on the cybernetic theory of Petrovic, who stated that the maxillary anterior-inferior growth was responsible for the anterior functional adaptation of the mandible followed by secondary growth of the condyles.

5. Low-angle class II deep bite malocclusion characteristics

McNamara and Moyers et al. have suggested that the fundamental problems in class II malocclusion are due not to maxillary prognathism but rather to mandibular retrognathism.

The characteristics of the class II deep bite malocclusion are the following: the mandible is small and retruded, the posterior maxillary occlusal plane is steep, presence of posterior occlusal interferences, upper incisors normally labially inclined with spaces between them, labial incompetence, low vertical dimension, lack of occlusal support, molar teeth slightly erupted (infra-eruption), deep overbite, low gonial angle (GOA), and small lower facial height (LFH) [10].

The APDI is less than 74.5°, and the overbite depth indicator (ODI) is quite high (1980s and 1990s). The angle of the cranial base is extended.

The skeletal characteristics of class II malocclusion are closely related to vertical occlusion deficiencies.

6. Treatment of class II low-angle malocclusion based on the control of occlusal plane

In the 1970s, several studies (Petrovic, Carlson, McNamara, and Woodside) showed the ability to change the growth pattern of the mandible according to its function. McNamara, Graber, Harvold, and Bass (1970) evidenced that the amount of changes in mandibular growth due to cell increase in the condyles was in conformity with the modifications of the occlusal function. Fushima et al. (1989) measured vertical height of molar and premolar teeth in patients with mandibular asymmetry. They verified that the vertical dimension of the posterior teeth of the displaced side was smaller than the contralateral dental height (nonshifted side).

The MEAW philosophy created by Dr. Young Kim and developed by Prof. Sadao Sato considers that the treatment of class II low-angle malocclusion should eliminate occlusal interferences, increase the vertical dimension (extruding the maxillary molars), and reconstruct the occlusal plane. Once the vertical dimension increases, the mandible moves anteriorly to a functional position [11–13].

The mandibular dentition, especially the premolars, is extruded to increase the vertical dimension and flatten the occlusal plane, creating conditions for the mandible to move to a forward position, more physiologically, and improving the occlusal function.

The forward adaptation of the mandible followed by adaptive remodeling of the TMJ is necessary for the success and stability of the treatment.

The objectives of class II deep bite treatment are:

- Increase of the vertical dimension
- Rebuilding and flattening of the upper posterior occlusal plane

- Correction of the differences of shape between the dental arches
- Mandibular advancement to obtain a physiological position
- Correction of deep bite
- Obtaining correct occlusion and improving the profile

Sequence of class II deep bite treatment:

(1) Alignment and leveling, (2) correction of occlusal interferences, (3) attaining a physiological mandibular position, (4) rebuilding the occlusal plane, and (5) attaining a physiological occlusion (**Figure 3**).

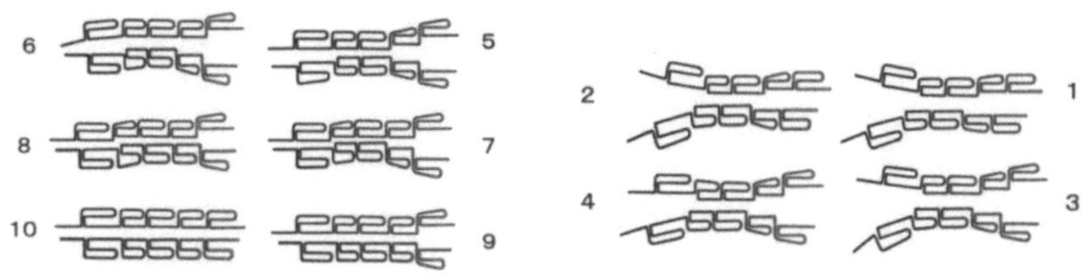

Figure 3. Sequence of low-angle class II deep bite treatment.

7. Case report 1

A male patient 14 years and 10 months old, with skeletal class II and dental class II/1 on a hypodivergent face pattern (FMA 17°), deep bite (8 mm), overjet (5 mm), steep posterior occlusal plane producing interferences in the posterior area, insufficient occlusal support on the posterior area, crossbite on the right side, crown fracture of 11, posterior discrepancy, and crowding on the anterior maxillary area. The patient began the treatment at the age of 14 years and 10 months old, and the treatment lasted 24 months. The type of appliance was an edgewise multi-bracket 0.022 × 0.028 slot, 0° torque, 0° angulation, and MEAWs arch wires along with short class II elastics.

The treatment objectives for this patient with class II deep bite were increasing the vertical dimension, elimination of the posterior interferences, reconstruction of posterior occlusal plane (flatten), coordination between both arches, production of anterior adaptation of the mandible, and secondarily induction condylar remodeling. The patient and their parents refused the extraction of 38 and 48 to eliminate the posterior mandibular discrepancy and were advised to the consequences of such refusal.

Sequence of treatment:

(a) Leveling, (b) correction of occlusal interferences, (c) achieving mandibular position, (d) rebuilding of the occlusal plane, and (e) achieving a physiological occlusion.

Step 1: Leveling (alignment), onset with 0.016″ ss arch wires.

Step 2: Elimination of occlusal interferences—0.017 × 0.025 multiloop edgewise arch wires were inserted in both arches, through the use of small class II (3/16 inch, 6 ounces) elastics bilaterally.

Step 3: Achieving a functional mandibular position: step-down bends (premolars) in the upper arch and step-up bends (premolars) in the lower arch were done to bite rising (to apply small class II, 3/16 inch, 6 ounces of elastics). When this phase is finished, the molar relationship is class I.

Steps 4 and 5: Rebuilding the posterior occlusal plane (flatten the posterior occlusal plane) and establishing a physiological occlusion.

The retention period was done with maxillary Hawley plate for nighttime use (12 months) and bonded lingual wire from 33 to 43.

The posttreatment results demonstrate an improved smile, profile, and facial balance.

The intraoral photos show a normal class I relationship, a correct overbite, and overjet. The cephalometric analysis shows a reduction of ANB angle of 4°, mandibular advancement (point B has advanced 3°), an AO-BO reduction of 3 mm, and a better profile. The APDI increased 7° (from 66 to 73°) showing an improvement of the skeletal class II malocclusion (**Figures 4–11**, **Tables 1** and **2**).

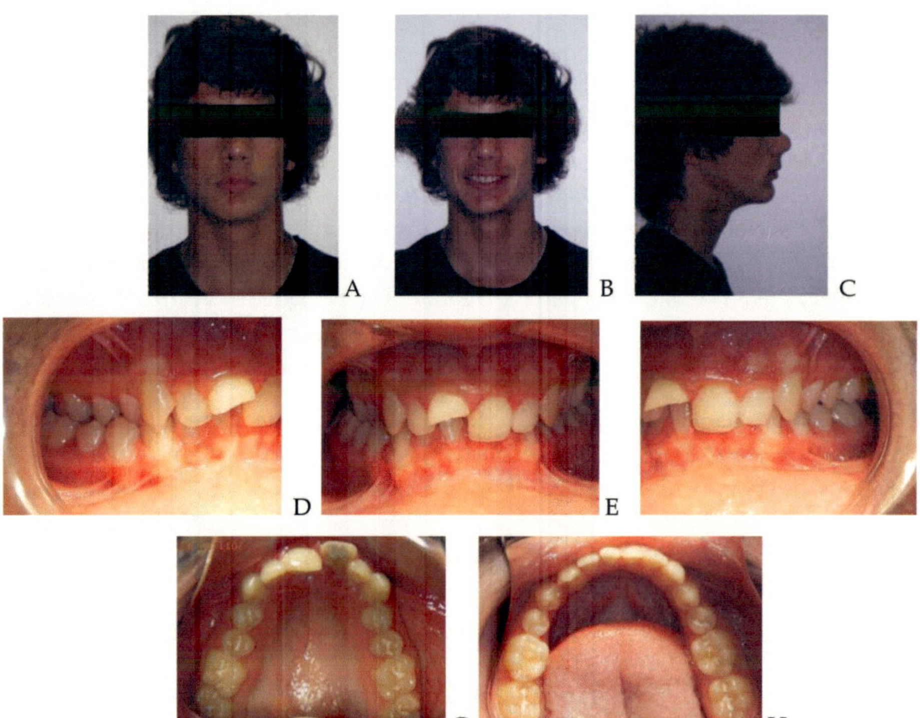

Figure 4. Pretreatment extraoral (A–C) and intraoral (D–H) photographs.

http://dx.doi.org/10.5772/intechopen.69331

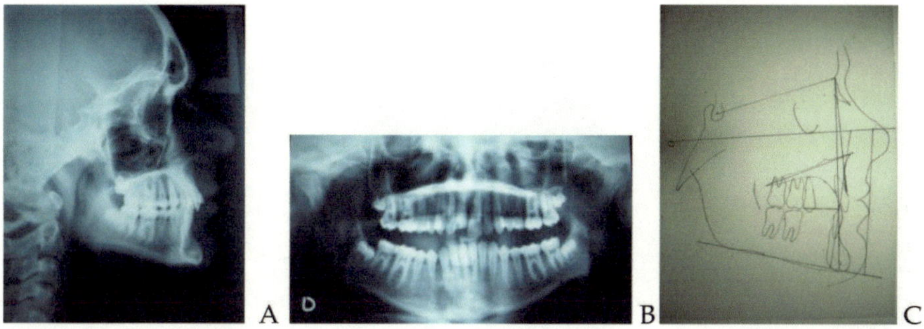

Figure 5. Pretreatment records (A–C).

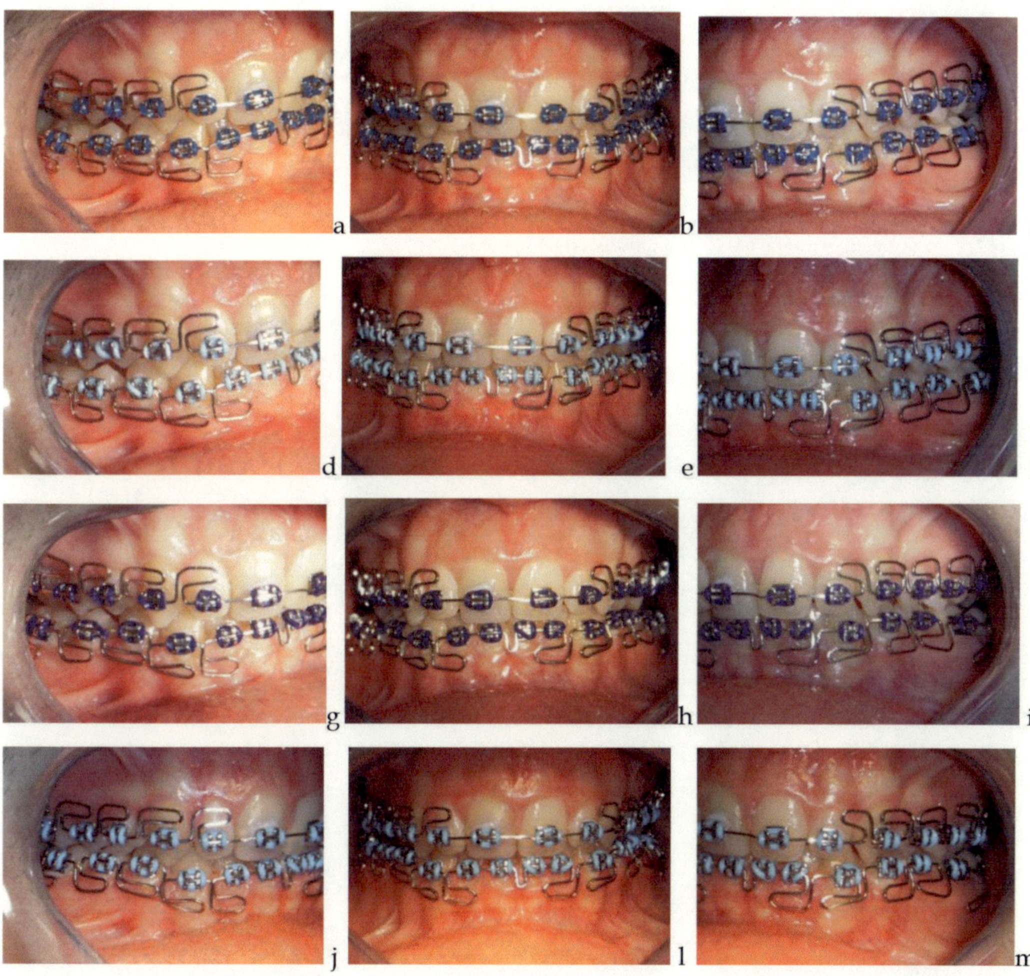

Figure 6. Photos during the treatment (a–m).

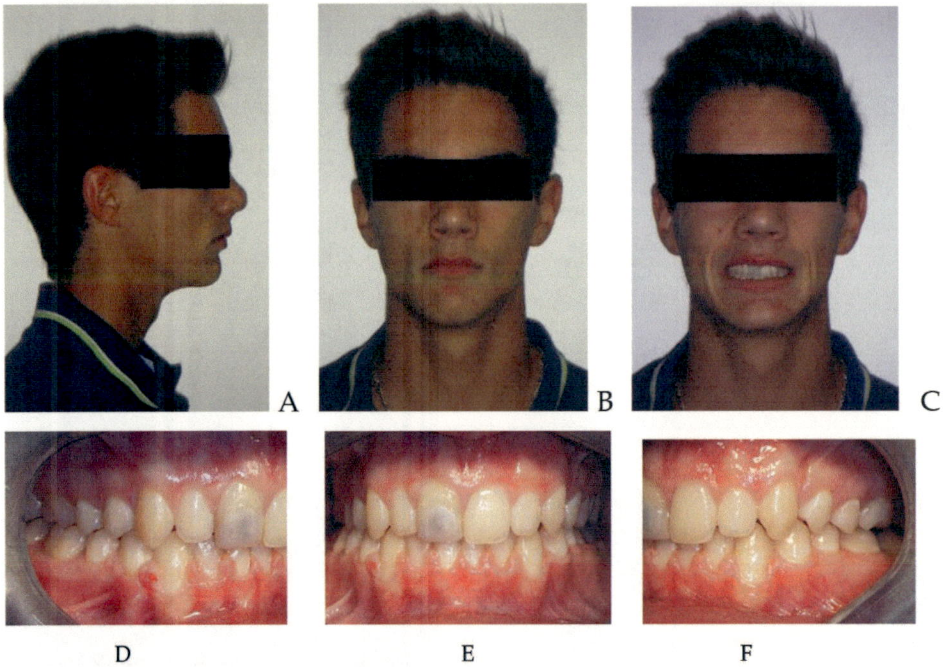

Figure 7. Posttreatment extraoral (A–C) and intraoral (D–F) photos.

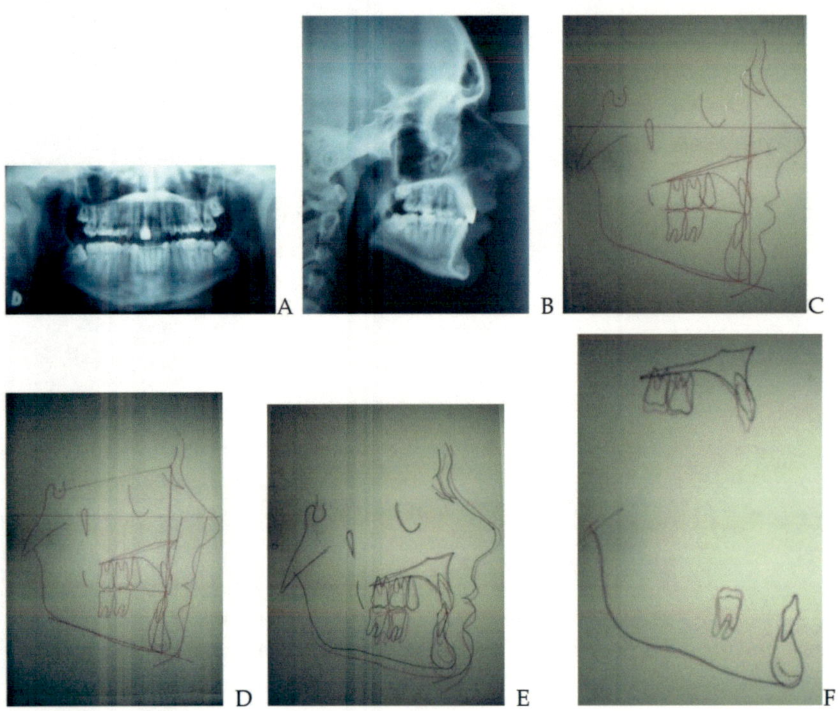

Figure 8. Posttreatment records (A–D) and superimpositions between pre- and posttreatment (E–F).

http://dx.doi.org/10.5772/intechopen.69331

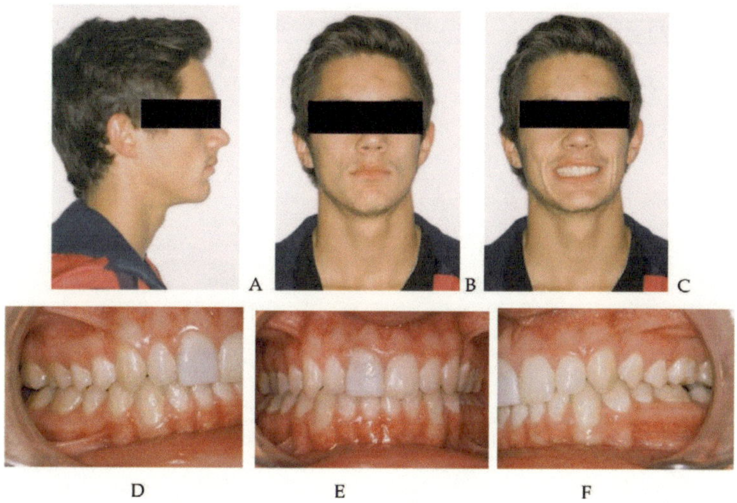

Figure 9. Postretention extraoral photos (A–C) and intraoral photos (D–F).

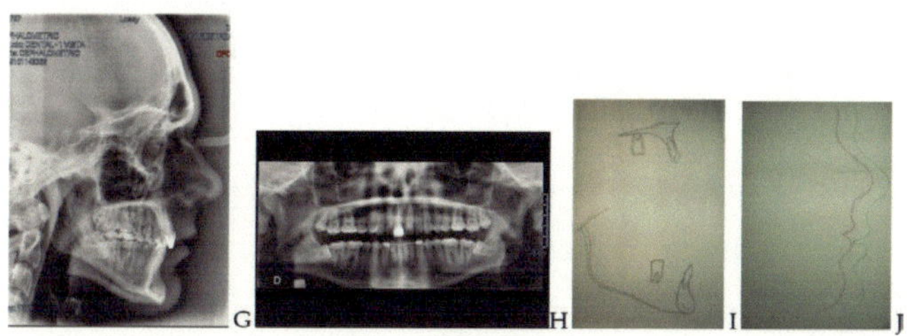

Figure 10. Postretention records (G–H) and postretention superimpositions.

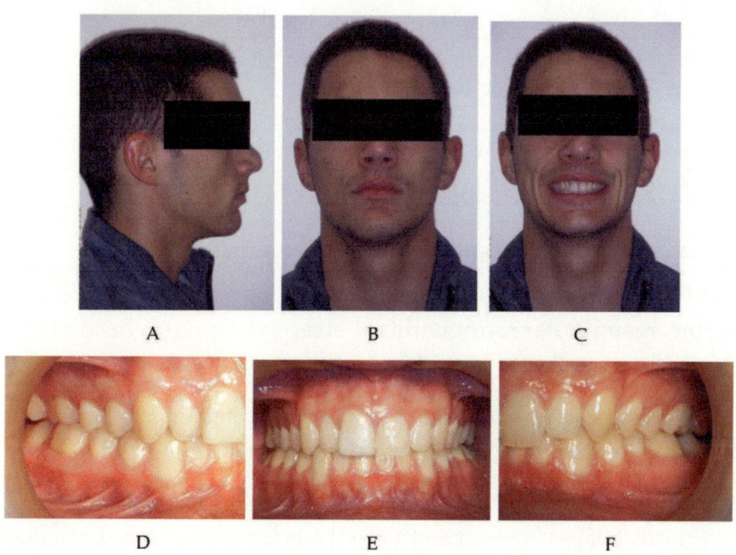

Figure 11. Three years after the end of treatment: extraoral photos (A–C) and intraoral photos (D–F).

	Pretreatment			Posttreatment		End of retention	
ODI	MP/AB	83	69	77	63	76	62
	FH/PP	−14		−14		−14	
APDI	HF/FP	90	66	91	73	91	74
	FP/AB	−10		-4		-3	
	HF/PP	−14		−14		−14	
CF	ODI + APDI		135		136		136

Table 1. Cephalometric analysis (Kim).

	Range	Pretreatment	Posttreatment	End of retention
FMIA	67 ± 3°	73	73	72
FMA	25 ± 3°	17	17	17
IMPA	88 ± 3°	90	90	91
SNA	82 ± 2°	78	78	78
SNB	80 ± 2°	73	77	76
ANB	2 ± 2°	05	01	02
AO-BO	2 mm	4 mm	1 mm	1 mm
OP	10–14°	7	5	5
Z	75 ± 5°	83	80	81
PFH	45 mm	45	47	48
AFH	65 mm	66	70	72
INDEX	0.69	0.68	0.67	0.67

Table 2. Cephalometric analysis (Tweed-Merrifield) [14, 15].

8. Case report 2

A young male patient 13 years and 10 months old, with small anterior facial height, skeletal class II (FMA = 18°), dental class II/1 with deep bite of 7 mm and an overjet of 10 mm, hypodivergent face scheme, mandibular retrognathism, steep posterior occlusal plane creating interferences in the molar area, and lack of occlusal support.

The z angle of 66° confirms an unbalanced face which is based on a rethrognatic chin, absence of crowding and shape of dental arches is different due to an old habit of thumb sucking.

According to Kim's cephalometric analysis, the patient shows a low-angle skeletal pattern (ODI = 86°), and removal of permanent teeth is not advised, due to the high potential for deep bite relapse. The APDI = 70° shows a class II skeletal pattern, and the combination factor = 156°

http://dx.doi.org/10.5772/intechopen.69331

indicates a skeletal pattern that has a capacity to accommodate the entire dentition. Onset of treatment with age of 13 years and 10 months, after 2 months a double arch wire (DAW) was placed to extrude maxillary molars and to align and intrude upper incisors [16]. After 5 months, MEAWs were inserted in both dental arches, along with small class II elastics (3/16 inch, 6 ounces).

The duration of the treatment was 24 months. The posttreatment photographs (**Figure 15**) show a better pleasant face, an improved facial profile, a pleasant wide smile, a stable class I molar occlusion, and overbite and overjet corrected.

The mandibular incisors were kept in its pretreatment position. The cephalometric superimposition between pretreatment and posttreatment displays the entire mandibular improvement in height and length. The APDI = 80 at the end of treatment is a guarantee to define this clinical case as stable and with little tendency to relapse (**Figures 12–20, Tables 3** and **4**).

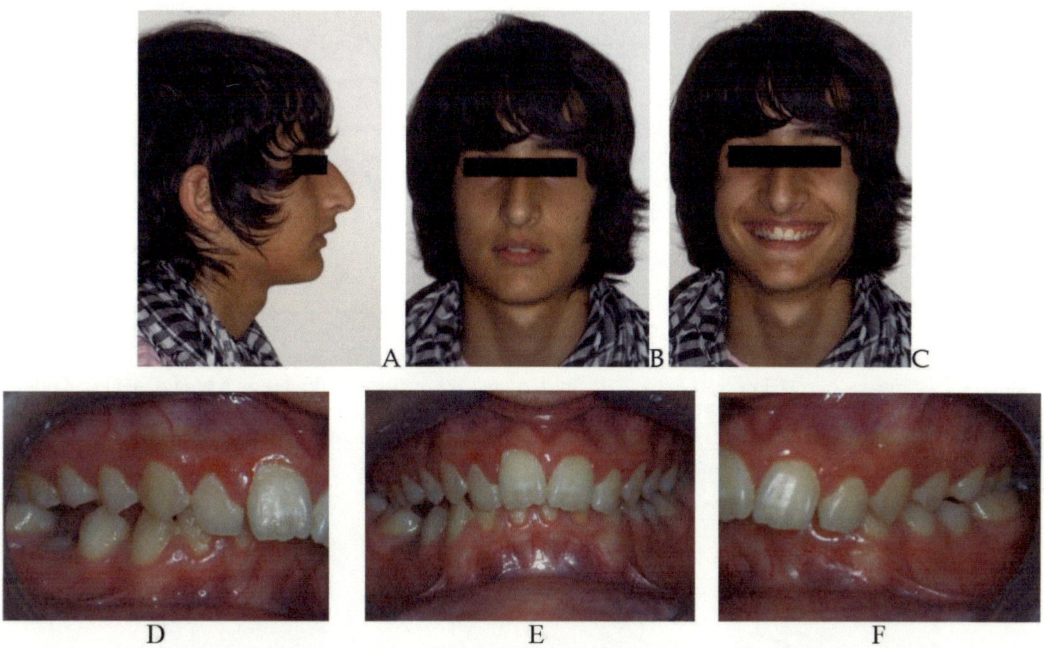

Figure 12. Pretreatment extraoral (A–C) and intraoral (D–F) photos.

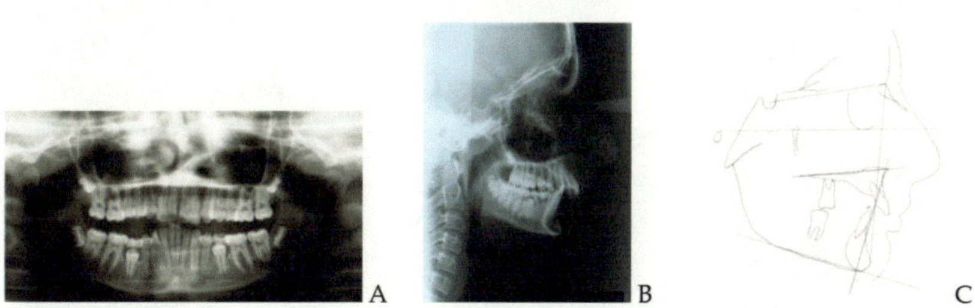

Figure 13. Pretreatment records (A–C).

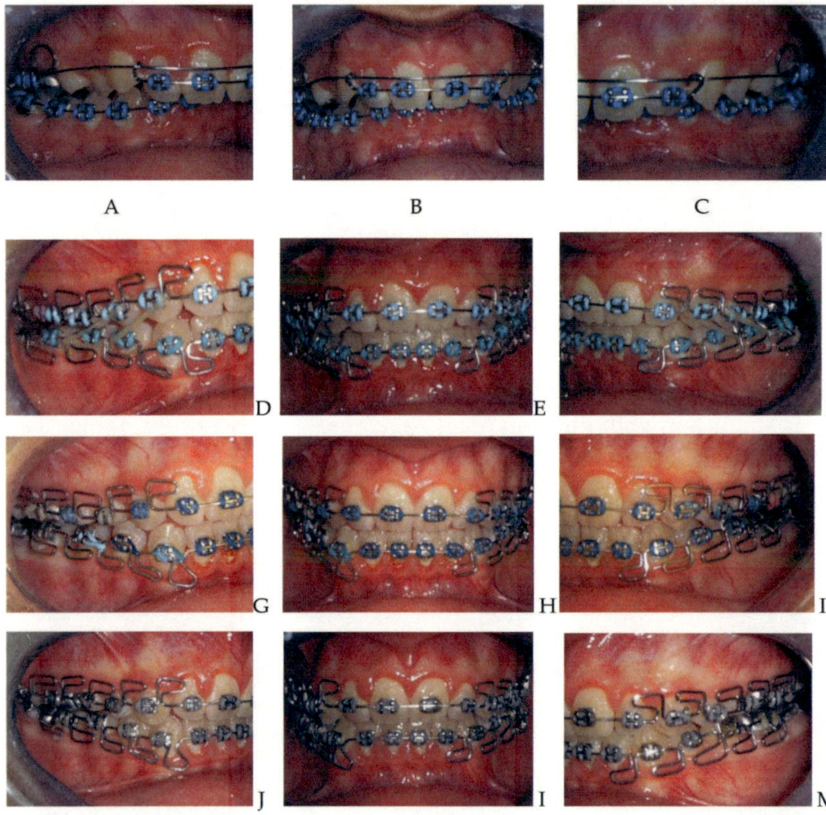

Figure 14. Treatment sequence images. (A–C) In the third month of treatment, a double arch wire (DAW) was placed and remained in mouth 5 months. (D–F) One year of treatment (5 months with MEAWs along with small class II elastics (6 ounces, 3/16 inch)). (G–I) Eighteenth month of treatment. (J–M) Twenty-second months of treatment.

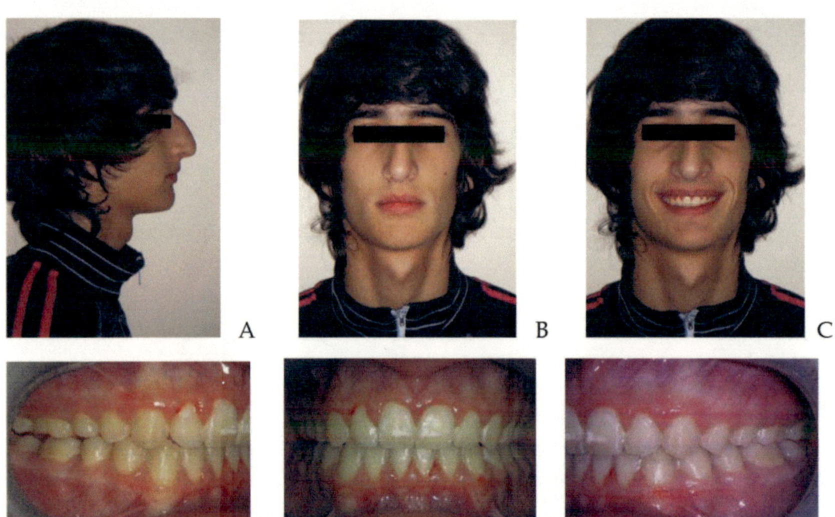

Figure 15. End of treatment: extraoral photos (A–C) and intraoral photos (D–F).

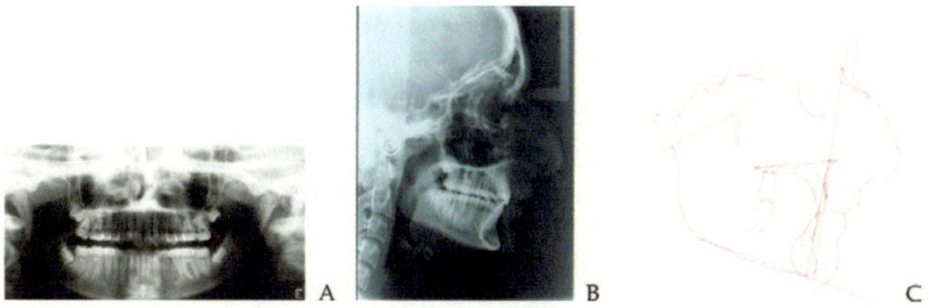

Figure 16. Posttreatment records (A–C).

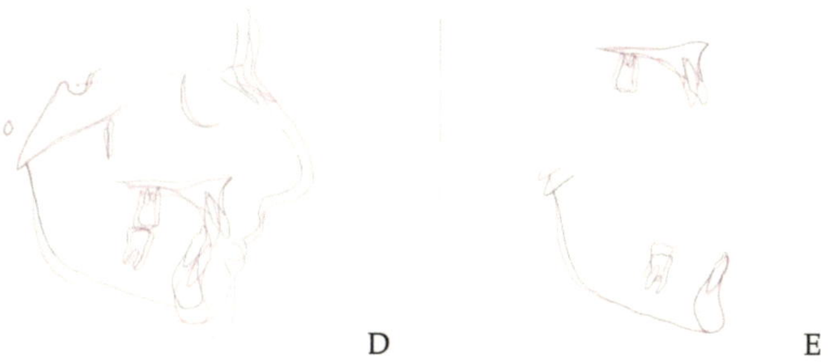

Figure 17. Superimpositions between pre- and posttreatment (D, E).

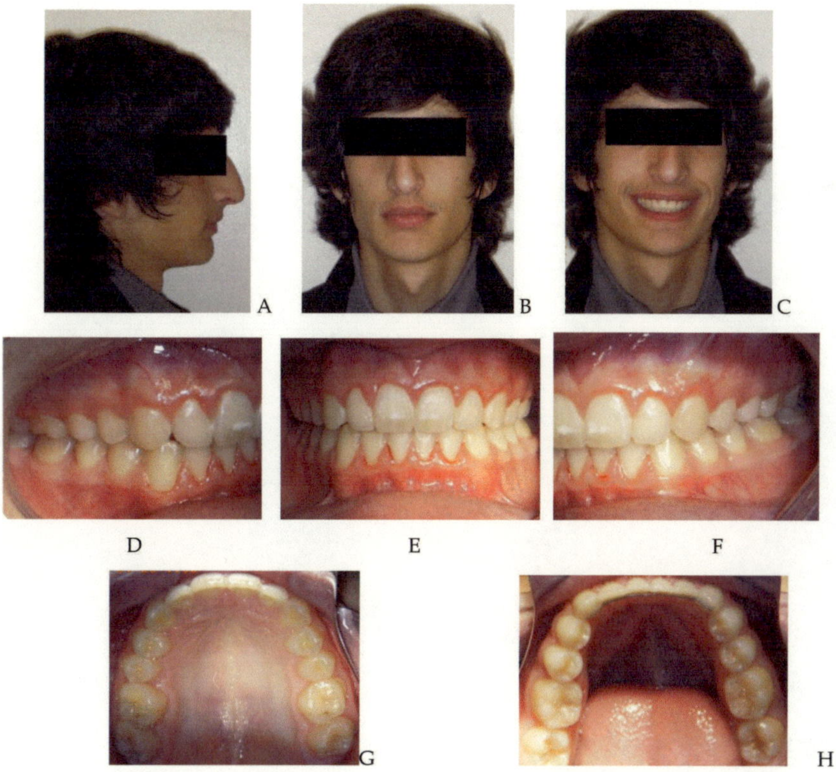

Figure 18. Postretention: extraoral photos (A–C) and intraoral photos (D–H).

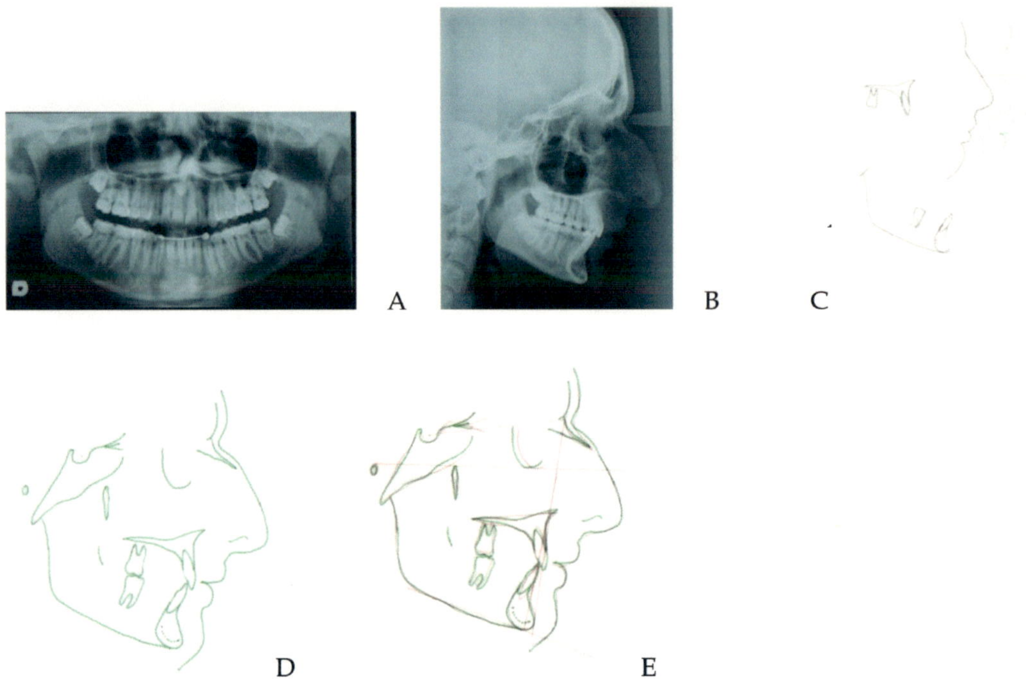

Figure 19. Postretention records (A–B) and superimpositions between posttreatment and postretention (C–E).

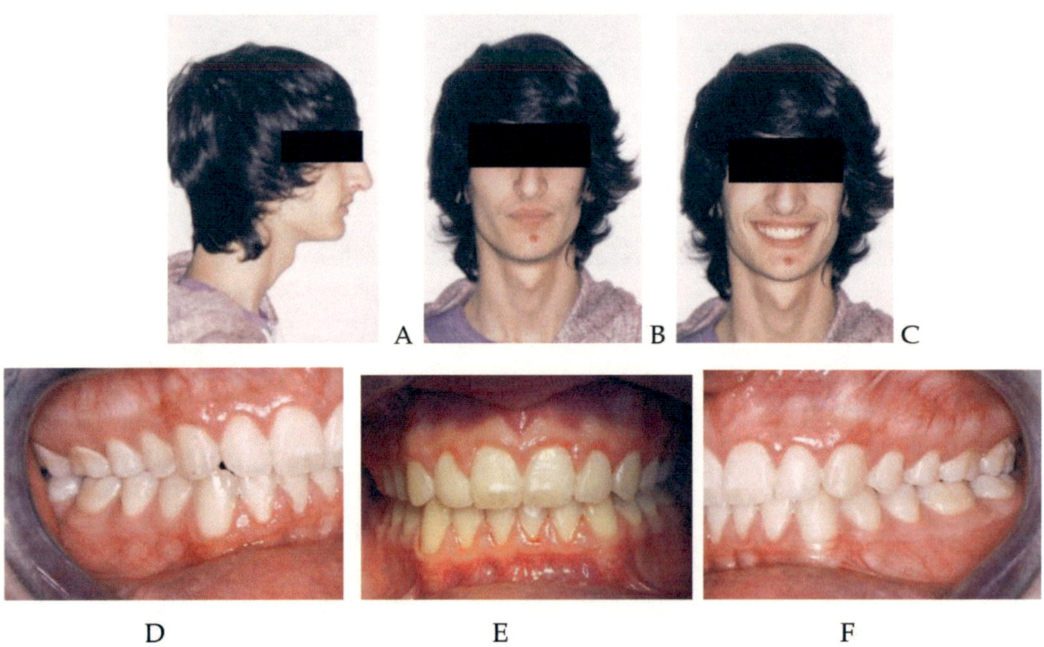

Figure 20. Three years after the end of treatment: extraoral photos (A–C) and intraoral photos (D–F).

http://dx.doi.org/10.5772/intechopen.69331

	Pretreatment			Posttreatment		Post-retention	
ODI	MP/AB	82	80	82	80	82	80
	FH/PP	−2		−2		−2	
APDI	HF/FP	80	73	84	80	84	80
	FP/AB	−5		−2		−2	
	HF/PP	−2		−2		−2	
CF	ODI + APDI		153		160		160

Table 3. Cephalometric analysis (Kim).

	Range	Pretreatment	Posttreatment	Post-retention
FMIA	67 ± 3°	64	61	60
FMA	25 ± 3°	18	20	20
IMPA	88 ± 3°	98	99	100
SNA	82 ± 2°	78	76	76
SNB	80 ± 2°	72	74	74
ANB	2 ± 2°	6	2	2
AO-BO	2 mm	7 mm	2 mm	2 mm
OP	10–14°	7	8	8
Z	75 ± 5°	67	73	72
PFH	45 mm	45	50	50
AFH	65 mm	60	65	65
INDEX	0.69	0.75	0.77	0.77

Table 4. Cephalometric analysis (Tweed-Merrifield).

9. Conclusion

The superimposed tracings confirm in both cases that the mandible shifted forward, the flattening of the posterior occlusal plane, and the vertical dimension increased during active appliance therapy.

The objectives of both treatments were successfully achieved by the use of MEAW therapy. A good functionally occlusion and an esthetic profile had been attained. The records 3 years after the end of treatment show the stability of the treatment and the occlusion.

The MEAW technique proved to be effective in the treatment of class II deep bite malocclusion.

Author details

Paulo Augusto de Sousa Beltrão

Address all correspondence to: paulobeltrao@sapo.pt

French Board of Orthodontics, Portugal

References

[1] Tanaka E, Sato S. Longitudinal alteration of the occlusal plane and development of different dentoskeletal frames during growth. American Journal of Orthodontics and Dentofacial Orthopedics. 2008;**134**(5):602.e1-602.e11

[2] Fushima K, Kitamura Y, Mita H, Sato S, Kim Y. The significance of the cant of occlusal plane in class II/1 malocclusion. European Journal of Orthodontics. 1996;**18**:27-40

[3] Kim H-S, Kim S-Y. Compensatory changes of a occlusal plane angles in relation to a skeletal factors. Korea Journal of Orthodontics. 2004;**34**(3):229-240

[4] McNamara JA Jr, Carlson DS. Quantitative analysis of temporomandibular joint adaptations to protrusive function. American Journal of Orthodontics. 1979;**76**:593-611

[5] Sato S. A Treatment Approach to Malocclusions Under the Consideration of Craniofacial Dynamics. Grace Printing Press, Philippines, inc; 2001

[6] Kim YH. Overbite depth indicator with particular reference to anterior open-bite. AJO. 1974;**65**:586-611

[7] Kim YH, Vietas JJ. Anteroposterior dysplasia indicator. American Journal of Orthodontics. 1978;**73**:619-633

[8] Kim YH. ODI/APDI combination factor. Angle Orthodontics. 1979;**49**:77-84

[9] Petrovic AG, Stutzaman J. Control process in the postnatal growth of the condylar cartilage. In: McNamara JA Jr, editor. Determinants of Mandibular Growth, Monograph 4: Craniofacial Growth Series. Ann Arbor: Center for Human Growth and Development, University of Michigan; 1975

[10] Kato S, Chung W-N, Sato S. Morphological characterization of different types of class II malocclusion. Bulletin of Kanagawa Dental College. September 2002;**30**(2):93-98

[11] Kim YH. Treatment of anterior openbite and deep overbite malocclusions with MEAW therapy. In: McNamara JA Jr, editor. The Enigma of Vertical Dimension-Craniofacial Growth Series. Vol. 36. Ann Arbor: Center for Human Growth and Development-University of Michigan; 1999

[12] Kim YH. Treatment of severe deep overbite in juveniles and in adults: An introduction to the reverse MEAW. International Journal of MEAW Technic and Research Foundation. 2004;**11**(1):12-32

http://dx.doi.org/10.5772/intechopen.69331

[13] Knierim RW. Diagnosis of openbite and deepbite problems: A clinician`s perspective on the Kim approach. In: McNamara JA Jr, editor. The Enigma of Vertical Dimension-Craniofacial Growth Series. Vol. 36. Ann Arbor: Center for Human Growth and Development-University of Michigan; 1999

[14] Merrifield LL. The profile line as an aid to critical evaluation of facial esthetics. American Journal of Orthodontics. 1966;**11**:804-822

[15] Ortial JP. Les modifications faciales par l`orthodontie. Journal de l`edgewise. 1989; **20**:53-86

[16] Beltrão P. Treatment of class II deep overbite with multiloop edgewise arch-wire (MEAW) therapy. In: Naretto S, editor. Principles in Contemporary Orthodontics. InTech; 2011

Section 3

Innovations in Dental Restorations

Chapter 8

Functional Biomimetic Dental Restoration

Elham M. Senan and Ahmed A. Madfa

Additional information is available at the end of the chapter

http://dx.doi.org/10.5772/intechopen.69534

Abstract

Bioinspired functionally graded approach is an innovative material technology, which has rapidly progressed both in terms of materials processing and computational modeling in recent years. Bioinspired functionally graded structure allows the integration of dissimilar materials without formation of severe internal stress and combines diverse properties into a single material system. It is a remarkable example of nature's ability to engineer functionally graded dental prostheses. Therefore, this novel technology is designed to improve the performance of the materials in medical and dental fields. Thus, this chapter book reviews the current status of the functionally graded dental prostheses and biomimetic process inspired by the human bone, enamel and dentin-enamel junction (DEJ) structures and the linear gradation in Young's modulus of the human bone, enamel and dentin-enamel junction, as a new material design approach, to improve the performance compared to traditional dental prostheses. Notable research is highlighted regarding application of biomimetic prostheses into various fields in dentistry. The current chapter book will open a new avenue for recent researches aimed at the further development of new dental prostheses for improving their clinical durability.

Keywords: functionally graded materials, dental restorations, dental implant, dental post, dental crown

1. Introduction

The biomechanical behavior of biologic structures as well as restorative systems is influenced by several factors that interact with one another other [1, 2]. In the oral environment, several variables contribute to the long term success of restorations. Some of them are dependent on the individual, just like occlusion, load intensity and direction, temperature, moisture, wear, presence of sound tooth structure and quality of supporting tissues, whereas other factors are not controllable, such as structural integrity, microleakage, fatigue and time. Furthermore, teeth and restorative materials are characterized by intrinsic physical characteristics which are responsible for their mechanical performances during functions over time [3].

Biomaterials are essential for life and health in certain cases. They generally have a high added value for their size. Biomaterials should simultaneously satisfy many requirements and possess properties such as non-toxicity, corrosion resistance, thermal conductivity, strength, fatigue durability, biocompatibility and sometimes aesthetics. However, a single composition with a uniform structure may not satisfy all such requirements. Therefore, materials scientists increasingly aim to engineer materials that are more damage-resistant than their conventional homogeneous counterparts. This is particularly important at surfaces or at interfaces between dissimilar materials, where contact failure commonly occurs.

Learning from nature, natural biomaterials often possess the structure of functionally graded materials (FGMs) which enables them to satisfy these requirements. Many engineered materials are graded in some manner, but FGMs are often characterized by a gradient purposefully formed using compositional or microstructural design. FGMs provide the structure with which synthetic biomaterials should essentially be formed.

Bioinspired functionally graded approach is an innovative material technology, which has rapidly progressed both in terms of materials processing and computational modeling in recent years [4]. Bioinspired functionally graded structure allows the integration of dissimilar materials without formation of severe internal stresses and combines diverse materials properties into a single material system. The graded structure eliminates the sharp interface resulting from traditional core-veneer fabrication, thus, eliminating the potential for delamination between layers. Reduced stress concentration at the intersection between an interface and a free surface is another advantage of this graded transition. Likewise, the local driving force for crack growth across an interface can be increased or decreased by altering the gradients in elastic and plastic properties across the interface [5, 6].

Many applications of this innovative technology are found in medical and dental fields [7–15]. Thus, this chapter book will review the current status of the functionally graded dental prostheses and biomimetic process inspired by the human bone, enamel and dentin-enamel junction (DEJ) structures and the linear gradation in Young's modulus of the human bone, enamel and DEJ, as a new material design approach, to improve the performance compared to traditional dental prostheses.

2. Dental implant

2.1. Overview

Dental implants are an effective treatment to replace the root part of the missing natural tooth [16], in order to restore patients' appearance, speech and health [17]. They are completely placed into the jaw bone and give support to a dental prosthesis [18].

During the last 10 years, dental implants had received an increasingly growing interest and focus worldwide. They are used to treat about one million individual per year around the globe [19]. Complete restoration of dentition, rise in the mean age of population, higher number of elderly individuals in population along with increased public awareness are all causes for the increasing demand for dental implants [19].

Basically, implants should be fabricated from biomaterials congruous with the human body environmental conditions. Titanium and its alloys have been reported as the materials of choice for most dental implants because of their inertness, biocompatibility and distinguished mechanical properties [20]. However, the Young's modulus of titanium alloys is higher than that of mineralized tissues. Moreover, the dense structure of titanium for biomedical implants can result in a divergence among the titanium implant Young's modulus (110 GPa) and that of human cortical (17–20 GPa) and cancellous bones (about 4 GPa) [21, 22].

The increased stiffness of titanium implants causes stress shielding with improper loading of the underlying bone tissue [23]. Human bone is a dynamic vital tissue that undergoes continuous modifications by bone-forming and bone-eating cells in response to applied external signals. This results in a reduced mechanical loading of bone which in turn leads to bone resorption, implant loosening and ultimate failure which has been a problem for implants in the past [9]. Overloading, on the other hand, also creates high stresses in local regions of bone which can also stimulate resorption [24]. For that reason, many trials have been performed to improve the mechanical properties of different biomaterials to be compatible with those of bone tissue. Most of these efforts have directed to develop certain significant interaction features at the implant surface and bone tissue interface. Recent developments in dental implant designs, and bone tissue engineering scaffolds, have all added to manufacturing novel porous titanium structures, and these fields utilize and benefit from each other's technologies.

Other issue is configuration of implant that represents an essential factor in bone-implant interface and can promote the process of osseointegration. For promotion of dental implant stability, various implant surface adjustments have been suggested to adapt the properties of dental implants [25]. Modifying the implant surface can upgrade the interaction of implant to bone; however, there is not always a clear explanation for the mechanism of interface improvement. For example, a morphological modification, such as roughening the implant surface, can also create alterations in the chemistry of dental implant surface [26]. Sand blasting with stiff particles such as alumina, TiO_2 and ceramic has also been proposed to roughen dental implant surface [19]. Chemical modification, such as plasma spraying with different powder particles such as titanium oxide, calcium phosphate and hydroxyapatite, has been used to coat dental implants surface [27]. In spite of being very successful, there are number of disadvantages related to the previous procedures; the bulk structure is still high-density titanium, the coating materials can dissolve away over a long period of time. Furthermore, coating particles that break away from the surface spray layer could have a negative biological effect on the adjacent tissue such as peri-implantitis [27]. Thus, various alternative approaches have been employed to overcome these shortcomings of coating materials by producing porous biomaterials as an alternative for the classical solid structure. Cellular structures can create a suitable biological environment for the host tissues to grow into these porous designs [28], establishing improved early implant stability. However, this technology is an expensive which may not be affordable to many individuals seeking dental implant treatments and, therefore, methods of providing a porous structure in titanium or a titanium alloy is of strong interest to the dental implant community [29].

2.2. Dental implant based on functionally graded concept

Presence of a porous surface or rough surface with macroscopic grooves and threads is one of the basic requirements of dental implants to establish a primarily mechanical stabilization between implants and bone tissues [30]. In addition, adequate support should be present mechanically between the radicular part of dental implant and its superstructure coronal part. This should be accomplished by forming a solid inner core and porous outer shell as a replacement to a completely porous structure [30]. A problematic issue is that high magnitude of stress could form at the implant shell and core junction area where the mechanical properties alter quickly [31]. Consequently, the bond between the implant covering layer and its core is weakened. Cook et al. [32] have suggested a post-sintering heat treatment in order to reduce the aforementioned problem that is related to residual accumulated stresses. This method showed an improvement in the fatigue strength of titanium alloy by about 15%. However, the concept of designing and manufacturing functionally graded structures can be useful to prevent stress concentrations between the interface layers where the elastic modulus changes suddenly [33].

Development of implants based on biocompatible FGMs for various applications in medical and dental fields has been emphasized [7–15]. FGM permits the integration of different materials without creating severe internal stresses and combines various unlike properties into a single material system (**Figure 1**). Materials in nature, such as bones and teeth, are the source to the development of FGM concept with its origin in regard to their sophisticated

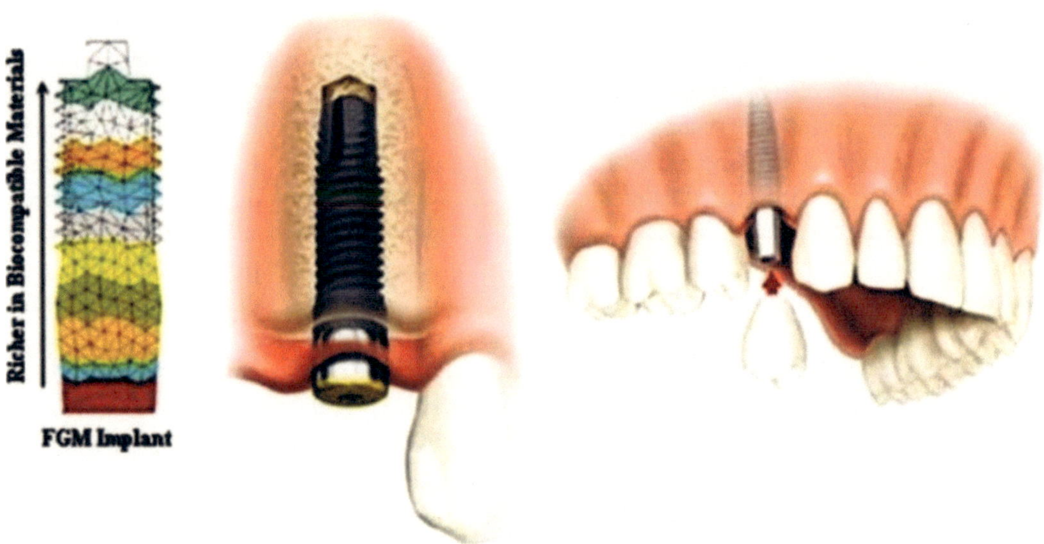

Figure 1. FGM dental implant with graded material composition.

properties [34, 35]. For example, bone design which gradually changes from a dense, stiff external structure (the cortical bone) to a porous internal one (the cancellous bone) reflects the idea that functional gradation has been utilized by biological adaptation [34]. This unique bony structure demonstrates biologic revolution and enhances the material's reaction to extrinsic loads. Thereby, improved structure for a synthetic implant must exhibit alike gradation. A similar trend has been noticed in the development of functionally graded dental implants with the suggestion of placing surface layer coatings, adding porosity gradients and composite materials formed basically of metal and ceramics (e.g. hydroxyapatite), which ought to promote implant performance with regard to stress distribution and biocompatibility issues [36, 37].

Hydroxyapatite/titanium FGM, based on the criterion of minimum residual thermal stress, was optimally designed and fabricated by Chu et al. [38]. Due to the gradual increase of the thermal expansion coefficient from the substrate to the coating outer layer, the titanium component enhanced the mechanical properties of the coating and also assisted in decreasing the residual stresses in the final coating. Additionally, Khor et al. [39] produced hydroxyapatite-titanium functionally graded coatings which result in improvements related to microstructure, density, porosity, micro-hardness, and Young's modulus. Hedia and Mahmoud [7] utilize the finite element method (FEM) to optimize the hydroxyapatite/titanium functionally graded dental implant, based on the criterion of minimum von Mises' stress. Improved analysis by including this effect in another numerical investigation was later made by Hedia [8]. Yang and Xiang [12] used FEM to study the biomechanical behavior of a threaded functionally graded biomaterials dental implant/surrounding bone system under both static and harmonic occlusal forces. They found that functionally graded biomaterials dental implant effectively diminishes the stress difference at the implant-bone interfaces where maximum stresses occur. Furthermore, Wang et al. [11] investigated the thermal-mechanical performance of hydroxyapatite/titanium functionally graded dental implants with the FEM. They concluded that the functionally graded implants with different hydroxyapatite fraction perform almost equally well, while the titanium yields much higher von Mises' stress. Functionally graded coatings containing hydroxyapatite and glass also were prepared by Yamada et al. [40].The concentration of glass increased from the innermost to the outermost. The glass phase was noticed to improve adhesion of the coating to the titanium substrate.

The concept of creation of functionally graded structures in porous materials by changing the structure of the lattice has also been investigated [41]. Tolochko et al. [30] used Laser-forming techniques with continuous wave and pulsed lasers to produce dental implants from Ti powders with two different zones. They made a compact core and irregular porous shell by incorporating selective laser sintering (SLS) for the porous surface and selective laser melting (SLM) for the solid core. Microscopical examination showed that the average pore size was 100–200 μm and the porosity 40–45%. Traini et al. [42] used a laser metal sintering technique to construct Ti alloy dental implant incorporating a gradient of porosity, from the inner core to the outer surface. The functionally graded materials were proven to give better approximate to the elastic properties of the bone (**Figure 2**). Mangano et al. [43] used direct laser fabrication that has potential to produce dental implants with irregular and narrow intercommunicating crevices and shallow depressions using Ti alloy powder. However, they noticed a residue of metal

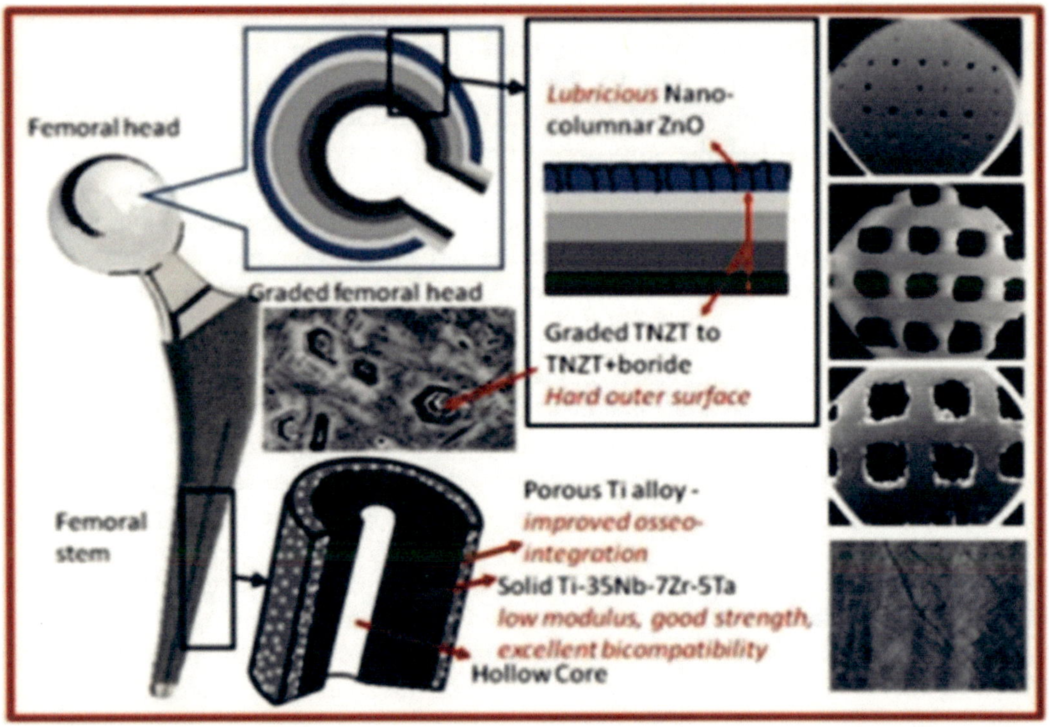

Figure 2. FGM implant with porous Ti alloy.

particles on the implant surface under stereo-scanning electron microscopy. As a result, they proposed acid etching procedure as a treatment to remove the surface adherent particles [43].

Murr et al. [44] used electron beam melting to produce Ti-6Al-4V open cellular foams with different cell wall structures (solid and hollow). The elastic moduli were decreased with increased porosity as widely known for porous metals of all types. On the other hand, the micro indentation hardness of the hollow cell wall structure was higher than that of the solid cell wall. Long term stability and mechanical properties of two types of porous dental implants were investigated under both dynamic and static circumstances [23]. Implants were coated by porous layers made from ammonium hydrogen-carbonate (NH_4) HCO_3 as space holder particles. Then testing these coated implant samples was performed in fatigue and finite element analysis was used to predict their fatigue behavior. It was determined that the melting process of the electron beam has the potential to process Ti-6Al-4V implants with wide range of pore geometry [45]. The compressive properties of porous implants varied with pore structure and can resemble those of human bone [46]. To improve the surface wear resistance of the titanium structures, Laoui et al. applied laser gas nitriding using a CW Nd:YAG laser, and consequently, the coating layer withstand more cycles without fracture [46].

Nomura et al. [47] recommended the vacuum infiltration technique with sintering to generate porous titanium/hydroxyapatite composites. The elastic modulus was rated utilizing the porosity percentage and then tailored to be in the scale of bone tissue (given by 24–34% porosity).

Porosity can be specified by adjusting and controlling the applied temperature and pressure in a hot-pressing stage. Likewise, Hanks' buffered salt solution was applied to reduce the elastic modulus of the sintered porous titanium/hydroxyapatite composites. The bone implant contact and removal torque of dental implants with a porous layer produced by laser sintering were measured and compared with sandblasted-acid etched implant (i.e., those with a rough, but not porous, surface) [48]. It was decided that resultant porous dental implants fabricated by the sintering process are better in terms of biocompatibility and biomechanical properties.

Basically, adequate combination of both mechanical properties and biocompatibility constitute important factors in the application of any biomaterial within the medical or dental field. Surface characteristics govern the material biocompatibility, while its mechanical strength is determined by the average mechanical strength of the materials. According to Chenglin et al. [49] and Lim et al. [50], the combinations of hydroxyapatite and Ti-6Al-4V can results in an excellent functionally graded material. Although the surface layer is essentially hydroxyapatite, the resultant functionally graded material exhibits excellent properties with regards to biocompatibility and bone-bonding ability or dental-bonding ability. Superior mechanical strength in the functionally graded material is accomplished by Ti-6Al-4V phase. Yokoyama et al. [51] analyzed the biocompatibility and mechanical properties of hydroxyapatite/titanium functionally graded implant synthesized by spark sintering technique and found that much enhancement was accomplished by this technique. Miyao et al. [52] manufactured titanium/hydroxyapatite functionally graded material utilizing spark plasma sintering method, and both biocompatibility and mechanical properties as an implant were investigated. They reported that the titanium/hydroxyapatite functionally graded material implants made by the spark plasma sintering method showed strength, excellent biocompatibility, and controllability for graded bioreaction. Watari et al. [53] fabricated the hydroxyapatite/titanium functionally graded dental implant and tested its biocompatibility in Wistar strain rat. They noticed that hydroxyapatite/titanium functionally graded dental implant had better biocompatibility than titanium implant. Foppiano et al. [54] evaluated in vitro the biocompatibility of functionally graded bioactive coating of novel glasses utilizing mouse osteoblast-like cells. Their results exhibited that functionally graded bioactive coating performed at least as well as tissue culture polystyrene and Ti-6Al-4V alloy in the performed biocompatibility tests. Also, functionally graded bioactive coating may influence gene expression favorably promoting osseointegration. Animal implantation tests have exhibited that the coexistence of the hydroxyapatite component in both titanium/hydroxyapatite implants and bone accelerates new bone formation from earlier stage without inflammation [55]. Hedia [9] introduced the optimal design of functionally graded material dental implant in the form of thin layer of cancellous bone around the implant. When compared with conventional titanium implants, stresses concentration in the cortical bone, cancellous bone, and implant were shown to be reduced with the optimal design of collagen/hydroxyapatite functionally graded material implant. In terms of biocompatibility and controllability, collagen/hydroxyapatite functionally graded material was excellent. Hedia claimed that the use of functionally graded material concept in dental implant materials achieve full integration of the implant with living bone, thus increasing the life span of implant. The computational results showed that the use of a functionally graded implant effectively reduces the stress difference at the implant-bone interfaces where the maximum stresses occurred.

2.3. Biomimetic process and biological interaction

Different biomimetic strategies were established to manufacture new materials, which are thought to promote the levels of biological and mechanical performance of biomaterials [56, 57].

A number of researchers utilized bovine and human sera in vitro to investigate protein adsorption on biomaterials [58, 59]. The observed reactions on the biomaterials surface which is in contact with these protein-containing solutions have also been studied using Dulbecco's Modified Eagle's minimum essential medium supplemented with 10% Nu-Serum [60], which includes growth factors, hormones and vitamins within their composition. Immersion in cell-containing solutions is a step further regarding *in vitro* method to mimic the real condition of biomaterials immersed into body fluids.

Most dental implant materials aim to support cell attachment by conferring a suitable an area for cell adhesion [61]. Mangano et al. seeded human dental pulp stem cells on direct laser metal sintered titanium scaffolds and acid etched surfaces. They observed that gene expression and protein secretion were faster on laser sintered scaffolds [62]. Cheng et al. proposed using a template from human trabecular bone to produce porous Ti-6Al-4V materials using particularly laser sintering method as additive manufacturing technology. Different porosities (low, medium and high) ranging from 15–70% with interconnected structure were manufactured to produce structures that simulated the human body trabecular bone. After certain surface treatment with calcium phosphate particles and acid etching, the trabecular bone structure revealed micro and nanoscale porosities which were able to boost osteoblast cell differentiation. Therefore, well-suited devices for dental and orthopedic implants can be produced using the potential of this trabecular structure [18].

Incorporation of a modified sponge replication method and anodization process represents another trial to promote the mechanical and biological properties of porous titanium structures as well. Titanium scaffolds with elongated pores were produced by coating a stretched polymeric sponge template with TiH_2. The anodization of the titanium can produce a nanoporous surface that can stimulate osteoblast cell proliferation and enhance attachment on implant surfaces [23]. Pore geometry has probably a potential strong effect on cell attachment and matrix formation [63]. However, different pore geometries within a single material and manufacturing process are rarely investigated by researchers. Recently, Markhoff et al. [64] evaluated the viability and proliferation of human osteoblast cells in porous Ti-6Al-4V using various scaffold designs and cultivation methods. They applied additive manufacturing technology to produce different pore geometries (cubic, diagonal, pyramidal), using both static and dynamic culture techniques which interestingly showed no significant differences in their results, however, the pyramidal pore design with a 400–620 μm pore size and 75% porosity showed the best results in regard to cell activity and its migration.

Crucial steps in the discovery of novel implant materials and structures include many in vitro studies. However, various inherent limitations are present in relation to the use of different cell culture methods to estimate the long-term service of an implant. Such limitations involve the lack of a three-dimensional environment that properly simulate both chemical and mechanical bone properties, the absence of exerted mechanical loads at the bone-implant interface after implantation procedure, the lack of proteins intricate matrix and different types of bone cells that are present at the bone-implant interface in vivo and the difficulty of preserving the culture for long time periods. Despite the researchers' efforts to improve the different in vitro studies using 3D environments and bioreactors, the in vivo studies represent the source to the current information regarding long-term implant stability.

Designing titanium dental implants with intertwined pores and irregular crevices using a laser sintering process was performed by Mangano et al *in vivo* studies [65] which showed 95% success rate on clinical observation after 1 year postoperatively. On the other hand, histological evaluations made by Shibli et al. who measured human bone tissue response to three types of dental implants: direct laser fabrication, sand-blasted acid-etched and machined commercially pure titanium under unloaded circumstances. Their results revealed that eight weeks post implant insertion, the bone-implant contact produced by the direct laser and sandblasted acid-etched processes was not significantly different but was higher than that of the machined implant, and there were no significant differences between the three types. These findings are explained and attributed to the surface roughness that was produced in both laser and sandblasting techniques, which improved the osseointegration process [66]. Another study using male Sprague-Dawley rats indicated that the biological fixation was affected by the percentage of titanium implants porosity (25, 11, 3%). Examinations after sixteen weeks showed that calcium ions concentration increased proportionally with increased percentage of porosity [67]. Laoui et al. inserted a Ti implant into a dog's lower jaw and their result showed a clear bone growth into the porous structure within the porous surface layer with no observed inflammation at the interface [46]. Tolochko et al. [30] inserted a prototype porous dental implant into the lower jaw of a cadaver which demonstrated a firm integration of the implant into the alveolar ridge of the lower jaw with a maximum gap width of 200–300 μm at the bone-implant interface. Another trial was made to decrease the required healing time for the dental implant and bone by covering a titanium dental implant with a layer of TiO_2 nanotubes, which was tested in a rat femur. Various diameter sizes of these nanotubes were used (30, 50, 70, and 100 nm), with the highest removal torque and osseointegration rate seen in the 30 nm implants after two weeks while the 70 nm implants exhibited the highest value after six weeks for both tests [23].

3. Dental restorations

The dental restorations categorize as dental post and crown.

3.1. Dental post

3.1.1. Overview

The primary role of teeth in the oral cavity is to serve as a mechanical device for mastication. Restoration of endodontically treated tooth presents a great challenge in everyday practice of dental clinicians. Despite the numerous developments in materials and techniques, patients' demand for improved aesthetics, function and longevity of such restoration drives researchers and practitioners to make further developments. This challenge is even greater in cases where there is massive tooth damage due to caries or trauma. This is explained by less fracture resistance of damaged tooth due to reduction in the number of cross-linked collagen fibers and loss of moisture within the tooth [68]. In such cases, there is often a need to compensate for the lack of tooth substance by additional restoration, which is achieved by placing a post in the root canal and core build up [69].

The main role of a post is to provide retention of the core of an endodontically treated tooth. When an occlusal force is applied coronally, the force is transferred to dentine through the core and post system. In such cases, stress tends to be concentrated at the coronal and apical regions (**Figure 3**). Stress concentrations at the coronal region of the root are likely to be due to the increased flexure of the compromised root structure, while stress concentrations at the apical region (**Figure 4**) are generally due to the root canal taper and post characteristics [70]. The regions of high stress concentration were also observed at the apical termination of the post [71]. In such cases, stress concentration which occurred at the apical end, could initiate a root fracture. This phenomenon is dependent on post geometry, material choice of the post and the adhesion between post and dentine. Considerable controversy exists with regards to the ideal choice of material and design of post and core.

Furthermore, as enamel and dentine reveal slightly mismatch coefficient of thermal expansion, thermal loads may even generate stresses in intact sound tooth [72].This problem is increased if the tooth is restored with various restorative materials. The effect of thermal stimuli may be further amplified during mastication as functional load could create tensile stresses on the buccal side of the teeth and compressive stresses on the lingual side.

Endodontically treated teeth are at higher risk of biomechanical failure than vital teeth [73]. The placement of a dental post creates an unnatural restored structure since it fills the root canal space with a material that has a defined stiffness unlike the pulp. Hence it is difficult to recreate the original stress distribution within the tooth in order to avoid fractures. Therefore, post systems must be carefully selected to reduce the incidence of root fractures and to preserve the root if failure occurs. Generally, there are significant mismatch between material properties of these types of posts, e.g. stiffness, and surrounding dental tissues resulting in the poor stress distribution and root fracture.

A widely discussed issue in the literature up to date is the most appropriate material for posts construction [74]. Flexible material that has a flexible dentine-like quality with a low Young's modulus, such as fiber-reinforced composite posts is the most highly recommended material for reducing the risk of root fracture [75, 76]. However, de-bonding of the post and movement of the core can occur due to stress concentrations focused at the post-dentine interface, which consequently results in microleakage [77]. On the other hand, rigid posts require minimal tooth preparation due to their smaller diameters but this may lead to root fracture [78, 79]. For the previous reasons, dental practitioners are left with two options: either continuing to use posts with a high modulus, which could lead to an irreparable failure or choosing low modulus posts that can result in a reparable failure [74].

3.1.2. Dental post based on functionally graded concept

Needless to say, dental post should be high modulus of elasticity at coronal part which is approximately similar to the crown/s and bridge abutment/s and it gradually reduced towards

http://dx.doi.org/10.5772/intechopen.69534

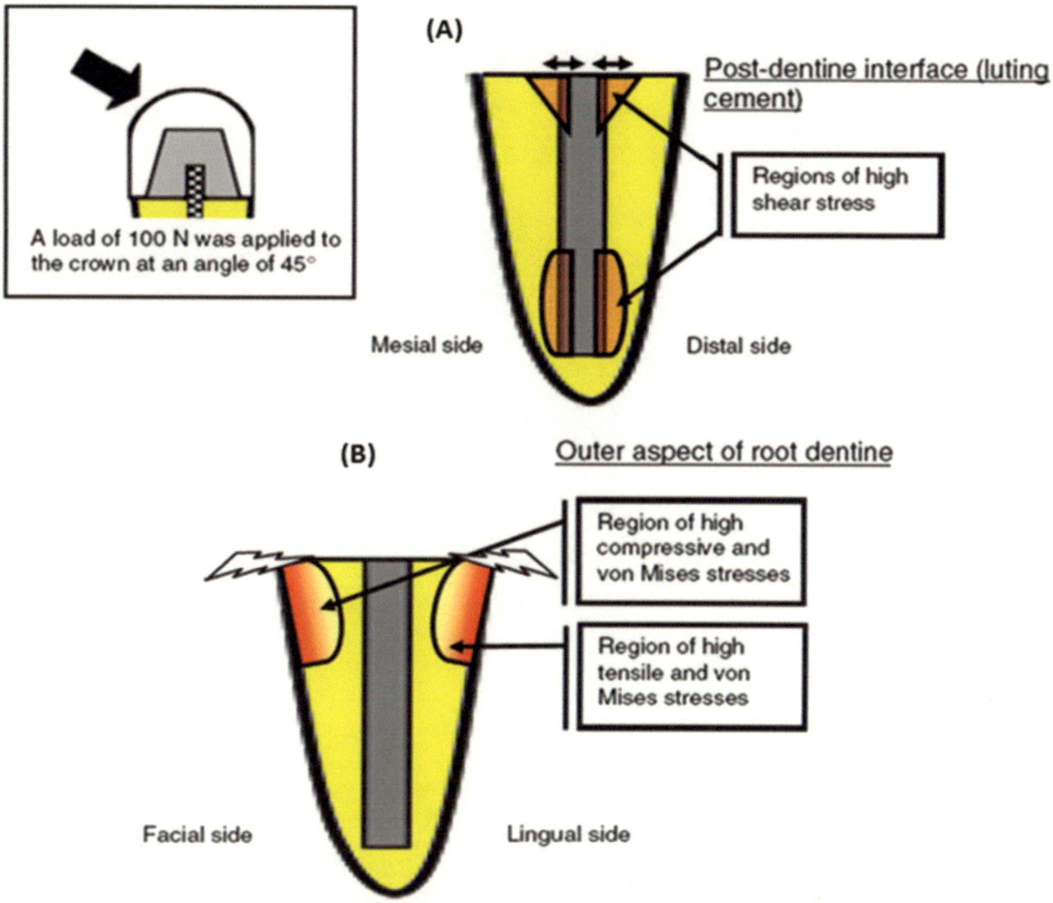

Figure 3. Schematic diagram obtained from FEM analysis showing the typical distribution of (A) shear and (B) tensile, compressive and von Mises stresses in a post and core restored teeth..

the apical part of the tooth (**Figure 5**). Ramakrishna et al. [80] suggested that ideal dental post should be stiff at the coronal region, i.e. in the region of the core, so that the core is not stressed excessively when occlusal force is applied to the crown and its stiffness should be reduced apically. The high stiffness eradicates the stress from the core and the gradual reduction of stiffness along the post would dissipate the stress from the post to the dentine uniformly. The gradual dissipation of stress would also help to eliminate local stress concentration areas and reduce the interfacial shear stress growth.

The problem of materials' properties mismatch can possibly be solved by compositional gradient of multilayer materials achieved in FGMs. Drake et al. The power distribution law was utilized to prove that significant stress and plastic strain reduction can be accomplished through increasing the ceramic materials thickness gradient and tailoring the exponent to create a compositional change gradient close to the parts showing high modulus and little plasticity [81].

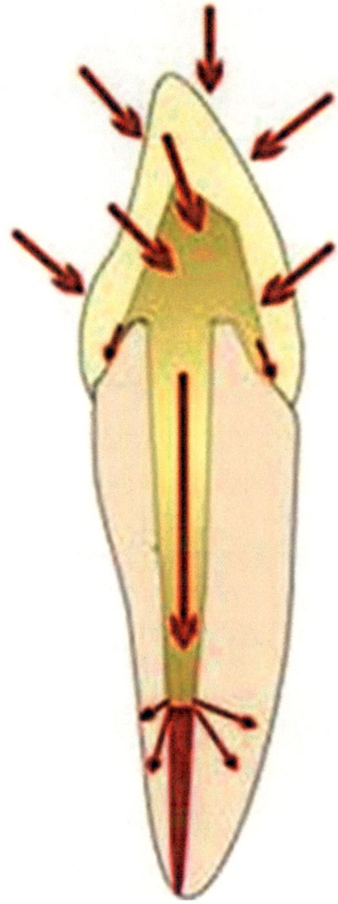

Figure 4. Stress concentration due to commercial dental post.

Matsuo et al. [82] fabricated functionally graded dental post (FGDP) using laser lithography, one of the photo-curing type computer-aided design/computer-aided manufacturing (CAD/CAM). The elastic modulus of the post could be changed longitudinally at its apical end by decreasing the filler content of ceramic powders from 64 to 0% in polymer matrix. They used FEM and showed that stress was reduced further by 30% in functionally graded dental post compared with the uniform one. Fujihara et al. [83] fabricated functionally graded dental post and analyzed the stress distribution by FEA. They showed that the peak tensile and shear stresses for a functionally graded dental post were less than that of stainless steel post. They suggested that the modulus of elasticity of post material should be as close as possible to the modulus of elasticity of dentine and crown at the apical part and the coronal part respectively, in order to minimize the chance of interfacial debonding. Lately, Abu Kasim et al. [84] patented three types of multilayered composite materials that were produced using powders of zirconia (ZrO_2), alumina (Al_2O_3), hydroxyapatite (HA), and titanium (Ti) to develop newly designed functionally graded dental post. The stress distribution of a newly constructed functionally

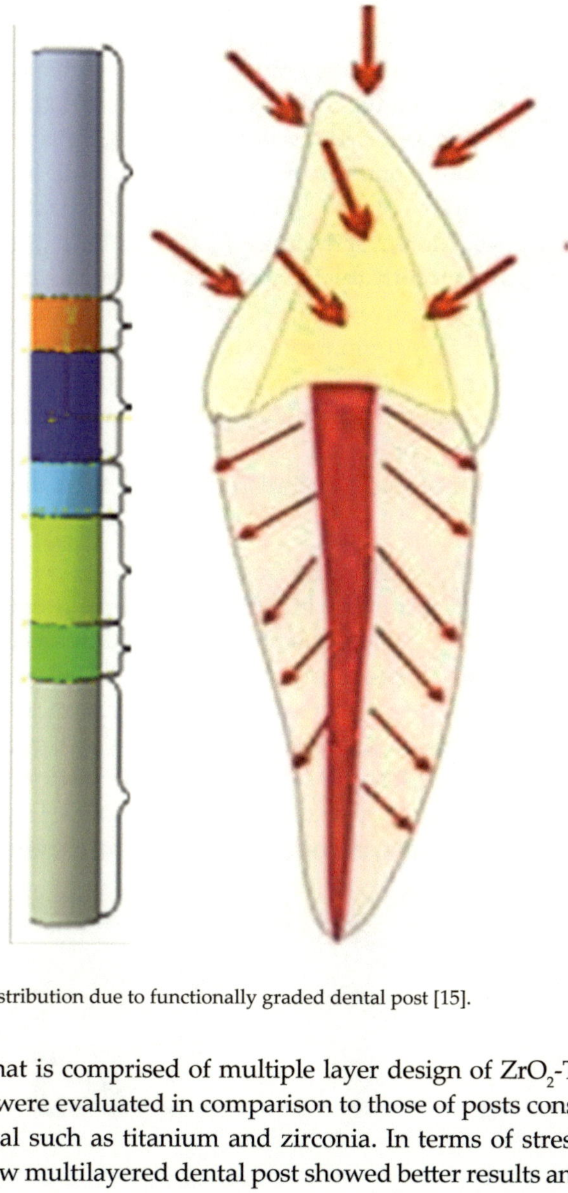

Figure 5. Uniform stress distribution due to functionally graded dental post [15].

graded dental post that is comprised of multiple layer design of ZrO_2-Ti-HA was studied in Ref. [85]. The results were evaluated in comparison to those of posts constructed from a single homogeneous material such as titanium and zirconia. In terms of stress distribution, it was concluded that the new multilayered dental post showed better results and advantages in comparison to homogenous posts with a better stress distribution at the post-dentine interface of functionally graded dental post (FGDP). Therefore, it is important to ascertain the thermal behavior of FGDP in order predict their performance in the oral environment. Madfa et al. [86] examined thermal stress in endodontically treated teeth restored with FGDP under cold and hot conditions using finite element analysis. They found that the magnitude of thermal stresses at the post and surrounding structures interface were greater in the zirconia and titanium posts especially at the middle third of the posts. In this study, thermal analysis showed that thermal stress level is closely related to the amount of temperature gradient. The peak stress by thermal stimuli for the zirconia and titanium posts are approximately three times higher than FGSP. This is due to that the FGDP possibly improved the heat flow into dentine because of the gradual change in thermal conductivity. Madfa [15] also investigated the shear stress distribution of a newly designed functionally graded dental post which consisted of multilayer design of ZrO_2-Ti-HA and was compared to posts fabricated from homogeneous material such as titanium and zirconia. They reported that shear stress of FGDP at posts and surrounding structures was lower than titanium and zirconia posts when tooth loaded obliquely. It was observed that the peak shear stress for the FGSP reduced approximately three times of those for titanium and zirconia posts. Moreover, Madfa [15] analyzed the strain distribution pattern in the natural tooth and endodontically treated teeth restored within either FGDP or titanium and zirconia posts. Strain mainly occurred at the coronal third of the root and gradually diminished towards the apical third. This strain may result from the increased displacement of the alveolar bone in the cervical region, relieving the apical third from any undue strain. The same authors found that FGDP and natural tooth models distributed strain uniformly in the tooth structure, the strain found to concentrate at the coronal third of the root, where the cemento-enamel junction (CEJ) creates a physiological discontinuity of the mechanical properties of natural tissue.

Furthermore, Madfa et al. [87] compared the fracture resistance and failure modes of endodontically treated bovine teeth restored with FGDP prototype, prefabricated titanium and cast posts. Their results found that there was no significant difference in the mean fracture resistance (N) for endodontically treated teeth restored with FGDP, titanium and cast posts. Surprisingly, the failure mode evaluation results exhibited significant differences between the groups. Most typically, fracture of the sample in all groups occurred initially at the crown margin on the palatal side where loading was applied. The fracture line then progressed towards the buccal surface of the root, above, below or at the simulated bone level. If the fracture terminates above or at the simulated bone level, this fracture mode was considered to be

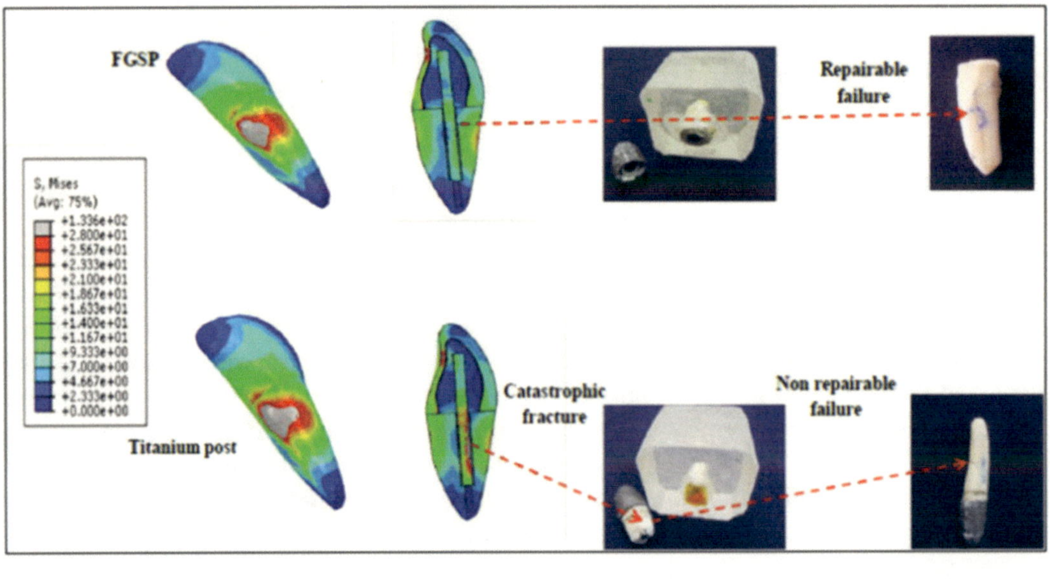

Figure 6. Relationship between failure mode and the finite element analysis [15].

repairable. The FGDP and the endodontically treated teeth without post showed more repairable failures compared to titanium and cast posts. The stress were concentrated at middle and apical thirds for endodontically treated teeth restored with titanium and cast posts compared to FGSPs and endodontically treated teeth without posts [15] as shown in **Figure 6**.

3.2. Dental crown

3.2.1. Overview

Ceramic dental restorations are designed to restore both function and esthetics of the compromised teeth. However, these materials showed somewhat poor flexural strength, particularly when exposed to fatigue loading in wet environments [88–90]. Consequently, this can result in severe discomfort to patients and can reduce the durability for ceramic prostheses due to their flexural fracture [91–93]. Furthermore, in metal-ceramic restorations, there are mismatches in the mechanical properties between the veneering porcelain and underlying metal core. The Young's modulus of the veneering porcelain is 60–80 GPa, while that of the metal core is in the range of 80–230 GPa [94]. Moreover, there are mismatches in the thermal properties between the veneering porcelain and metal core, where thermal expansion coefficient for metal core is usually higher than that of veneering porcelain (**Figure 7**). These significant mismatches between both materials properties result in stresses concentration at the metal-ceramic interfaces which may cause interface cracking and consequently lead to restoration failure [95, 96].

In spite of the continuous improvement in dental prostheses such as using a strong zirconia or alumina core to support the esthetic porcelain veneer, ceramic prostheses are still susceptible to failure at a rate of about 1–3% each year [97]. Also, ceramics prostheses have a dense, high purity crystalline structure at the cementation surface that cannot be adhesively bonded to tooth dentin support [98]. Although some authors recommended particles abrasion as surface roughening treatment to improve the bond of ceramic-resin-based cements utilizing mechanical interlocking, particles abrasion further causes surface defects or microcracks which could result in deterioration of flexural strength of ceramic prostheses on the long-term service [99–105]. Furthermore, the white opaque appearance of the zirconia cores

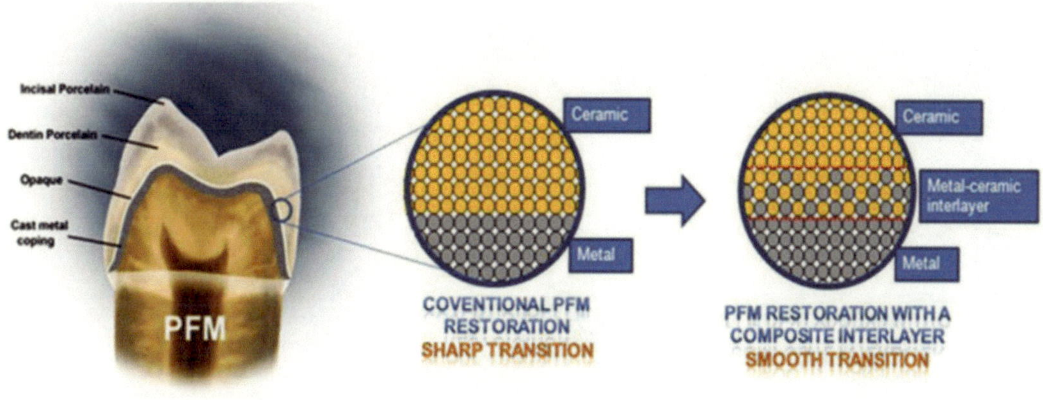

Figure 7. Schematic of the conventional sharp restoration and the new graded approach.

necessitates placing a thick layer of porcelain veneer with stepwise change in translucency to cover zirconia core thereby achieving better esthetic results [106]. In addition, dental crowns generate over $2 billion in revenues each year, with 20% of crowns being all ceramic units. Aging populations will drive the demand for all types of dental restorations even higher [107]. Moreover, occlusal contacts induce deformation and cracking of dental crowns leading to structure failure [108].

For the above reasons, it is highly advisable to develop ceramic prostheses that are more resistant to cracking under occlusal contact in recent decade for long term service and success [109, 110]. Composite ceramics have been designed in an effort to improve strength and toughness while enhancing functionality. For many years, simple laminate materials have been developed, where a number of materials with different properties are bonded into a layered structure [111]. Even though these composites combine varying properties, the abrupt interfaces between the two materials often reserve residual stresses [10, 112] and perhaps delaminate under load [113].

3.2.2. Dental crown based on functionally graded concept

Natural teeth are composed of layered structures, dentin and enamel, that are bonded by a functionally graded dentin-enamel junction (DEJ) layer that is about 10–100 micrometers thick [114, 115]. The DEJ acts as a bridge between the hard brittle enamel (E~70 GPa) and the softer durable dentin layer (E~20 GPa), allowing a smooth Young modulus transition between the two structures [115] as shown in **Figure 8**. He and Swain [35] investigated the nanoindentation mechanical behavior of the inner and outer regions of human enamel. They reported that inner enamel has lower stiffness and hardness but higher creep and stress redistribution abilities than their outer counterpart. They attributed this observation to the gradual compositional change throughout

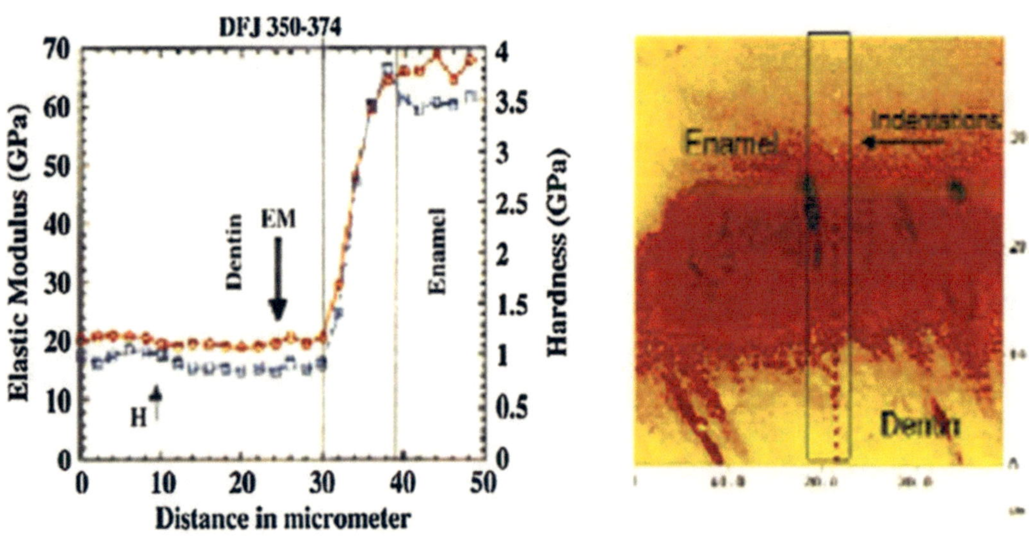

Figure 8. Elastic modulus distribution in natural DEJ [10].

the enamel from the outer region near the occlusal surface to the inner region near DEJ. They suggested that enamel can be regarded as a functionally graded natural bio-composite.

Inspired by the microstructure and mechanical properties of natural teeth, synthetic functionally graded materials were proposed to mimic the DEJ. Recently, functionally graded dental prostheses inspired by the DEJ structures and the linear gradation in Young's modulus of the DEJ have been recommended, as an alternative technique, aiming to enhance the overall performance of metal-ceramic and all-ceramic dental restorative systems. This technique permits the production of a material with very different characteristics within the same material at various interfaces [4].

Francis et al. [115] introduced a procedure to create a DEJ-like interface and enamel coating involved depositing slurries of oxide or glass powder by a draw-down blade method, drying at then higher temperature heating. They used alumina-glass or alumina-polymer composite to mimic the dentin and a calcium phosphate-based coating to mimic the enamel. Bonding between the two materials was accomplished by a eutectic melt in the $CaO-Al_2O_3-SiO_2$ system. The interpenetration in this DEJ-like interface originates from a solidified melt phase penetrating into the dentin. Huang et al. [10] added a FGM layer forming an enamel-like dental ceramic layer. FE simulations of the structure showed that the addition of FGM adhesive layer could significantly reduce the stress concentrations in the sub-surface of ceramic. This increases the resistance of the structure to radial cracking. This suggests the possibility of building synthetic bio-inspired functionally graded dental multilayers that have comparable or better durability than those of natural teeth. Consequently, also showed similar reductions in stress concentrations in simulations using a bio-inspired functionally graded material layer have been shown also by Niu et al. [14]. Their experimental study demonstrated the processing of such functionally graded multi-layers and the increased critical loads in dental multilayer structures with FGM structures.

Rahbar and Soboyejo [13] used computational and experimental effort to develop crack-resistant multilayered crowns that are inspired by the functionally graded DEJ structure. The calculated stress distributions revealed that the highest stress was concentrated at the ceramic outer layer of crown which then was reduced significantly toward the DEJ with the use of bioinspired functionally graded architecture. In addition, promotion of improvements in the critical crack size was reported because of these bioinspired functionally graded layers. Du et al. [116] also found that the bioinspired functionally graded layers were also shown to promote improvements in the critical crack size. Suresh [117] established that controlled gradients in mechanical properties offer unprecedented opportunities for the design of surfaces with resistance to contact deformation and damage that cannot be realized in conventional homogeneous materials.

Graded dental crowns have been shown to display improved features relative to conventional ones, namely higher resistance to contact and sliding [118, 119]; higher adhesion of porcelain to the substructure (metal or ceramic) [120–122]; improved esthetical properties and improved behavior under fatigue conditions [122]. FGM design can address another important point related to diminishing the thermal residual stresses which persist at the metal-ceramic interface after firing of porcelain throughout its cooling cycles. Such stresses are additionally exaggerated due to the presence of a prominent mismatch between the metal and porcelain thermal expansion behavior. Basing on the remnant thermal residual stress level in the crown and along with those originating from occlusal functional loads, a disastrous restoration failure can follow. It was revealed that FGMs reduce dramatically the remnants of thermal stresses raised at the metals and ceramics interface in other fields of applications [123]. Some studies demonstrated that when the contact surface of alumina or silicon nitride was infiltrated with aluminosilicate or oxynitride glass, respectively, they noticed that the graded glass/ceramic surfaces produced in this manner offered much better resistance to contact damage with and without a sliding action than either constituent ceramic or glass [124, 125].

A number of the studies investigated the effects of increasing elasticity as a function of depth from the surface on the resistance to contact damage. They established that mass fracture and failure of veneer may be considerably diminished by specific gradual inclination of the modulus of elasticity through the veneer material thickness. These graded layers show a noticeable increased resistance to fatigue sliding-contact and flexural damage regarding veneered and monolithic core ceramics. This is due to the reduction of the tensile stresses intensity as a result of this gradient and, at the same time, transfers these stresses from the surface layer toward the interior, away from the source of failure-inducing surface defects [126–133] as shown in **Figure 9**.

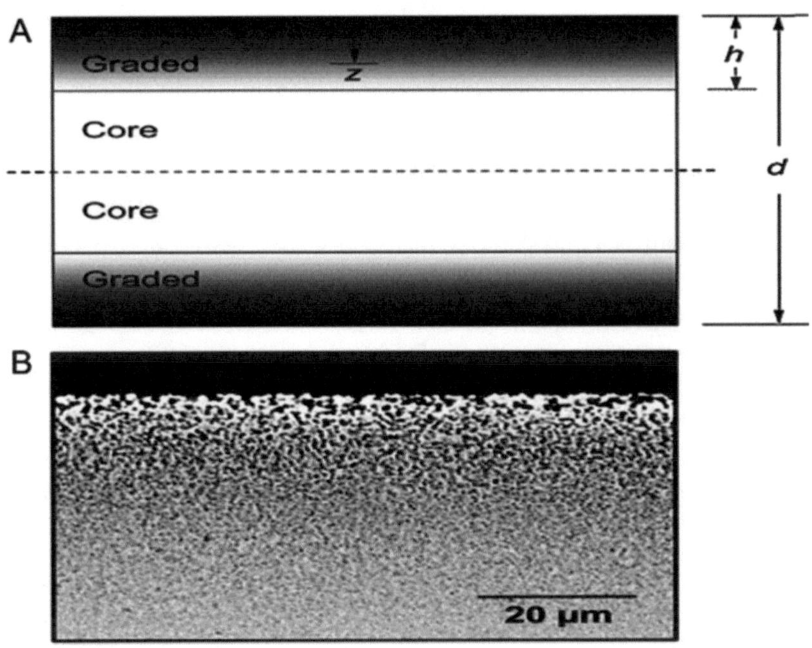

Figure 9. Morphology of the graded zone. (A) Schematic of graded structure, (B) Section view of graded zone of glass-infiltrated yttria stabilized zirconia [126].

4. Conclusions and future perspectives

The development and selection of biocompatible, long-lasting, direct-filling tooth restoratives and indirectly prosthetic materials capable of withstand the aggressive environment of the oral cavity, have been a challenge for practitioners of dentistry since the beginning of dental practice. In order to replace the mechanical function of tooth from a restorative perspective, it is not only important to study its localized tissue properties but also its bulk structural behavior. Therefore, this chapter highlights functionally graded dental implant and restorations inspired from nature. The bioinspired functionally graded structure can be seen as the precursor to recent studies. This is a remarkable example of nature's ability to engineer functionally graded dental prostheses. These dental prostheses mimic the biological and mechanical behavior of natural bone and tooth. These prostheses could potentially lead to superior long-term clinical performance for dental prostheses.

Work in this area is promising and provides a basis for exciting improvements in dental implant and restorations for patients. However, the body of research to date has still not clearly identified the optimal graduation for the most effective biomechanical and biological properties and their behaviors. Therefore, further studies are necessary to evaluate the potential of advanced manufacturing methods to optimize the graduation structure of dental prostheses. The present chapter opens a new avenue for recent researches aimed at further development of new direct filling tooth restoratives and indirect prosthetic materials for improving their clinical durability.

Author details

Elham M. Senan[1] and Ahmed A. Madfa[1,2]*

*Address all correspondence to: ahmed_um_2011@yahoo.com

1 Restorative and Prosthodontic Department, College of Dentistry, University of Science and Technology, Sana'a, Yemen

2 Department of Conservative Dentistry, Faculty of Dentistry, Thamar University, Dhamar, Yemen

References

[1] Zarone F, Apicella D, Sorrentino R, et al. Influence of tooth preparation design on the stress distribution in maxillary central incisors restored by means of alumina porcelain veneers: A 3D-finite element analysis. Dental Materials. 2005;**21**:1178-1188

[2] Zarone F, Sorrentino R, Apicella D, et al. Evaluation of the biomechanical behavior of maxillary central incisors restored by means of endocrowns compared to a natural tooth: A 3D static linear finite elements analysis. Dental Materials. 2006;**22**:1035-1044

[3] Van Noort R. Introduction to Dental Materials. 2nd ed. Mosby Ltd., London, United Kingdom; 2002

[4] Madfa AA, Yue XG. Dental prostheses mimic the natural enamel behavior under functional loading: A review article. Japanese Dental Science Review. 2016;**52**:2-13

[5] Hsueh C-H, Luttrell CR, Becher PF. Analyses of multilayered dental ceramics subjected to biaxial flexure tests. Dental Materials. 2006;**22**:460-469

[6] Hsueh CH, Latrell CR, Becher PF. Modeling of multilayered disks subjected to biaxial flexure tests. International Journal of Solids and Structures. 2006;**43**:6014-6025

[7] Hedia H, Mahmoud NA. Design optimization of functionally graded dental implant. Bio-Medical Materials and Engineering. 2004;**14**:133-143

[8] Hedia H. Design of functionally graded dental implant in the presence of cancellous bone. Journal of Biomedical Materials Research Part B: Applied Biomaterials. 2005;**75**:74-80

[9] Hedia H. Effect of cancellous bone on the functionally graded dental implant concept. Bio-Medical Materials and Engineering. 2005;**15**:199-209

[10] Huang M, Rahbar N, Wang R, Thompson V, Rekow D, Soboyejo W. Bioinspired design of dental multilayers. Materials Science and Engineering A. 2007;**464**:315-320

[11] Wang F, Lee H, Lu C. Thermal-mechanical study of functionally graded dental implants with the finite element method. Journal of Biomedial Materials Research Part A. 2007;**80**:146-158

[12] Yang J, Xiang H-J. A three-dimensional finite element study on the biomechanical behavior of an FGBM dental implant in surrounding bone. Journal of Biomechanics. 2007;**40**:2377-2385

[13] Rahbar N, Soboyejo W. Design of functionally graded dental multilayers. Fatigue & Fracture of Engineering Materials & Structures. 2011;**34**:887-897

[14] Niu X, Rahbar N, Farias S, Soboyejo W. Bio-inspired design of dental multilayers: Experiments and model. Journal of the Mechanical Behavior of Biomedical Materials. 2009;**2**:596-602

[15] Madfa AA. Development of Functionally Graded Composite for Fabrication of Dental Post. University of Malaya, Kuala Lumpur, Malaysia; 2011

[16] Elias CN. Factors affecting the success of dental implants. In: Turkyilmaz I, editor. New York, NY, USA: InTech; 2011

[17] Esposito M, Hirsch J, Lekholm U, et al. Differential diagnosis and treatment strategies for biologic complications and failing oral implants: A Review of the literature. The International Journal of Oral & Maxillofacial Implants. 1999;**14**:473-490

[18] Cheng A, Humayun A, Cohen DJ, et al. Additively manufactured 3D porous Ti-6Al-4V constructs mimic trabecular bone structure and regulate osteoblast proliferation, differentiation and local factor production in a porosity and surface roughness dependent manner. Biofabrication. 2014;**6**:045007

[19] Le Guéhennec L, Soueidan A, Layrolle P, Amouriq Y. Surface treatments of titanium dental implants for rapid osseointegration. Dental Materials. 2007;**23**:844-854

[20] Özcan M, Hämmerle C. Titanium as a reconstruction and implant material in dentistry: Advantages and pitfalls. Materials. 2012;**5**:1528-1545

[21] Nomura N, Kohama T, Oh H, et al. Mechanical properties of porous Ti-15Mo-5Zr-3Al compacts prepared by powder sintering. Materials Science and Engineering C. 2005;**25**:330-335

[22] Krishna BV, Bose S, Bandyopadhyay A. Low stiffness porous Ti structures for load-bearing implants. Acta Biomaterialia. 2007;**3**:997-1006

[23] Schiefer H, Bram M, Buchkremer HP, Stöver D. Mechanical examinations on dental implants with porous titanium coating. Journal of Materials Science Materials in Medicine. 2009;**20**:1763-1770

[24] Isidor F. Influence of forces on peri-implant bone. Clinical Oral Implants Research. 2006;**17**:8-18

[25] Mangano F, Chambrone L, van Noort R, et al. Direct metal laser sintering titanium dental implants. International Journal of Biomaterials. 2014;**2014**:461534

[26] Junker R, Dimakis A, Thoneick M, et al. Effects of implant surface coatings and composition on bone integration: A systematic review. Clinical Oral Implants Research. 2009;**20**:185-206

[27] Gaviria L, Salcido JP, Guda T, et al. Current trends in dental implants. Journal of the Korean Association of Oral and Maxillofacial Surgeons. 2014;**40**:50-60

[28] Teixeira LN, Crippa GE, Lefebvre L-P, et al. The influence of pore size on osteoblast phenotype expression in cultures grown on porous titanium. International Journal of Oral and Maxillofacial Surgery. 2012;**41**:1097-1101

[29] Mohandas G, Oskolkov N, McMahon MT, et al. Porous tantalum and tantalum oxide nanoparticles for regenerative medicine. Acta Neurobiologiae Experimentalis. 2014;**74**:188-196

[30] Tolochko NK, Savich VV, Laoui T, et al. Dental root implants produced by the combined selective laser sintering/melting of titanium powders. Journal of Materials: Design and Applications. 2002;**216**:267-270

[31] Ryan G, Pandit A, Apatsidis DP. Fabrication methods of porous metals for use in orthopaedic applications. Biomaterials. 2006;**27**:2651-2670

[32] Cook SD, Thongpreda N, Anderson RC, et al. The effect of post-sintering heat treatments on the fatigue properties of porous coated Ti-6Al-4V alloy. Journal of Biomedial Materials Research. 1988;**22**:287-302

[33] Joshi GV, Duan Y, Neidigh J, et al. Fatigue testing of electron beam-melted Ti-6Al-4V ELI alloy for dental implants. Journal of Biomedical Materials Research Part B: Applied Biomaterials. 2013;**101**:124-130

[34] Pompe W, Worch H, Epple M, et al. Functionally graded materials for biomedical applications. Materials Science and Engineering A. 2003;**362**:40-60

[35] He LH, Swain MV. Enamel—A functionally graded natural coating. Journal of Dentistry. 2009;**37**:596-603

[36] Sadollah A, Bahreininejad A. Optimum gradient material for a functionally graded dental implant using metaheuristic algorithms. Journal of the Mechanical Behavior of Biomedical Materials. 2011;**4**:1384-1395

[37] Lin D, Li Q, Li W, et al. Design optimization of functionally graded dental implant for bone remodeling. Composites Part B: Engineering. 2009;**40**:668-675

[38] Chu C, Zhu J, Yin Z, and Lin P. Optimal design and fabrication of hydroxyapatite-Ti asymmetrical functionally graded biomaterial. Materials Science and Engineering A. 2003;**348**:244-250

[39] Khor KA, Gu YW, Quek CH, et al. Plasma spraying of functionally graded hydroxyapatite/Ti-6Al-4V coatings. Surface and Coatings Technology. 2003;**168**:195-201

[40] Yamada K, Imamura K, Itoh H, et al. Bone bonding behavior of the hydroxyapatite containing glasstitanium composite prepared by the Culletmethod. Biomaterials. 2001;**22**:2207-2214

[41] Van Grunsven W, Hernandez-Nava E, Reilly G, et al. Fabrication and mechanical characterisation of titanium lattices with graded porosity. Metals. 2014;**4**:401-409

[42] Traini T, Mangano C, Sammons RL, et al. Direct laser metal sintering as a new approach to fabrication of an isoelastic functionally graded material for manufacture of porous titanium dental implants. Direct laser metal sintering as a new approach to fabrication of an isoelastic functionally grad. Dental Materials. 2008;**24**:1525-1533

[43] Mangano C, Raspanti M, Traini T, et al. Stereo imaging and cytocompatibility of a model dental implant surface formed by direct laser fabrication. Journal of Biomedical Materials Research. Part A. 2009;**88**:823-831

[44] Murr LE, Gaytan SM, Medina F, et al. Next-generation biomedical implants using additive manufacturing of complex, cellular and functional mesh arrays. Philosophical Transactions of the Royal Society of London A: Mathematical, Physical and Engineering SciencesPhilosophical Transactions of the Royal Society of London A: Mathematical, Physical and Engineering Sciences. 2010;**368**:1999-2032

[45] Li X, Wang C, Zhang W, et al. Fabrication and compressive properties of Ti6Al4V implant with honeycomb-like structure for biomedical applications. Rapid Prototyping Journal. 2010;**16**:44-49

[46] Laoui T, Santos E, Osakada K, et al. Properties of titanium dental implant models made by laser processing. Journal of Mechanical Engineering Science. 2006;**220**:857-863

[47] Nomura N, Sakamoto K, Takahashi K, et al. Fabrication and mechanical properties of porous Ti/HA composites for bone fixation devices. Materials Transactions. 2010;**51**:1449-1454

[48] Witek L, Marin C, Granato R, et al. Characterization and *in vivo* evaluation of laser sintered dental endosseous implants in dogs. Journal of Biomedical Materials Research Part B: Applied Biomaterials. 2012;**100**:1566-1573

[49] Chenglin C, Jingchuan Z, Zhongda Y, et al. Hydroxyapatite-ti functionally graded biomaterial fabricated by powdermetallurgy. Materials Science and Engineering A. 1999;**271**:95-100

[50] Lim YM, Park YJ, Yun YH, et al. Functionally graded Ti/HAP coatings on Ti-6Al-4V obtained by chemical solution deposition. Ceramics International. 2002;**28**:37-41

[51] Yokoyama A, Watari F, Miyao R, et al. Mechanical properties and biocompatibility of titanium-hydroxyapatite implant material prepared by spark plasma sintering method. Key Engineering Materials. 2001;**192-195**:445-448

[52] Miyao R, Yokoyama A, Watari F, et al. Properties of titanium/hydroxyapatite functionally graded implants by spark plasma sintering and their biocompatibility. Dental Materials Journal. 2001;**20**:344-355

[53] Watari F, Yokoyama A, Saso F, et al. Fabrication and properties of functionally graded dental implant. Composites B. 1997;**28**:5-11

[54] Foppiano S, Tomsia A, Marshall G, et al. In vitro Biocompatibility of Novel Functionally Graded Bioactive Coatings, IADR/AADR/CADR, Hawaii, USA; 82nd General Session; 2004

[55] Watari F, Yokoyama A, Omori M, et al. Biocompatibility of materials and development to functionally graded implant for bio-medical application. Composites Science and Technology. 2004;**64**:893-908

[56] Yuan XY, Mak AF, Li J. Formation of bone-like apatite on poly (L-lactic acid) fibers by a biomimetic process. Journal of Biomedial Materials Research. 2001;**57**:140-150

[57] Takeuchi A, Ohtsuki C, Miyazaki T, et al. Deposition of bone-like apatite on silk fiber in a solution that mimics extracellular fluid. Journal of Biomedical Materials Research. Part A. 2003;**65**:283-289

[58] Bosetti M, Verne E, Ferraris M, et al. In vitro characterisation of zirconia coated by bioactive glass. Biomaterials. 2001;**22**:987-994

[59] Rosengren A, Oscarsson S, Mazzocchi M, et al. Protein adsorption onto two bioactive glass ceramics. Biomaterials. 2003;**24**:147-155

[60] Kaufmann EA, Ducheyne P, Radin S, et al. Initial events at the bioactive glass surface in contact with protein-containing solutions. Journal of Biomedial Materials Research. 2000;**52**:825-830

[61] Bidan CM, Kommareddy KP, Rumpler M, et al. Geometry as a factor for tissue growth: Towards shape optimization of tissue engineering scaffolds. Advanced Healthcare Materials. 2013;**2**:186-194

[62] Mangano C, Piattelli A, d'Avila S, et al. Early human bone response to laser metal sintering surface topography: A histologic report. The Journal of Oral Implantology. 2010;**36**:91-96

[63] Rumpler M, Woesz A, Dunlop JWC, et al. The effect of geometry on three-dimensional tissue growth. Journal of the Royal Society Interface. 2008;**5**:1173-1180

[64] Markhoff J, Wieding J, Weissmann V, et al. Influence of different three-dimensional open porous titanium scaffold designs on human osteoblasts behavior in static and dynamic cell investigations. Materials.. 2015;**8**:5490-5507

[65] Mangano C, Mangano FG, Shibli JA, et al. Immediate loading of mandibular overdentures supported by unsplinted direct laser metal-forming implants: Results from a 1-year prospective study. The Journal of Periodontology. 2012;**83**:70-78

[66] Shibli JA, Mangano C, D'avila S, et al. Influence of direct laser fabrication implant topography on type IV bone: A histomorphometric study in humans. Journal of Biomedical Materials Research. Part A. 2010;**93**:607-614

[67] Bandyopadhyay A, Espana F, Balla VK, et al. Influence of porosity on mechanical properties and *in vivo* response of Ti6Al4V implants. Acta Biomaterialia. 2010;**6**:1640-1648

[68] Gutmann JL. The dentin-root complex: Anatomic and biologic considerations in restoring endodontically treated teeth. Journal of Prosthetic Dentistry. 1992;**67**:458-467

[69] Morgano SM. Restoration of pulpless teeth: Application of traditional principles in present and future contexts. Journal of Prosthetic Dentistry. 1996;**75**:375-380

[70] Kishen A. Mechanisms and risk factors for fracture predilection in endodontically treated teeth. Endodontic Topics. 2006;**13**:57-83

[71] Kishen A, Asundi A. Photomechanical investigations on post-endodontically rehabilitated teeth. Journal of Biomedial Optics. 2002;**7**:262-270

[72] Magne P, Versluis A, Douglas WH. Effect of luting composite shrinkage and thermal loads on the stress distribution in porcelain laminate veneers. Journal of Prosthetic Dentistry. 1999;**81**:335-344

[73] Llena-Puy MC, Forner-Navarro L, Barbero-Navarro I. Vertical root fracture in endodontically treated teeth: A review of 25 cases. Oral Medicine, Oral Pathology, Oral Radiology & Endodontics. 2001;**92**:553-555

[74] Torbjörner A, Fransson B. A literature review on the prosthetic treatment of structurally compromised teeth. International Journal of Prosthodontics. 2004;**17**:369-376

[75] Asmussen E, Peutzfeldt A, Heitmann T. Stiffness, elastic limit and strength of newer types of endodontic posts. Journal of Dentistry. 1999;**27**:275-280

[76] King PA, Setchell DJ. An in vitro evaluation of a prototype CFRC prefabricated post developed for the restoration of pulpless teeth. Journal of Oral Rehabilitation. 1990;**17**:599-609

[77] Schwartz RS, Robbins JW. Post placement and restoration of endodontically treated teeth: A literature review. Journal of Endodontics. 2004;**30**:289-301

[78] Raygot GG, Chai J, Jameson DL. Fracture resistance and primary failure mode of endodontically treated teeth restored with a carbon fiber-reinforced resin post system in vitro. International Journal of Prosthodontics. 2001;**14**:141-145

[79] Sorensen J, Ahn S, Berge H, Edelhoff D. Selection criteria for post core materials in the restoration of endodontically treated teeth. Proceedings of Conference on Scientific Criteria for Selecting Materials and Technique in Clinical Dentistry; 2001. pp. 67-84

[80] Ramakrishna S, Mayer J, Wintermantel E, et al. Biomedical applications of polymer-composite materials: A review. Composites Science and Technology. 2001;**61**:1189-1224

[81] Drake JT, Williamson RL, Rabin BH. Finite element analysis of thermal residual stresses at graded ceramic-metal interfaces. Part II. Interface optimization for residual stress reduction. Journal of Applied Physics. 1993;**74**:1321-1326

[82] Matsuo S, Watari F, Ohata N. Fabrication of a functionally graded dental composite resin post and core by laser lithography and finite element analysis of its stress relaxation effect on tooth root. Dental Materials Journal. 2001;**20**:257-274

[83] Fujihara K, Teo K, Gopal R, et al. Fibrous composite materials in dentistry and orthopaedics: Review and applications. Composites Science and Technology. 2004;**64**:775-788

[84] Abu Kasim NH, Madfa AA, Abd Shukor MH, et al. Metal-ceramic dental post. Patent no. WO2013043039 (A2); 2013

[85] Abu Kasim NH, Madfa AA, Abd Shukor MH, et al. FE Analysis of functionally graded structured dental posts. Dental Materials Journal. 2011;**30**:869-880

[86] Madfa AA, Abu Kasim NH, Abd Shukor MH, et al. Thermo-mechanical stress in multi-layered dental post due to temperature gradient. Journal of Dental Research. 2010;**89C**: Abstr. 086

[87] Madfa AA, Abu Kasim NH, Abd Shukor MH, et al. Fracture resistance of endodontically teeth restored with functionally graded posts. Journal of Dental Research. 2011;**90B**: Abstr. 086

[88] Lawn BR, Deng Y, Thompson VP. Use of contact testing in the characterization and design of all-ceramic crownlike layer structures: A review. Journal of Prosthetic Dentistry. 2001;**86**:495-510

[89] Studart A, Filser F, Kocher P, Gauckler L. In vitro lifetime of dental ceramics under cyclic loading in water. Biomaterials. 2007;**28**:2695-2705

[90] Rahaman MN, Li Y, Bal BS, Huang W. Functionally graded bioactive glass coating on magnesia partially stabilized zirconia (Mg-PSZ) for enhanced biocompatibility. Journal of Materials Science Materials in Medicine. 2008;**19**:2325-2333

[91] Jarrett CA, Ranawat AS, Bruzzone M, Blum YC, Rodriguez JA, Ranawat CS. The squeaking hip: A phenomenon of ceramic-on-ceramic total hip arthroplasty. The Journal of Bone and Joint Surgery. 2009;**91**:1344-1349

[92] Kelly JR. Clinically relevant approach to failure testing of all-ceramic restorations. Journal of Prosthetic Dentistry. 1999;**81**:652-661

[93] Lawn B, Bhowmick S, Bush MB, Qasim T, Rekow ED, Zhang Y. Failure modes in ceramic-based layer structures: A basis for materials design of dental crowns. Journal of the American Ceramic Society. 2007;**90**:1671-1683

[94] Rizkalla AS, Jones DW. Indentation fracture toughness and dynamic elastic moduli for commercial feldspathic dental porcelain materials. Dental Materials. 2004;**20**:198-206

[95] Lawn B, Deng Y, Lloyd I, Janal M, Rekow E, Thompson V. Materials design of ceramic-based layer structures for crowns. Journal of Dental Research. 2002;**81**:433-438

[96] Soboyejo WO, Wang RJ, Katsube N, Seghi R, Pagedas C, Skraba P, et al. Contact Damage of Model Dental Multilayers: Experiments and Finite Element Simulations. Key Engineering Materials. 2001;**198-199**:135-178

[97] Burke F, Fleming GJ, Nathanson D, Marquis PM. Are adhesive technologies needed to support ceramics? An assessment of the current evidence. The Journal of Adhesive Dentistry. 2002;**4**:7-22

[98] Blatz MB, Sadan A, Kern M. Resin-ceramic bonding: A review of the literature. Journal of Prosthetic Dentistry. 2003;**89**:268-274

[99] Zhang Y, Lawn BR, Malament KA, Thompson VP, Rekow ED. Damage accumulation and fatigue life of particle-abraded ceramics. International Journal of Prosthodontics. 2006;**19**:442-448

[100] Zhang Y, Lawn BR, Rekow ED, Thompson VP. Effect of sandblasting on the long-term performance of dental ceramics. Journal of Biomedical Materials Research Part B: Applied Biomaterials. 2004;**71**:381-386

[101] Barrack R, Burak C, Skinner H. Concerns about ceramics inTHA. Clinical Orthopaedics and Related Research. 2004;**429**:73-79

[102] Vasanthavel S, Kannan S. Development of ageing resistant and bioactive t-ZrO_2 polymorph by the combined additions of Ca^{2+}, PO_4^{3-} and SiO_2. Journal of the American Ceramic Society. 2016;**99**:1212-1220

[103] Tinschert J, Schulze KA, Natt G, Latzke P, Heussen N, Spiekermann H. Clinical behavior of zirconia-based fixed partial dentures made of DC-Zirkon: 3-year results. International Journal of Prosthodontics. 2008;**21**:217-222

[104] Sailer I, Pjetursson BE, Zwahlen M, Hammerle CH. A systematic review of the survival and complication rates of all-ceramic and metal-ceramic reconstructions after an observation period of at least 3 years. Part II: Fixed dental prostheses. Clinical Oral Implants Research. 2007;**18**(Suppl 3):86-96

[105] Sailer I, Fehér A, Filser F, Gauckler LJ, Luthy H, Hammerle CHF. Five-year clinical results of zirconia frameworks for posterior fixed partial dentures. International Journal of Prosthodontics. 2007;**20**:383

[106] Sailer I, Holderegger C, Jung RE, Suter A, Thiévent B, Pietrobon N, et al. Clinical study of the color stability of veneering ceramics for zirconia frameworks. International Journal of Prosthodontics. 2007;**20**:263-269

[107] Rekow D, Thompson VP. Engineering long term clinical success of advanced ceramic prostheses. Journal of Materials Science Materials in Medicine. 2007;**18**:47-56

[108] Kelly JR. Ceramics in restorative and prosthetic dentistry 1. Annual Review of Materials Science. 1997;**27**:443-468

[109] Özcan M. Fracture reasons in ceramic-fused-to-metal restorations. Journal of Oral Rehabilitation. 2003;**30**:265-269

[110] Anusavice KJ. Standardizing failure, success, and survival decisions in clinical studies of ceramic and metal-ceramic fixed dental prostheses. Dental Materials. 2012;**28**:102-111

[111] Lawn BR, Deng Y, Miranda P, Pajares A, Chai H, Kim DK. Overview: Damage in brittle layer structures from concentrated loads. Journal of Materials Research. 2002;**17**:3019-3036

[112] Taskonak B, Mecholsky JJ, Anusavice KJ. Residual stresses in bilayer dental ceramics. Biomaterials. 2005;**26**:3235-3241

[113] Aboushelib MN, Feilzer AJ, de Jager N, Kleverlaan CJ. Prestresses in bilayered all-ceramic restorations. Journal of Biomedical Materials Research Part B: Applied Biomaterials. 2008;**87**:139-145

[114] Lin CP, Douglas WH, Erlandsen SL. Scanning electron microscopy of type I collagen at the dentin-enamel junction of human teeth. Journal of Histochemistry and Cytochemistry. 1993;**41**:381-388

[115] Francis LF, Vaidya KJ, Huang HY, et al. Design and processing of ceramic based analogs to the dental crown. Materials Science and Engineering C. 1995;**3**:63-74

[116] Du J, Niu X, Rahbar N, Soboyejo W. Bio-inspired dental multilayers: Effects of layer architecture on the contact induced deformation. Acta Biomaterialia. 2013;**9**:5273-5279

[117] Suresh S. Graded materials for resistance to contact deformation and damage. Science. 2001;**292**:2447-2451

[118] Ren L, Zhang Y. Sliding contact fracture of dental ceramics: Principles and validation. Acta Biomaterialia. 2014;**10**:3243-3253

[119] Zhang Y. Overview: Damage resistance of graded ceramic restorative materials. Journal of the European Ceramic Society. 2012;**32**:2623-2632

[120] Henriques B, Soares D, Silva F. Optimization of bond strength between gold alloy and porcelain through a composite inter-layer obtained by powder metallurgy. Materials Science and Engineering: A. 2011;**528**:1415-1420

[121] Henriques B, Gasik M, Soares D, Silva FS. Experimental evaluation of the bond strength between a CoCrMo dental alloy and porcelain through a composite metal-ceramic graded transition interlayer. Journal of the Mechanical Behavior of Biomedical Materials. 2012;**13**:206-214

[122] Henriques B, Felix S, Soares D, Silva FS. Shear bond strength comparison between conventional porcelain fused to metal and new functionally graded dental restorations after thermal-mechanical cycling. Journal of the Mechanical Behavior of Biomedical Materials. 2012;**13**:194-205

[123] Gasik M. Micromechanical modeling of functionally graded materials. Computational Materials Science. 1998;**13**:42-55

[124] Pender DC, Padture NP, Giannakopoulos AE, Suresh S. Gradients in elastic modulus for improved contact-damage resistance. Part I: The silicon nitride-oxynitride glass system. Acta Materialia. 2001;**49**:3255-3262

[125] Suresh S, Olsson M, Giannakopoulos AE, Padture NP, Jitcharoen J. Engineering the resistance to sliding-contact damage through controlled gradients in elastic properties at contact surfaces. Acta Materialia. 1999;**47**:3915-3926

[126] Zhang Y, Chai H, Lawn BR. Graded structures for all-ceramic restorations. Journal of Dental Research. 2010;**89**:417-421

[127] Ren L, Janal MN, Zhang Y. Sliding contact fatigue of graded zirconia with external esthetic glass. Journal of Dental Research. 2011;**90**:1116-1121

[128] Zhang Y, Kim JW. Graded zirconia glass for resistance to veneer fracture. Journal of Dental Research. 2010;**89**:1057-1062

[129] Zhang Y, Ma L. Optimization of ceramic strength using elastic gradients. Acta Materialia. 2009;**57**:2721-2729

[130] Piascik JR, Thompson JY, Bower CA, Stoner BR. Stress evolution as a function of substrate bias in rf magnetron sputtered yttria-stabilized zirconia films. Journal of Vacuum Science & Technology A. 2006;**24**:1091-1095

[131] Cannillo V, Manfredini T, Montorsi M, Siligardi C, Sola A. Microstructure-based modelling and experimental investigation of crack propagation in glass-alumina functionally graded materials. Journal of the European Ceramic Society. 2006;**26**:3067-3073

[132] Dorthé E, Zhang Y. Load-bearing increase in alumina evoked by introduction of a functional glass gradient. Journal of the European Ceramic Society. 2012;**32**:1213-1220

[133] Jitcharoen J, Padture NP, Giannakopoulos AE, Suresh S. Hertzian-crack suppression in ceramics with elastic-modulus-graded surfaces. Journal of the American Ceramic Society. 1998;**81**:2301-2308

Chapter 9

Assessment of All-Ceramic Dental Restorations Behavior by Development of Simulation-Based Experimental Methods

Liliana Porojan, Florin Topală and Sorin Porojan

Additional information is available at the end of the chapter

http://dx.doi.org/10.5772/intechopen.69162

Abstract

New dental materials are often introduced into the market and especially in the current practice, without a basic understanding of their clinical performance because long-term controlled clinical trials are required, which are both time consuming and expensive. Ceramic materials are known for their relatively high fracture resistance and improved aesthetics, but brittleness remains a concern. The stressed areas of the materials are key factors for the failure analysis, and numerical simulations may play an important role in the understanding of the behavior of all-ceramic restorations. Simulation-based medicine and the development of complex computer models of biological structures are becoming ubiquitous for advancing biomedical engineering and clinical research. The studies have to be focused on the analysis of all-ceramic restorations failures, investigating several parameters involved in the tooth structure–restoration complex, in order to improve clinical performances. The experiments have to be conducted and interpreted reported to the brittle behavior of ceramic systems. Varied simulation methods are promising to assess the biomechanical behavior of all-ceramic systems, and first principal stress criterion is an alternative for ceramic materials investigations. The development of well-designed experiments could be useful to help to predict the clinical behavior of these new all-ceramic restorative techniques and materials.

Keywords: all-ceramic restorations, design parameters, simulation methods, stress, biomechanical behavior

1. Introduction

Ceramic materials and their technologies applied in dental field are in continuous development, but the clinical performance of all-ceramic restorations has to be improved due to the brittle nature of these materials.

As a consequence of brittle behavior, crack initiations and propagations in the materials can result in compromise of the restorations during functions and will be reflected in a poor clinical performance. In order to minimize clinical failures, restorations should be fabricated with consideration of their constituent material properties. Ceramic materials are known for their relatively high fracture resistance and improved aesthetics, but brittleness remains a concern [1]. The stressed areas of the materials are key factors for the failure analysis, and numerical simulations may play an important role in the understanding of the behavior of all-ceramic restorations.

New materials are often introduced into the market and especially in the current practice, without a basic understanding of their clinical performance because long-term controlled clinical trials are required, which are both time consuming and expensive. Simulation-based medicine and the development of complex computer models of biological structures are becoming ubiquitous for advancing biomedical engineering and clinical research [2–4].

In order to improve clinical performances of new all-ceramic restorations, studies have to be focused on the analysis of their failures, investigating different parameters involved in the tooth-restoration complex. Some of these parameters, like framework design, depend on the manufacturing technique and can be easily modified, influencing the failure rates and fracture modes of the restorations. How different designs may influence the fracture load and the mode of fracture of all-ceramic restorations is a topic of interest.

Finite element analysis (FEA) is a simulation method, widely used to understand and predict biomechanical phenomena in different areas of interest. Because modeling and simulation in dental field are complex, they involve skilled developers. With the advances in modeling and simulation, the clinical simulation becomes more real. FEA is a powerful and flexible computational tool to model dental structures and devices simulate the occlusal loading conditions and predict the stress and strain distribution. Establishing guidelines for model development and simulation, particularly for complex structures and different materials, pose a challenge in the field of dental technology.

Further studies are required to assess the durability of such restorations by different experimental methods before clinical use [5–7].

2. Digital design for all-ceramic crowns

The use of computer-aided design/computer-aided manufacturing (CAD/CAM) technology has grown in the last 30 years with the development of data acquisition technologies and computing technology. This led to improved quality restorations in terms of both resistance and adaptation to preparation and accuracy of occlusal morphology.

The evolution of these technologies has led to the widespread use of materials with superior mechanical and esthetic properties, like zirconia ceramics, which has the advantage that it can be used for almost any type of fixed prosthetic restoration.

It has been shown that resistance to fracture of ceramic restorations is not influenced only by the mechanical properties of the used material but also by the design of the preparations and the proper thickness of the restoration [8].

Traditionally, zirconia frameworks were fabricated at 0.5 mm thickness. Introduction of new types of zirconia served to reduce their thickness to 0.3 mm, allowing more conservative preparations [9]. Recommended finishing lines for these restorations are shoulder with rounded internal angles and slight chamfer, as a minimally invasive preparation designs, acceptable from both mechanical and periodontal reasons [8]. A point of interest is the effect of zirconia copings design on the resistance to load in posterior area, in order to prevent "chipping." In current practice, the framework is obtained by milling even thickness copies, rather than using a scientific-based design [2]. The main reason for zirconia restoration failures is veneering ceramic fracture and chipping. These are caused by an inappropriate framework design, which cannot provide a proper support and thickness for porcelain veneer layer [10–12].

The following example suggests various designs for the framework of zirconia-ceramic molar crowns [13]. For the experiments, a maxillary right first molar prepared for all-ceramic crown was used. The tooth was prepared leaving a chamfer finishing line; with anatomical occlusal reduction, a 6° occlusal convergence angle and the palatal surface of the functional cusp were reduced in two planes.

The master die, the antagonist stone cast, and bite-registration were scanned using the Cercon Eye scanner (Degudent, Hanau, Germany) (**Figure 1**).

Scanned data were computed, and frameworks for all-ceramic crowns were designed using Cercon Art 3.2 software (Degudent, Hanau, Germany). Three different framework designs were chosen: first, a 0.6-mm-thick framework was prepared, second, a cutback design was prepared as same as that for metal-ceramic crowns, in order to obtain a uniform, adequate thickness for the veneering porcelain, and third, a buccal reduction from the anatomic framework, for esthetic purposes (**Figures 2–4**).

All steps indicated from the manufacturer have been completed for each type of framework design. Cercon Art allows obtaining different designs for lateral single crowns frameworks due to the continuous improvements of the software. Hence, the design of the framework and the future veneer can be controlled.

Cercon Art soft allows also the possibility to scan the bite-registration and therefore an improved digital design of the framework (**Figures 5** and **6**), concerning the control of the veneer thickness in case of the cutback design and also of the contacts with the antagonists in case of a buccal veneering.

In case of the uniform framework thickness, the veneer design can be also digitized and have an overview of the finished restoration. Beginning from the final morphology of the restoration, the cutback design provides a uniform thickness of the veneer and a digital control of the

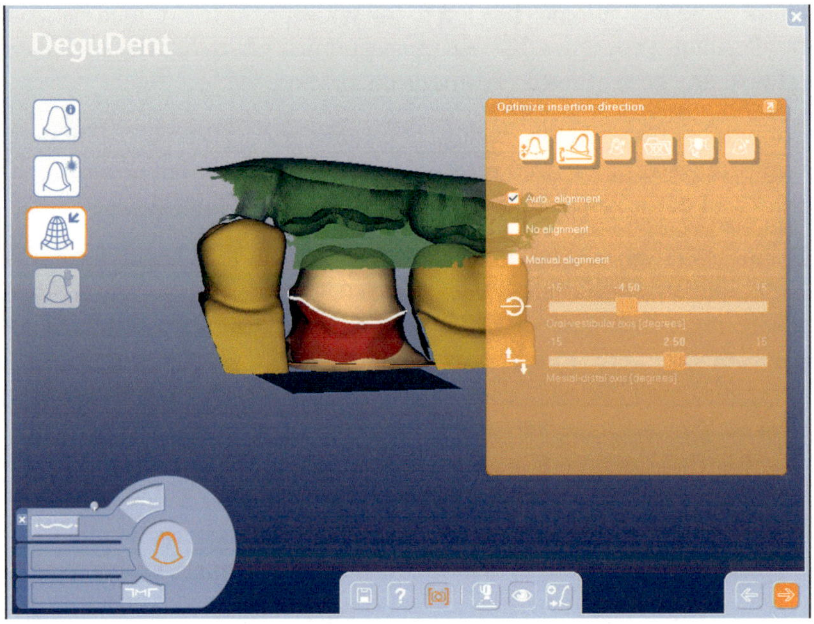

Figure 1. Scanned preparation, adjacent teeth, antagonists, and occlusion.

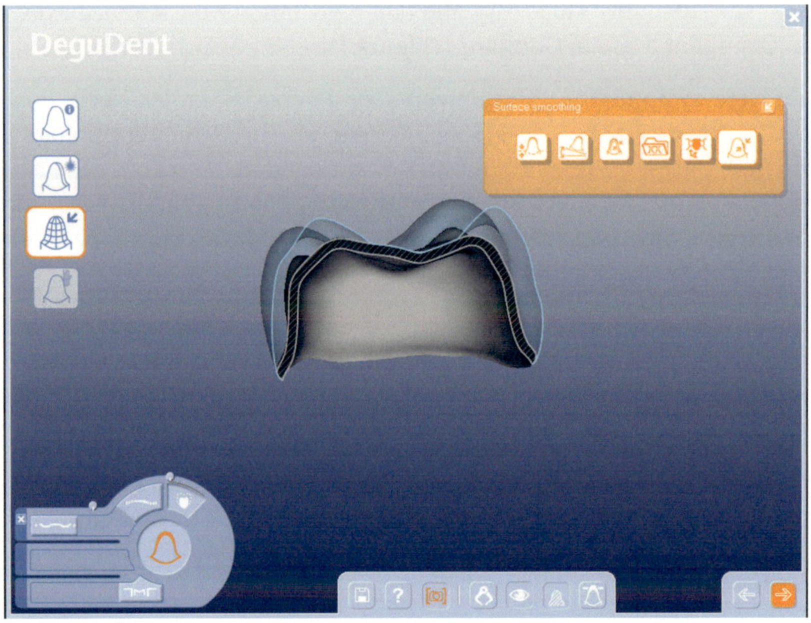

Figure 2. Uniform thickness of zirconia framework and digital control of the veneer design.

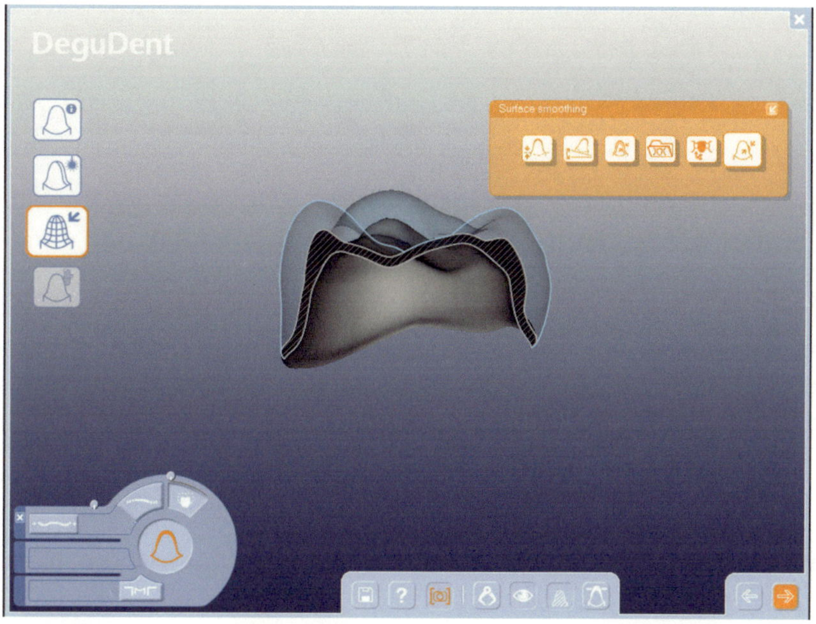

Figure 3. Uniform thickness of veneering ceramic when the framework is obtained with cutback design.

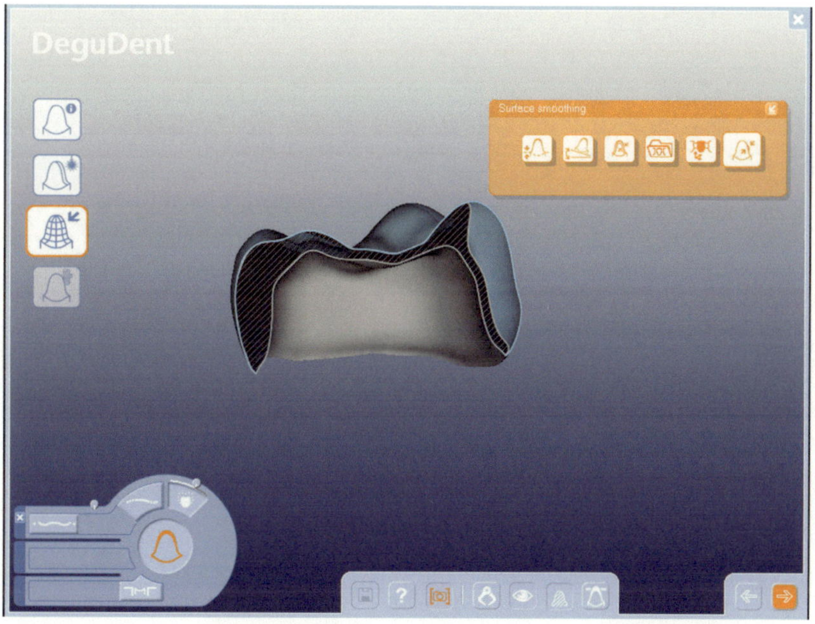

Figure 4. Full anatomic contour of the zirconia framework, with buccal reduction of the veneer.

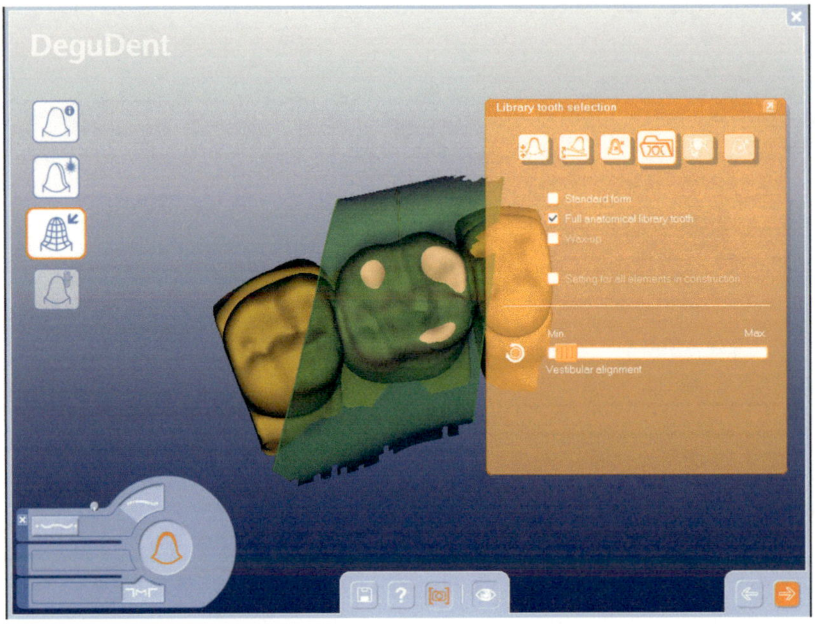

Figure 5. Zirconia anatomical framework design.

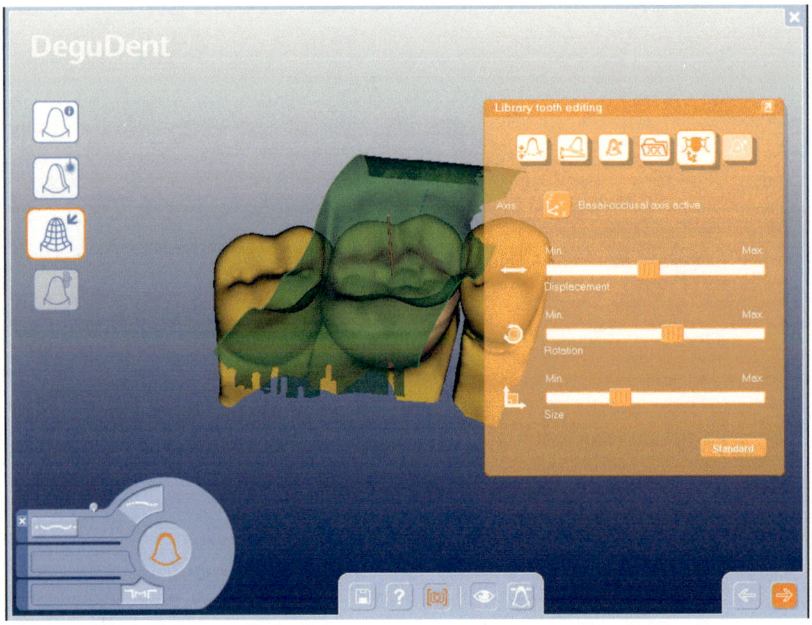

Figure 6. Zirconia anatomical framework design after optimization of the contact points with the adjacent teeth and antagonists.

framework thickness. The vestibular veneer became possible also due bite registration, allowing accurate and individualized modeling of the occlusal morphology. A facility of the soft is to have diagnostic tools, regarding thicknesses and distances, which allow a better control of the design (**Figure 7**).

Literature concerning the clinical performance of all-ceramic systems is inconclusive regarding the relative performance of different materials and physical configurations. Proper studies investigated modified designs and showed the benefits of additional porcelain support compared with a standard design by improving the reliability of all-ceramic crown systems [14]. Clinical studies on zirconia fixed partial dentures with anatomic framework design showed promising survival rates [15].

Improper framework designs cause an inadequate substrate for the veneering material and also its inadequate thickness. The improvement of the framework design, by creating an appropriate support, allows a proper thickness of the veneer proved to reduce the chipping rates [16]. The cutback design of the zirconia framework for all-ceramic crowns is thus a promising way to reduce veneer chipping failures [10].

The design of the substructure, especially the zirconia frameworks, provided different support of the veneering. Veneering porcelain with improved strength and fracture toughness may be one aspect to reduce chipping effects, but only with the change in the design of the supporting substructure, the number of chipping should be effectively reduced [17].

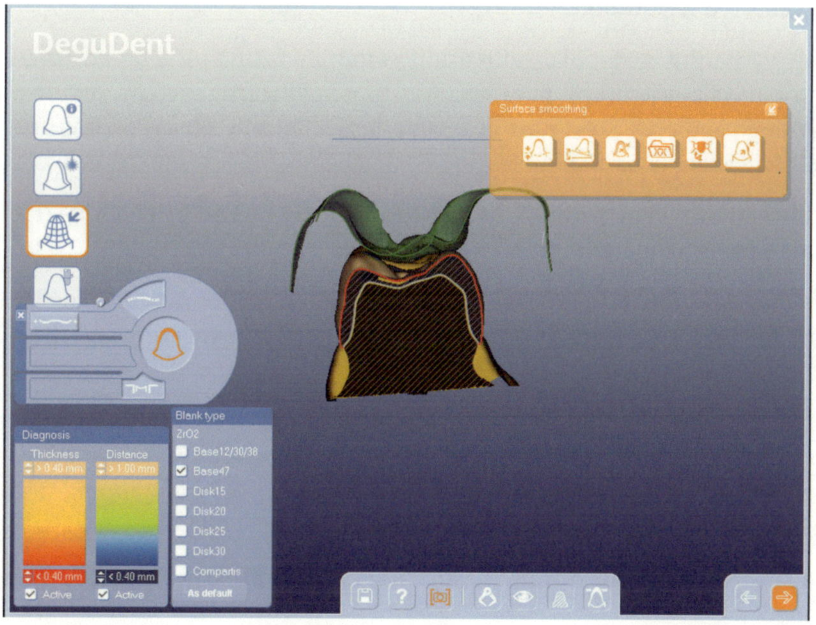

Figure 7. Diagnostic tools of the soft regarding thicknesses and distances.

Various influencing factors have been reported, such as the support and thickness of the veneer, the morphology of the circular finishing line, the adhesive forces between substructure and veneering, the mismatch of coefficients of thermal expansion, or the firing protocol during the veneering process [17–20].

Optimization of the zirconia substructure design has been proven as a considerable factor in reducing chipping failures, and coping modifications are still a topic of current investigations [14, 21].

Experiments using finite element analysis may help to predict the fracture behavior of specific material combinations, but failure types and patterns are notably influenced by clinical variables, such as an individual crown design with its occlusal variations, the patients chewing behavior, and functioning in an oral environment [22, 23].

3. Simulation methods applied in all-ceramic bilayered crowns

For restoring teeth with single crowns, yttria-stabilized zirconia cores veneered with dental porcelains are highly esthetic alternatives to conventional metal-ceramic crowns. Zirconia ceramics can be processed only with computer-aided design/computer-aided manufacturing technologies, and its properties were proven under in vitro and in vivo conditions over the past years [24–27].

The application of full-contour zirconia restorations is currently discussed as alternative to commonly veneered restorations [27–29].

By applying veneering materials, esthetically superior results can be achieved, but these materials have mechanical properties inferior to those of the frameworks. Because the veneering glass ceramic is the weakest part in this system, clinically observed failures are mainly restricted to the veneer layer [30].

Failure of all-ceramic dental restorations is predominately caused by cohesive fractures of the glass ceramic veneering material [31].

Failure rates were reported due to this "chipping" called failure mode. Some investigations showed an influence of the firing process of the glass ceramic veneering and the difference in the coefficients of thermal expansion [32–34].

Another important factor influencing the chipping behavior of veneered zirconia restorations is the framework design. An anatomical shape of the framework results in a low and nearly constant veneering thickness. This design is considered to prevent chipping in contrast to a thin framework with a thick and irregularly shaped veneering [35, 17].

Mechanical stresses that occur during mastication can also be strongly affected by the framework design [36].

Laboratory tests such as finite element analysis may help to predict fracture behavior of specific material combinations. It was demonstrated that failure types and patterns are mainly

http://dx.doi.org/10.5772/intechopen.69162

influenced by clinically determined reasons, such as preparation design, internal and marginal fit, cement thickness, and also technological reasons, like the individual crowns design with occlusal morphology and therefore different effects on stress distribution. Simulations imitating clinical situations during fatigue and thermal variations may help to study the behavior of the restorations under clinically approximated conditions. Failures resulted after simulation should be combined with clinically observed failures. Fractographic methods provide additional information to describe ceramic failures [26].

FEA can be used to evaluate the effect of core design on stress distribution in all-ceramic crowns [37]. A maxillary first premolar tooth was used as primary 3D model. The design of the prepared tooth was according to the clinical rules listed as follows: occlusal 2 mm reduction, 0.8 mm deep reduction chamfer margin, 6° convergence angle. The nonparametric modeling software (Blender 2.57b) was used to obtain the tooth shape. The collected data were used to construct three dimensional models using Rhinoceros (McNeel North America) Nonuniform Rational B-Splines (NURBS) modeling program (**Figure 8**).

A digital model of the bilayer crown was designed to occupy the space between the original tooth form and the prepared tooth form. Two different framework designs were constructed: model 1—a coping with a constant framework thickness of 0.6 mm and model 2—an anatomically modified shaped cusp-supporting framework with a constant veneering thickness (**Figure 9**). The geometric models were imported in the finite element analysis software Ansys and meshed using curvature-based mesh software. Finite element calculations were carried out.

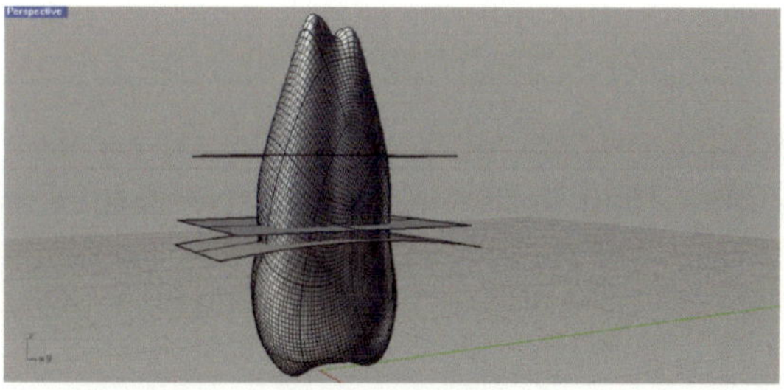

Figure 8. 3D model of the premolar.

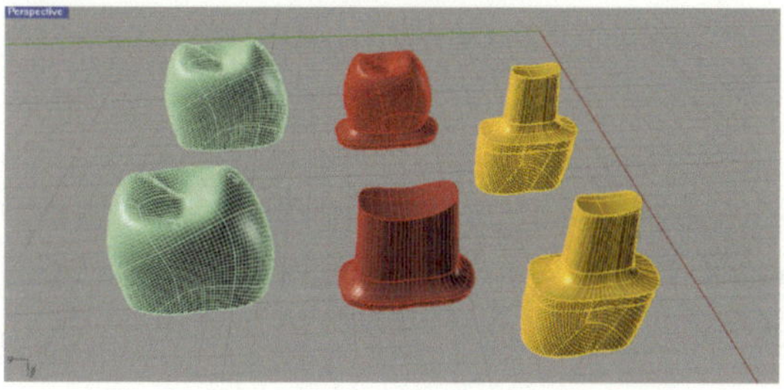

Figure 9. Tooth preparations and overlying restorations.

For the structural simulations, the Young's modulus and Poisson's ratio were entered into the computer soft: Young's modulus (GPa): 18 for dentin, 64 for veneering ceramics, and 205 for zirconia; Poisson's ratio 0.27 for dentin, 0.21 for veneering ceramics, and 0.31 for zirconia. Five loading areas were defined on the occlusal surface, each with a diameter of 0.5 mm. A total force of 600 N was applied as pressure load normal to the surface in each point. The bottom of the teeth models was constrained in all directions, for all simulations.

A static structural analysis was performed, in order to generate stress distribution for all designs taken into the study. Maximal equivalent stresses were recorded in the tooth structures and in the restorations for all preparation types (**Figures 10** and **11**).

For all cases, the stress values were higher in the veneers. Regarding the distribution, in the veneers, stresses were located around the contact areas with the antagonists. In the frameworks, maximal equivalent stress values were higher for the cutback design, but for interpretation, they have to be correlated with the thicknesses of the frameworks. The outer geometry of all-ceramic restorations is strongly defined by anatomical and physiological circumstances, and therefore, the thickness is variable.

However, a modification of the framework design does not affect the outer shape and thickness of the restoration which means that a thicker framework automatically results in a thinner veneering and vice versa.

Therefore, the models were created with constant outer shape, where the framework thickness was chosen to be either constant or anatomically optimized [38].

Different studies indicated core and veneer designs that minimize tensile loading of porcelain. They investigated the effect of differential coping designs on the stress distribution of all-ceramic crowns under varying loads. The hypothesis of whether a customized coping design could reduce the stress on veneers is partially accepted [39].

Mechanical testing of anatomic core design modification revealed a significant increase in the reliability of the coping design and resulted in reduced chip sizes in the veneer porcelain [40].

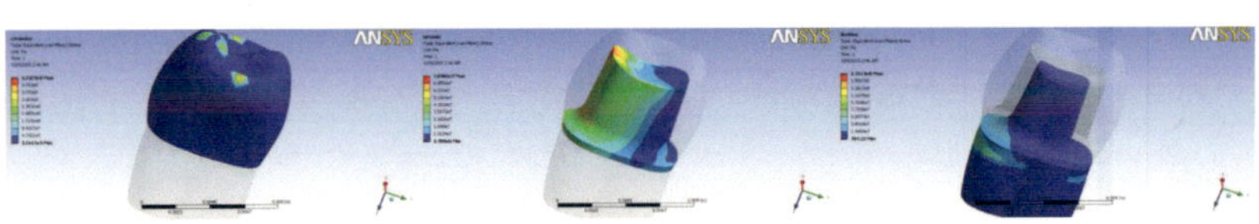

Figure 10. Von Mises equivalent stress distribution in model 1.

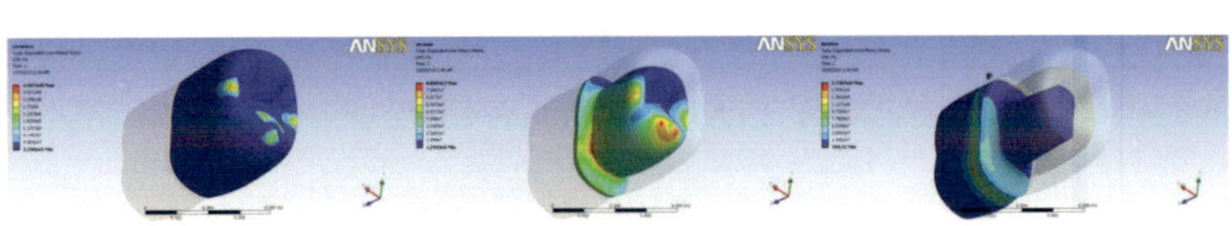

Figure 11. Von Mises equivalent stress distribution in model 2.

Based on the results, chipping seems to be a phenomenon, which is not limited to zirconia restorations, but to the design of the substructure. The chipping failures of all-ceramic zirconia crowns can be significantly reduced in number and surface by fabricating optimized zirconia substructures. These have to provide occlusal support and similar layer thickness for the veneering porcelain [17].

The results showed that not only the substructure design but also the application technique and type of veneering material influenced the chipping behavior of zirconia molar crowns [41].

Some authors investigated the influence of framework design and framework material on the stress distribution in a single tooth restoration, also under different mastication scenarios using the finite element method. The results presented here show that a cusp-supporting framework design can significantly decrease maximum tensile stresses in the veneering material of single crowns. Therefore, it can be expected that such a design could decrease the risk of chipping in all-ceramic restorations in vivo [38].

Use of controlled veneer application techniques, such as the press technique, as well as minimizing stress during the firing conditions may constitute one possibility to reduce cracking and chipping failures. However, only in combination with an anatomically reduced substructure design and a constant layer of the veneering porcelain, the number and dimension of failures (chippings, cracks) are likely to be effectively reduced [41].

4. Simulation methods applied in monolithic ceramic crowns

Zirconia is considered a proper material for posterior teeth restoration, because of the excellent esthetic quality, biocompatibility, and mechanical properties. Thus, zirconia is getting attention to replace existing ceramic systems. Processing of zirconia is closely linked to the development of CAD/CAM systems [42–44]. CAD/CAM technology has been increasingly used to fabricate dental crowns in recent years. It resulted in new restorative materials that would otherwise have been infeasible to use in the dental market, like Yttria-Stabilized Tetragonal Zirconia Polycrystals (Y-TZP). Recently, the introduction of new computerized milling technologies and new zirconia made it possible to manufacture full-contour zirconia crowns with higher strength [45–47]. Several manufacturers have improved the aesthetics of the zirconia materials mainly by reducing the opacity of the material and by addition of coloring pigments. It might also be assumed that, by omitting the veneering, a more solid framework can be made and a conservative preparation similar to full-cast metal-alloy restorations can be performed [48].

Monolithic crowns offer advantages compared to bilayered crowns like reduced production time and related improved cost effectiveness. Because crown preparation involves traumatization to the vital tooth, eliminating the veneering material in monolithic crowns allows to achieve minimally invasive preparations and subsequent restorations [49–51].

Finite element analysis is a specific method for stress analyses. Since it was developed, it has been a popular option to analyze stresses in engineering field. In dentistry, FEA has been introduced to study stress distributions in the teeth structures and all kind of restorations [52–54]. Even computer-controlled techniques are used in producing dental crowns in order to improve the accuracy during the manufacturing process, not enough studies have been conducted on stresses in esthetic monolithic crowns regarding the load values. Therefore, it is advisable to compare the stresses in anatomic contour zirconia crown to that of glass ceramic crown regarding the load values, from biomechanical point of view [55]. For the experimental analyses, first upper molars were chosen in order to simulate the biomechanical behavior of the teeth restored with complete esthetic monolithic crowns made of yttria-stabilized tetragonal zirconia polycrystals and glass ceramic. The prepared dies were designed with a chamfer finishing line and an 6° occlusal convergence angle of the axial walls.

Geometric models of monolithic crowns were designed to occupy the space between the original obtained tooth form and the modeled prepared tooth form. At first, a nonparametric modeling software (Blender 2.57b) was used to obtain the 3D tooth shapes. The collected data were used to construct 3D models using Rhinoceros modeling program (McNeel North America) (Nonuniform Rational B-Splines). These were imported in the FEA software ANSYS; meshed and finite element calculations were carried out. In order to simulate stress distribution and calculate stress values, the Young's modulus and Poisson's ratio were introduced: Young's modulus (GPa) 18 for dentin, 64 for glass ceramic, and 205 for zirconia and Poisson's ratio 0.27 for dentin, 0.21 for glass ceramic, and 0.31 for zirconia. Five loading areas were defined on the occlusal surface, in order to simulate physiological mastication behavior. Each defined loading area had a diameter of 0.5 mm. A total force between 200 N, respective 800 N was allocated to these areas as pressure load normal to the surface in each point. For all simulations, the bottom of the abutment teeth models was constrained in all directions. A static structural analysis was performed using the computer-aided engineering software, to calculate stress values and highlight stress distribution. First principal stresses were recorded in the tooth structures and in the restorations for all load values and all geometries. Stresses were calculated in the crowns for both materials and in the teeth structures, under different load values (**Figures 12** and **13**).

Between the materials, the highest stresses were recorded in glass ceramic, followed by zirconia. In the dentin, the lowest stresses were recorded for the teeth restored with glass ceramic, followed by zirconia. Compared to the tensile strength of the materials, 745 MPa for zirconia,

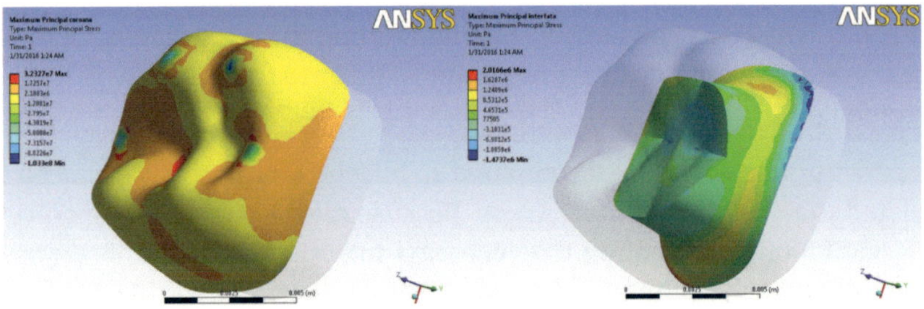

Figure 12. First principal stress distribution in the zirconia crowns and subjacent dentin (for 200 N load).

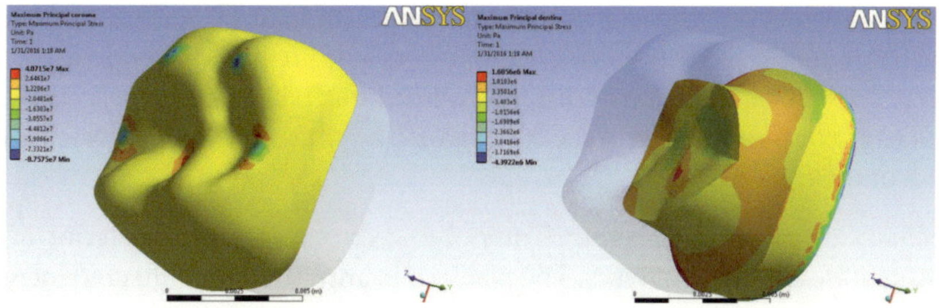

Figure 13. First principal stress distribution in the glass ceramic crowns and subjacent dentin (for 200 N load).

and 48.8 MPa for glass ceramic, the maximal principal stresses in the crowns exceed them for 600 N and 800 N load for zirconia crowns, respective for 400 N, 600 N, and 800 N load for glass ceramic crowns. The maximal principal stresses in the crowns do not exceed the strength of the materials in case of 200 N load for both studied materials. For glass ceramic at a load of 400 N, maximal principal stresses exceed the tensile strength value of the material.

Regarding stress distribution in the crowns, high stresses are concentrated around the contact areas with the antagonists, and they are larger for the zirconia crowns. In the dentin for molars, high stresses were distributed around the shoulder, and under the preparation line for all type of restorations.

The material is important to withstand increased loads which occur during functions. Reported loads during normal function in vivo vary considerably. It is not stated how these loads should be replicated in vitro. Some authors use lower loads, 100–200 N, others use loads in the range of 500–800 N [56].

According to the literature data [57] that the tensile strengths of dentin ranged from 44.4 to 97.8 MPa, no harmful effects occur in hard teeth structures, because in all cases, first principal stresses in dentin are much lower.

When compared with some reported clinical failure rates, it can be stated that the theoretical predictions showed relevant quantitative values for some materials. Even though there are some differences in assumptions between clinical and theoretical models, they can be justified and an even more accurate prediction tool for single crowns may be developed by incorporating better mechanical models in the future [58].

5. Conclusions and perspectives

In current practice, frameworks of all-ceramic restorations are obtained by milling even thickness copies, rather than using a scientific-based design. The recent possibility of the softs of the CAD/CAM systems to scan the bite-registration allows achieving an improved digital design for the framework, through the control of the final veneer thickness in case of cutback design and of the contacts with the antagonists in case of buccal veneering.

The effect of zirconia copings design on the resistance to load in posterior crowns in order to prevent "chipping" is very important. Finite element analyses provide a biomechanical explanation of the clinical behavior of different all-ceramic bilayer crowns. A cusp-supporting design reduces maximum stresses in the framework, but these have to be correlated also with the thickness of the framework.

The biomechanical behavior of ceramic monolithic crowns for the posterior areas can be assessed using finite element analyses. The material is important to withstand increased loads which occur during functions.

Stress values and distribution results can provide design guidelines for new and varied esthetic crowns, in order to withstand functional loads in the posterior areas. The development of well-designed experiments could be useful to help to predict clinical survival of these new all-ceramic restorative techniques and materials. The experiments have to be conducted and interpreted reported to the brittle behavior of ceramic systems. Varied simulation methods are promising to assess the biomechanical behavior of all-ceramic systems and first principal stress criterion is an alternative for ceramic materials investigations.

Acknowledgements

This work was supported by a grant of the Romanian National Authority for Scientific Research and Innovation CNCS-UEFISCDI, project number PN-II-RU-TE-2014-4-0476.

Author details

Liliana Porojan[1*], Florin Topală[2] and Sorin Porojan[3]

*Address all correspondence to: lilianasandu@gmail.com

1 Department of Dental Prostheses Technology, School of Dentistry, "V. Babes" University of Medicine and Pharmacy, Timisoara, Romania

2 Department of Dental Prosthodontics, School of Dentistry, "V. Babes" University of Medicine and Pharmacy, Timisoara, Romania

3 Department of Oral Rehabilitation, School of Dentistry, "V. Babes" University of Medicine and Pharmacy, Timisoara, Romania

References

[1] Zhang Y, Mai Z, Barani A, Bush M, Lawn B. Fracture-resistant monolithic dental crowns. Dental Materials Journal. 2016;**32**(3):442-449. DOI: 10.1016/j.dental.2015.12.010

[2] Kokubo Y, Tsumita M, Kano T, Fukushima S. The influence of zirconia coping designs on the fracture load of all-ceramic molar crowns. Dental Materials Journal. 2011;**30**(3):281-285. DOI: 10.4012/dmj.2010-130

[3] Sornsuwan T, Ellakwa A, Swain MV. Occlusal geometrical considerations in all-ceramic pre-molar crown failure testing. Dental Materials Journal. 2011;**27**(11):1127-1134. DOI: 10.1016/j.dental.2011.08.005

[4] Ferrari M, Giovannetti A, Carrabba M, Bonadeo G, Rengo C, Monticelli F, Vichi A. Fracture resistance of three porcelain-layered CAD/CAM zirconia frame designs. Dental Materials Journal. 2014;**30**(7):e163–e168. DOI: 10.1016/j.dental.2014.02.004

[5] Erdemir A, Guess TM, Halloran J, Tadepalli SC, Morrison TM. Considerations for reporting finite element analysis studies in biomechanics. Journal of Biomechanics. 2012;**45**(4):625-633. DOI: 10.1016/j.jbiomech.2011.11.038

[6] Ehrenberg D, Weiner GI, Weiner S. Long-term effects of storage and thermal cycling on the marginal adaptation of provisional resin crowns: A pilot study. Journal of Prosthetic Dentistry. 2006;**95**:230-236. DOI: 10.1016/j.prosdent.2005.12.012

[7] Porojan L, Porojan S, Cernescu A, Savencu C. Fracture behaviour of hot-pressed glass ceramic dental crowns. International Journal of Systems Applications, Engineering & Development. 2016;**10**:266-269

[8] Beuer F, Aggstaller H, Edelhoff D, Gernet W. Effect of preparation design on the fracture resistance of zirconia crown copings. Dental Materials Journal. 2008;**27**(3):362-367. DOI: 10.4012/dmj.27.362

[9] Omori S, Komada W, Yoshida K, Miura H. Effect of thickness of zirconia-ceramic crown frameworks on strength and fracture pattern. Dental Materials Journal. 2013;**32**(1):189-194. DOI: 10.4012/dmj.2012-255

[10] Urapepon S, Taenguthai P. The effect of zirconia framework design on the failure of all-ceramic crown under static loading. Journal of Advanced Prosthodontics. 2015;**7**:146-150. DOI: 10.4047/jap.2015.7.2.146

[11] Quinn GD, Giuseppetti AA, Hoffman KH. Chipping fracture resistance of dental CAD/CAM restorative materials: Part 2. Phenomenological model and the effect of indenter type. Dental Materials. 2014;**30**(5):99-111. DOI: 10.1016/j.dental.2014.02.014

[12] Fan R, Jin X. Controllable edge feature sharpening for dental applications. Computational and Mathematical Methods in Medicine. 2014;**2014**:873635. DOI: 10.1155/2014/873635

[13] Porojan S, Porojan L, Savencu C. Improved core design for CAD/CAM all ceramic crowns. International Journal of Chemical and Environmental Engineering. 2015;**6**:386-390

[14] Silva NR, Bonfante EA, Rafferty BT, Zavanelli RA, Rekow ED, Thompson VP, et al. Modified Y-TZP core design improves all-ceramic crown reliability. Journal of Dental Research. 2011;**90**(1):104-108. DOI: 10.1177/0022034510384617

[15] Tinschert J, Schulze KA, Natt G, Latzke P, Heussen N, Spiekermann H. Clinical behavior of zirconia-based fixed partial dentures made of DC-Zirkon: 3-year results. International Journal of Prosthodontics. 2008;**21**:217-222

[16] Marchack BW, Futatsuki Y, Marchack CB, White SN. Customization of milled zirconia copings for all-ceramic crowns: A clinical report. Journal of Prosthetic Dentistry. 2008;**99**:169-173. DOI: 10.1016/S0022-3913(08)00028-0

[17] Rosentritt M, Steiger D, Behr M, Handel G, Kolbeck C. Influence of substructure design and spacer settings on the in vitro performance of molar zirconia crowns. Journal of Dentistry. 2009;**37**:978-983. DOI: 10.1016/j.jdent.2009.08.003

[18] Silva NR, Bonfante EA, Zavanelli RA, Thompson VP, Ferencz JL, Coelho PG. Reliability of metalloceramic and zirconia-based ceramic crowns. Journal of Dental Research. 2010;**89**:1051-1056. DOI: 10.1177/0022034510375826

[19] Fischer J, Stawarzcyk B, Trottmann A, Hämmerle CH. Impact of thermal misfit onshear strength of veneering ceramic/zirconia composites. Dental Materials. 2009;**25**:419-423. DOI: 10.1016/j.dental.2008.09.003

[20] Rues S, Kröger E, Müller D, Schmitter M. Effect of firing protocols on cohesive failure of all-ceramic crowns. Journal of Dentistry. 2010;**38**:987-994. DOI: 10.1016/j.jdent.2010.08.014

[21] Silva NR, Bonfante E, Rafferty BT, Zavanelli RA, Martins LL, Rekow ED, et al. Conventional and modified veneered zirconia vs. metalloceramic: Fatigue and finite element analysis. Journal of Prosthodontics. 2012;**21**:433-439. DOI: 10.1111/j.1532-849X.2012.00861.x

[22] Coelho PG, Bonfante EA, Silva NR, Rekow ED, Thompson VP. Laboratory simulation of Y-TZP all-ceramic crown clinical failures. Journal of Dental Research. 2009;**88**:382-386. DOI: 10.1177/0022034509333968

[23] Rosentritt M, Siavikis G, Behr M, Kolbeck C, Handel G. Approach for evaluating the significance of laboratory simulation. Journal of Dentistry. 2008;**36**:1048-1053. DOI: 10.1016/j.dental.2008.08.009

[24] Fehér A, Filser F, Gauckler LJ, Lüthy H, Hämmerle CH. Five-year clinical results of zirconia frameworks for posterior fixed partial dentures. International Journal of Prosthodontics. 2007;**20**(4):383-388. DOI: 10.1007/s00784-011-0575-2

[25] Beuer F, Edelhoff D, Gernet W, Sorensen JA. Three-year clinical prospective evaluation of zirconia-based posterior fixed dental prostheses (FDPs). Clinical Oral Investigations. 2009;**13**(4):445-451. DOI: 10.1007/s00784-009-0249-5

[26] Rosentritt M, Behr M, van der Zel JM, Feilzer AJ. Approach for evaluating the influence of laboratory simulation. Dental Materials. 2009;**25**(3):348-352. DOI: 10.1016/j.dental.2008.08.009

[27] Preis V, Behr M, Hahnel S, Handel G, Rosentritt M. In vitro failure and fracture resistance of veneered and full-contour zirconia restorations. Journal of Dentistry. 2012;**40**:921-928. DOI: 10.1016/j.jdent.2012.07.010

[28] Preis V, Behr M, Handel G, Schneider-Feyrer S, Hahnel S, Rosentritt M. Wear performance of dental ceramics after grinding and polishing treatments. Journal of the Mechanical Behavior of Biomedical Materials. 2012;**10**:13-22. DOI: 10.1016/j.jmbbm.2012.03.002

[29] Beuer F, Stimmelmayr M, Gueth JF, Edelhoff D, Naumann M. In vitro performance of full-contour zirconia single crowns. Dental Materials. 2011;**28**:449-456. DOI: 10.1016/j.dental.2011.11.024

[30] Sailer I, Gottnerb J, Kanelb S, Hammerle CH. Randomized controlled clinical trial of zirconia-ceramic and metal-ceramic posterior fixed dental prostheses: A 3-year follow-up. Journal of Prosthodontics. 2009;**22**:553-560

[31] Pjetursson BE, Sailer I, Zwahlen M, Hämmerle CH. A systematic review of the survival and complication rates of all-ceramic and metal-ceramic reconstructions after an observation period of at least 3 years. Part I: Single crowns. Clinical Oral Implants Research. 2007;**18**:73-85. DOI: 10.1111/j.1600-0501.2007.01467.x

[32] Swain MV. Unstable cracking (chipping) of veneering porcelain on all-ceramic dental crowns and fixed partial dentures. Acta Biomaterialia. 2009;**5**:1668-1677. DOI: 10.1016/j.actbio.2008.12.016

[33] Taskonak B, Borges GA, Mecholsky JJ Jr, Anusavice KJ, Moore BK, Yan J. The effects of viscoelastic parameters on residual stress development in a zirconia/glass bilayer dental ceramic. Dental Materials. 2008;**24**:1149-1155. DOI: 10.1016/j.dental.2008.01.004

[34] Guazzato M, Walton TR, Franklin W, Davis G, Bohl C, Klineberg I. Influence of thickness and cooling rate on development of spontaneous cracks in porcelain/zirconia structures. Australian Dental Journal. 2010;**55**:306-310. DOI: 10.1111/j.1834-7819.2010.01239.x

[35] Zarone F, Russo S, Sorrentino R. From porcelain-fused-to-metal to zirconia: Clinical and experimental considerations. Dental Materials. 2011;**27**:83-96. DOI: 10.1016/j.dental.2010.10.024

[36] Möllers K, Pätzold W, Parkot D, Kirsten A, Güth JF, Edelhoff D, Fischer H. Influence of connector design and material composition and veneering on the stress distribution of all-ceramic fixed dental prostheses: A finite element study. Dental Materials. 2011;**27**:171-175

[37] Porojan L, Topală F, Porojan S. Effect of 3D core design on stresses in all ceramic crowns. International Journal of Chemical and Environmental Engineering. 2015;**6**:381-385

[38] Kirsten A, Parkot D, Raith S, Fischer H. A cusp supporting framework design can decrease critical stresses in veneered molar crowns. Dental Materials. 2014;**30**:321-326. DOI: 10.1016/j.dental.2013.12.004

[39] Hua J, Daib N, Baob Y, Gua W, Maa J, Zhanga FM. Effect of different coping designs on all-ceramic crown stress distribution: A finite element analysis. Dental Materials. 2013;**29**:291-298. DOI: 10.1016/j.dental.2013.09.001

[40] Guess PC, Bonfante EA, Silva NR, Coelho PG, Thompson VP. Effect of core design and veneering technique on damage and reliability of Y-TZP-supported crowns. Dental Materials. 2013;**29**(3):307-316. DOI: 10.1016/j.dental.2012.11.012

[41] Preis V, Letsch C, Handel G, Behr M, Schneider-Feyrer S, Rosentritt M. Influence of substructure design, veneer application technique, and firing regime on the in vitro performance of molar zirconia crowns. Dental Materials. 2013;**29**:113-121. DOI: 10.1016/j.dental.2013.04.011

[42] Ji MK, Park JH, Park SW, Yun KD, Oh GJ, Lim HP. Evaluation of marginal fit of 2 CAD-CAM anatomic contour zirconia crown systems and lithium disilicate glass-ceramic crown. Journal of Advanced Prosthodontics. 2015;**7**(4):271-277. DOI: 10.4047/jap.2015.7.4.271

[43] Filser F, Kocher P, Weibel F, Lüthy H, Schärer P, Gauckler LJ. Reliability and strength of all-ceramic dental restorations fabricated by direct ceramic machining (DCM). International Journal of Computerized Dentistry. 2001;**4**:89-106

[44] Conrad HJ, Seong WJ, Pesun IJ. Current ceramic materials and systems with clinical recommendations: A systematic review. Journal of Prosthetic Dentistry. 2007;**98**:389-404. DOI: 10.1016/S0022-3913(07)60124-3

[45] Baig MR, Tan KB, Nicholls JI. Evaluation of the marginal fit of a zirconia ceramic computer-aided machined (CAM) crown system. Journal of Prosthetic Dentistry. 2010;**104**:216-227. DOI: 10.1016/S0022-3913(10)60128-X

[46] Preis V, Behr M, Kolbeck C, Hahnel S, Handel G, Rosentritt M. Wear performance of substructure ceramics and veneering porcelains. Dental Materials. 2011;**27**:796-804. DOI: 10.1016/j.dental.2011.04.001

[47] Jung YS, Lee JW, Choi YJ, Ahn JS, Shin SW, Huh JB. A study on the in-vitro wear of the natural tooth structure by opposing zirconia or dental porcelain. Journal of Advanced Prosthodontics. 2010;**2**:111-115. DOI: 10.4047/jap.2010.2.3.111

[48] Mitov G, Anastassova-Yoshida Y, Nothdurft FP, von See C, Pospiech P. Influence of the preparation design and artificial aging on the fracture resistance of monolithic zirconia crowns. Journal of Advanced Prosthodontics. 2016;**8**(1):30-36. DOI: 10.4047/jap.2016.8.1.30

[49] Nordahl N, Vult von Steyern P, Larsson C. Fracture strength of ceramic monolithic crown systems of different thickness. Journal of Oral Science. 2015;**57**(3):255-261. DOI: 10.2334/josnusd.57.255

[50] Johansson C, Kmet G, Rivera J, Larsson C, Vult von Steyern P. Fracture strength of monolithic all-ceramic crowns made of high translucent yttrium oxide-stabilized zirconium dioxide compared to porcelain-veneered crowns and lithium disilicate crowns. Acta Odontologica Scandinavica. 2014;**72**:145-153. DOI: 10.3109/00016357.2013.822098

[51] Mjör IA. Pulp-dentin biology in restorative dentistry. Part 2: Initial reactions to preparation of teeth for restorative procedures. Quintessence International. 2001;**32**:537-551

[52] Ha SR. Biomechanical three-dimensional finite element analysis of monolithic zirconia crown with different cement type. Journal of Advanced Prosthodontics. 2015;**7**(6):475-483. DOI: 10.4047/jap.2015.7.6.475

[53] Ha SR, Kim SH, Han JS, Yoo SH, Jeong SC, Lee JB, Yeo IS. The influence of various core designs on stress distribution in the veneered zirconia crown: A finite element analysis study. Journal of Advanced Prosthodontics. 2013;**5**:187-197. DOI: 10.4047/jap.2013.5.2.187

[54] Li X, Cao Z, Qiu X, Tang Z, Gong L, Wang D. Does matching relation exist between the length and the tilting angle of terminal implants in the all-on-four protocol? Stress distributions by 3D finite element analysis. Journal of Advanced Prosthodontics. 2015;**7**:240-248. DOI: 10.4047/jap.2015.7.3.240

[55] Porojan L, Topală F, Porojan S. Load values influence on stresses in monolithic ceramic molar crowns. International Journal of Theoretical and Applied Mechanics. 2016;**1**:165-169

[56] Kohorst P, Dittmer MP, Borchers L, Stiesch-Scholz M. Influence of cyclic fatigue in water on the load-bearing capacity of dental bridges made of zirconia. Acta Biomaterialia. 2008;**4**:1440-1447. DOI: 10.1016/j.actbio.2008.04.012

[57] Staninec M, Marshall GW, Hilton JF, Pashley DH, Gansky SA, Marshall SJ, Kinney JH. Ultimate tensile strength of dentin: Evidence for a damage mechanics approach to dentin failure. Journal of Biomedical Materials Research. 2002;**63**(3):342-345. DOI: 10.1002/jbm.10230

[58] Lekesiz H. Reliability estimation for single-unit ceramic crown restorations. Journal of Dental Research. 2014;**93**(9):923-928. DOI: 10.1177/0022034514544215

Section 4

Research Guidelines on Oral Health Promotion

Chapter 10

Oral Health Promotion: Evidences and Strategies

Vikram R. Niranjan, Vikas Kathuria,
Venkatraman J and Arpana Salve

Additional information is available at the end of the chapter

http://dx.doi.org/10.5772/intechopen.69330

Abstract

Oral health promotion is for upliftment of oral health of community rather than an individual and has long-term impact. Since Ottawa Charter for health promotion is implemented, significant advancements have happened in oral health promotion. Under comprehensive health programs, India has been running oral health promotion programs, and these evidences are shared here. Such examples are apt learning and execution to any part of world having similarities. The chapter put forward the strategic view points to consider further oral health promotion aspects and based on the needs. The authors have gathered various examples from national programs implemented in India. The authors discuss how these programs are linked to the Oral health promotion concept. For example, National tobacco control program which currently running across many states in India, how the banning on tobacco products near school premises helped to reduce the incidence is discussed. The worldwide literature and evidences of oral health promotion strategies are explained. The evidences and strategies mentioned can be significant for another region of world. Unless published, many programs remain hidden and are loss of valuable evidences to oral health science.

Keywords: oral health, oral health promotion, fluorosis, school health, dental health

1. Introduction

The twentieth century was noteworthy in dentistry for many epidemiologic advances that occurred in the study of oral diseases and conditions. These combined efforts of optimum personal, social, biological, behavioral and environmental factors contributed to better oral health. Hence, oral health promotion is a planned effort to build public policies, create supportive environments, strengthen community action, develop personal skills or reorient health services pertaining to influence above factors. Following are enlisted examples of effective oral health promotion:

- Promotion of healthy eating
- Training of relevant oral hygiene methods
- Access to preventive oral health services at the earliest
- Promotion of topical fluoride application [1].

Ottawa Charter principles form a sound base for oral health promotion. This suggest that individuals alone are not at risk but the entire population, which needs to be involved in directing action towards the causes of ill health. Importantly, three principles, that is, partnership, participation and protection, are taken into consideration while planning a public health program or intervention. Empowerment than compelling is the key for successful Oral health promotion while achieving good oral health [2].

The purpose of this article is threefold. First, it reviews the relevance of need of oral health promotion particularly through the public health surveillance of oral disease burden. Second, it puts forward the evidences from the various examples of oral health promotion programs integrated into general health promotion carried across the India. Finally, the authors briefly discuss the strategies for expanding frame of oral health promotion.

2. Oral health promotion through Ottawa Charter

Health promotion programs achieve success through actions that influence the social, physical, economic and political determinants of health. Health promotion irrefutably acknowledges the broader health determinants and focuses on risk reduction via sensitive policies and actions. Ideally, promotion of health in a day-to-day life setting having people live, work, learn and play is credible for efficacious and cost-effective way of improving oral health and indeed the quality of life. Imperatively, actions that address the determinants of health should not be progressed in isolation. Research evidences suggests that isolated activities can have limited impact, particularly over the long term. For this reason, we suggest using the logic model based on Ottawa Charter to develop a comprehensive oral health promotion program, involving a range of interventions.

The Ottawa Charter was developed by the World Health Organization[1] (WHO) as a framework for constructing health promotion programs that address the wider determinants of health. The charter suggests that programs be built around the following five action areas:

- Building healthy public policy
- Creating supportive environments

[1]WHO = World Health Organization.

http://dx.doi.org/10.5772/intechopen.69330

- Strengthening community action
- Developing personal skills
- Reorientating health services [2].

3. Need for oral health promotion

The remarkable improvements in oral health over the past half century reflect the strong science base for prevention of oral diseases that has been developed and applied in the community, in clinical practice and in the home. Yet, despite the remarkable achievements in recent decades, millions of people worldwide have been excluded from the benefits of socioeconomic development and the scientific advances that have improved health care and quality of life. Social and cultural determinants comprising poverty, lack of education, unsupportive traditions, cultures and beliefs increase the relative risk of oral disease and conditions. For instance, lack of safe water and sanitary facilities are the environmental risk factors for both oral and general health. While, access to high sugar containing foods and unhealthy dietary habits may lead to higher risk of dental caries in certain communities. Improvement in availability, accessibility and feasibility of oral health services can definitely cure and control oral diseases. However, strong evidences suggest that limiting the risks to disease is best possible when health services are primary care and prevention oriented. Clinically, oral health status is measured in terms of causal factors, that is, tobacco, sugar, micro-flora, which have negative impact on quality of life. Emphasizing the risk behavior modifications, such as curbing use of tobacco and alcohol; restraining sugar intake in terms of quantity, intake frequency and nature; proper oral hygiene practices, is equally important incongruent to social and cultural determinants [3].

The Global Burden of Disease (GBD) 2010 Study produced comparable estimates of the burden of 291 diseases and injuries in 1990, 2005 and 2010. Pertaining to oral health, dental caries, aggressive periodontitis and tooth loss are considered as global burden, which compared from 1990 to 2010. Criteria used were disability adjusted life-years (DALYs) and years lived with disability (YLDs) metrics to quantify burden. These oral diseases/conditions encroached 3.9 billion. Among all, prevalence of dental caries in permanent teeth was among the highest prevalent condition evaluated for the entire GBD 2010 study (global prevalence of 35% for all ages combined). Among the top 100 ranking as causes of DALYs, oral diseases also secured a ranking after some serious diseases. Oral diseases altogether affected 15 million DALYs globally with the breakdown as 1.9% of all YLDs; 0.6% of all DALYs. Statistical calculations imply that could be average health loss of 224 years *per* 100,000 populations. While there was reduction observed for other diseases from 1990 to 2010, DALYs due to oral conditions increased by 20.8%. This was due to population overgrowth and aging. DALYs due to aggressive periodontitis and dental caries increased, however due to extensive tooth loss has decreased. While DALYs differed by age groups and regions, those not by genders. The report revealed the challenging scenario of diversified oral health needs across the globe, with alarming needs in developing countries. Further, the burden of oral diseases has unevenly risen in the past 20 years.

As the noted prevalence of oral diseases is very high and has association with disability, it accounted for a substantial number of DALYs. Dental caries without any treatment was the most prevalent condition among all 291 conditions. Moreover, the disability weight in connection with extensive tooth loss (0.073) was marginally neared to those reported for moderate heart failure (0.068) and moderate consequences of stroke (0.074). Oral diseases received ranking of 31st, 34th and 35th of health outcomes causing YLDs in the category of non-fatal outcomes. Compared to other non-communicable diseases/conditions, such as maternal conditions, hypertensive heart disease, schizophrenia, hemoglobinopathies and hemolytic anemias, oral diseases/conditions were ranked higher. While oral conditions scored high index for more YLDs than 25 of 28 categories of cancer, shows its significance in terms of affecting individuals equal to lethal diseases. The other organ cancers, such as stomach, liver and trachea, and bronchus and lung cancers ranked higher than oral diseases [4].

The global burden of oral conditions is shifting from extensive tooth loss toward aggressive periodontitis and untreated dental caries. Tooth loss is a final common pathway when preventive or conservative treatments to alleviate pain fail or are unavailable. The social, economic, political and cultural determinants of health are significant, and it may be argued that better health can be achieved by reducing poverty. Poverty, poor education and inequality not only result in poor oral health but also affect the way in which people think about their oral health. In spite of excellent oral health care, oral diseases are prevalent. This suggests that improving healthcare services merely will not address the issue, oral health promotion is mandatory. Hence, health policymakers should be made aware of these evidences and directs themselves to restructure the policy framework. Health promotion policy acknowledges complimentary measures such as legislation, fiscal measures, taxation and organizational change altogether. These are best example of a coordinated effort towards creating supportive environments and strengthening community action. Ottawa Charter implementation for health promotion through establishing concrete and effective community actions in setting priorities, making decisions, planning strategies leads to achieve better health. Communities facilitate themselves with self-help, social support, participation and ownership for development and empowerment. They are the best possible existing human and material resources of community and for community.

Oral health promotion through sensitive health policies and actions which already exist in some parts of world can address the global burden of oral diseases, essentially to improve oral health and quality of life.

4. Evidences: country examples from India

Identifying a significant health issue on the basis of prevalence, incidence, severity, cost, or impact on quality of life is preliminary step to design prevention programs. A combination of community, professional and individual strategies is the cost-effective and creative methods for oral disease prevention. Incorporating public, practitioners and policymakers into strategic development of oral disease prevention and health promotion intervention is necessary. They should be liable to create a healthy setting, limit risk factors, inform target groups, generate knowledge and thus improve behaviors. This section includes a discussion of knowledge and practices of the public and healthcare providers regarding the oral health promotion. The purpose of this discussion is not to outline specific health promotion strategies to enhance knowledge and practices but to indicate the opportunities and needs for both broad-based and targeted health promotion programs and activities.

4.1. Oral health promotion in health promoting schools (HPS)

Oral health education has been considered as one of the fundamentals in oral health promotion [5, 6]. With education, a child receives training and encouragement especially to stimulate development of skills, aptitude formation and creation of values, which lead to act positively in relation to his oral health and other people's oral health on a daily basis. High caries risk, change in dentition, ability to change bad habits and facilities to learn make oral health promotion for children a priority. The importance of oral health education programs in schools is significantly reported predominantly in the form of positive learning and behavior in children [5–11].

One-fifth of the world's population is adolescent, defined by WHO as a person between 10 and 19 years of age. The oral health promotion programs should primarily focus on this age group who become easy victims of excessive consumption of sweets, sugary beverages, tobacco and alcohol. Commonly, their main association is with home, school and community organizations. These three along with oral health professionals can form an effective alliance to control risks to oral diseases and form oral health promotion programs for young people [12]. Prevalence of dental caries and gingivitis is high in human populations throughout the world, and over 80% of schoolchildren are affected in some parts of the world. Dental erosion due to excessive carbonated beverages consumption is on rise, which was earlier noticed only among the late adulthood. Enamel defects due to malnourishments, dental trauma due to negligence and safety barriers are some of the increasing evidences in children. Moreover, youth became the easy targets of tobacco-containing products. Eventually and unknowingly, early start of tobacco consumption manifolds risks of oral precancerous lesions and cancer in life ahead [8, 10, 13].

Strong arguments for oral health promotion through schools include the following:

- Personal and social education aimed at developing life skills—Pupils and students can be accessed during their formative years, from childhood to adolescence. Students develop lifelong oral health-related behavior, as well as beliefs and attitudes are being developed.
- Schools can provide a supportive environment for promoting oral health. Access to safe water, for example, may allow for general and oral hygiene programs. Also, provision of mouth guards—accessible and affordable sports protection, a safe physical environment and school policy on bullying and violence between students reduce the risk of dental trauma.
- The burden of oral disease in children is significant. Most established oral diseases are irreversible, will last for a lifetime and have an impact on quality of life and general health.
- School policies on control of risk behaviors, such as intake of sugary foods and drinks, tobacco use and alcohol consumption.

- Schools can provide a platform for the provision of oral health care, that is, preventive and curative services [14–18].
- Common risk factor approach-based oral health promotion policies in schools can lead to improvement in oral health and reduce oral health inequality [10, 16].

The need to set up oral health promotion programs in schools is evident, and it can easily be integrated into general health promotion, school curricula and activities. One of the proposed examples has been shown in **Figure 1** [13].

Using the structures and systems already in place as a competent setting for the installation of vital facilities such as safe water and sanitation can instigate oral health promotion in schools. The HPS strategies are effective, leading to potential long-term cost savings. For instance, Each key components of an HPS, that is, *healthy school environment, school health education, school heath services, nutrition and food services, physical exercise and leisure activities, mental health and well-being, health promotion for staff and community relationships and collaboration,* incorporate equal opportunities oral health promotion as well as general health promotion. While oral health issue is specifically addressed, it can be admixed in general health promotion strategy. It is well illustrated in following examples of school health policies as shown in **Table 1** [13].

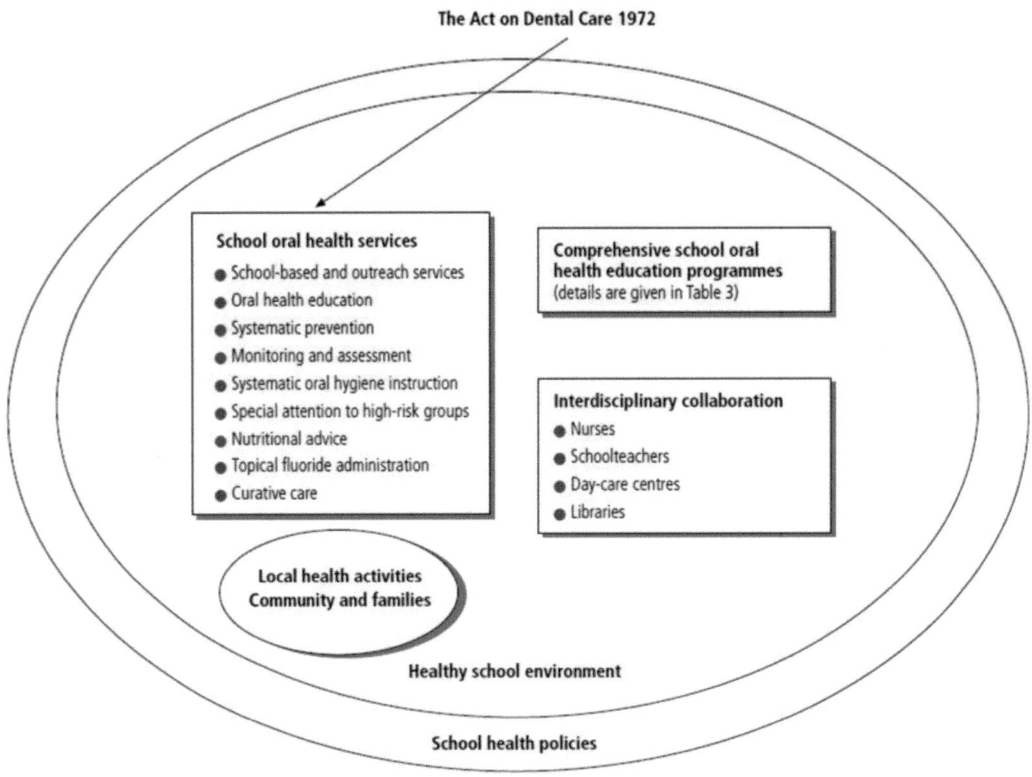
The Act on Dental Care 1972
School oral health services
School-based and outreach services
Oral health education
Systematic prevention
Monitoring and assessment
Systematic oral hygiene instruction
Special attention to high-risk groups
Nutritional advice
Topical fluoride administration
Curative care
Comprehensive school oral health education programmes
(details are given in Table 3)
Interdisciplinary collaboration
Nurses
Schoolteachers
Day-care centres
Libraries
Local health activities
Community and families
Healthy school environment
School health policies

Figure 1. Integration of oral health in health-promoting schools: an example from Denmark.

http://dx.doi.org/10.5772/intechopen.69330

Areas	Cause	Health promoting school measures
Trauma	Sports injury, violence/fights and unsafe playgrounds	*Healthy school environment* • Safe and well-designed school buildings and playgrounds to prevent injuries and avoid "sick building syndrome" • A caring and respectful psychosocial environment • A protocol for dealing with bullying and violent behavior, as well as interpersonal conflicts *Oral injury* • Accident prevention • Clear protocol of vital actions to be taken without delay • Monitoring incidence of oral trauma • A protocol on safe sport, for example, use of mouth guards
Dental caries/ periodontal disease	Sugary diet, lack of oral hygiene	*No sugar* • A ban on sugary foods and drinks on the school premises Policy developmen • The role of school in supporting local health issues, for example, water fluoridation *Oral health education* • Oral health education should form part of all subjects in the school curriculum • Daily supervised tooth brushing drills • Training for parents about good oral health and encouragement for them to take part in health promotion activities at school • Training for school staff
Areas	Cause	Health promoting school measures
Nutritional deficiency/ infections	Malnutrition, lack of adequate food/ knowledge	*Healthy eating* • Healthy foods must be made available in the school canteen, tuck shop, kiosks and vending machines • Only nutritious meals are served in the school canteen • Promotion of 5-a-day (fruit and vegetables) • Drinking water fountains throughout the school • Training for cooks and food providers • Assessment and surveillance of nutritional status • Support for school- or community-based health promotion activities such as breakfast clubs *Control of cross-infection* • Clear guidelines on how to control cross-infection • Training for school staff

Areas	Cause	Health promoting school measures
Areas	Cause	Health promoting school measures
General and oral health	Lack of knowledge, habits, social environment	*Oral health service* • Working closely with central or local oral health service providers • Dealing with dental emergencies • Role of teachers in oral health surveillance, screening and basic treatment, for example, ART • Monitoring of oral health-related complaints and absenteeism. • Training for school staff *Physical exercise* • Commitment to provide safe facilities for training in sport and leisure activities • Exercise and physical education are a compulsory part of the school curriculum

Table 1. Examples of oral health-related school health policies to be promoted in HPS.

There is an association of socio-economic, geographic factors and type of schools with school based health promoting activities. On an average, students attending private schools belong to more advantaged backgrounds than their counterparts in public schools. Privately managed schools achieve greater efficiency or academic value-added than publicly-managed schools [18]. According to one study, ten out of eleven participated countries (including India) had the large socio-economic gap between private and public school pupils except Chile [19]. Moreover, students going to city/town schools generally belonged to more privileged backgrounds than their counterparts in village schools. All the school headmasters in this study reported that primary school student's absenteeism rate decreased when the students received support in the form of school uniforms, textbooks, meals and various financial assistance schemes. For example, urban schools tend to have greater resources than those in rural. Also, students in private schools had higher levels of positive behavior than those in public schools, and these results were statistically significant for most countries [19]. Public and private school differ from each other in many ways as better amenities in school, extra-curricular activities, outdoor and indoor sports, etc. The private school allots more fees from students for such activities/facilities. Consequently, children from upper and high middle socioeconomic status prefer private schools, while children with low socioeconomic strata attend public schools [20]. Students gain more attention when the student to teacher ratio is higher. Bruneforth et al. [19] also reported inferior pupil-teacher ratios in village schools than in city/town schools in India. The children who do not have adult supervision after school are more vulnerable to indulge them into health hazarding habits like smoking, drugs and substance abuse and behavioral problems. The schools providing self care activities after school were found more effective in reducing the prevalence of smoking among ninth-grade students in Los Angeles and San Diego Counties [21]. Smoking and chewing tobacco are systematically associated with socioeconomic markers [20].

4.2. Healthy food at school: Mid Day Meal Scheme of India

The whole school approach with availability of healthy food in school canteen, tuck shops, instructing parents for healthy food and school staff involved in planning for food and curriculum has amplified student's knowledge. However, it has not led to change in behavior [22, 23].

Providing healthy food in schools can meet the nutritional requirement of students and also guide the parents to deal with healthy diet chart for their children. In UK, campaigns like the ones conducted by famous chef, Jamie Oliver, are one example of actions in this area.

In India, Mid Day Meal Scheme in school started in 1925 from a single city, Madras (now Chennai) and now spread to all States. From April 1st, 2008, the program covers all children studying in Government, Local Body and Government-aided primary and upper primary schools across the country. The Mid Day Meal Scheme is the world's largest school feeding program reaching out to 0.84 billion primary students and 0.33 billion upper primary Students, in total about 1.2 billion children in over 9.50 ten thousands schools across the country during 2009–2010 [24].

Unhealthy eating habits and sedentary lifestyles are closely bound not only to various socio-economic indicators such as the parent's education levels, financial resources and professional situations, but also to living in economically deprived areas. This suggests significant contributions of gender, age and religion belief to the eating habit. Therefore, Schools should introduce healthy food policy and activity after consulting with school authority, nutrition expert and parents so as to maintain good eating habits among students [25].

4.3. National tobacco control program of India

Tobacco consumption either in smoke form or smokeless form has deleterious effect general and oral health. Tobacco abuse is the leading preventable cause of death and disease so far. Long list of diseases caused by tobacco abuse includes different cancers – lung cancer, oral cancer, cardiovascular disease, stroke and chronic lung disease. Pertaining to oral health, it causes aggressive periodontitis, tooth loss, wound healing complications and mainly pre-cancerous or cancerous lesion leading to disfigurement of face. Risk of oral cancer is 10-fold in smokers than no-smokers and 11-fold risk in smokeless tobacco users than non-users. One can expect a normal life expectancy with early acknowledgement of tobacco health hazards and culminating tobacco use especially below 35 years. Prevention is the prime key factors, and at initial stage, most of the adverse effects of tobacco are reversible. This fact can be used to motivate tobacco using people to curb the use of tobacco [26].

India is the second largest consumer and producer of tobacco. India accounts for 10% of the world tobacco area and 9% of the production. 30% of cancer deaths, majority of cardiovascular and lung disorders; 40% of tuberculosis and other related diseases are attributed to tobacco consumption. Over 80% of oral cancers are caused due to tobacco use. As per the WHO Global Report on "Tobacco Attributable Mortality" 2012, 7% of all deaths (for ages 30 and over) in India are attributable to tobacco. Ministry of Health and Family Welfare

(MoHFW), Government of India inaugurated *The National Tobacco Control Program (NTCP)* in 2007–2008, as included in 11th five year plan. The program includes objectives as:

- Nationwide awareness regarding tobacco use harms and following tobacco control laws.
- Necessary actions for strong implementation of the Tobacco Control Laws.
    - Effective primordial and primary level prevention strategies are planned under the *National Tobacco Control Program (NTCP).*

The prime areas under the NTCP as targets are:

- Training of trainers, that is, health and social workers, NGOs, school teachers and enforcement officers.
- Information, Education and Communication (IEC) activities.
- School Programs.
- Monitoring tobacco control laws.
- Co-ordination at village level activities.
- Medicinal treatment facility for cessation at district level.

Indian government implemented Cigarette and Other Tobacco Products Act (COTPA; addressing tobacco use in public places, tobacco advertising and sale and packaging regulations) since 2003 with comprehensive action in 2005 following the Framework Convention of Tobacco Control (FCTC). Following laws through the lobbying of anti-tobacco advocates were successfully established by Indian judiciary.

- *Section 4: Prohibition of smoking in public places.*
- *Section 5: Prohibition of direct and indirect advertisement, promotion and sponsorship of cigarette and other tobacco products.*
- *Section 6a: Prohibition of sale of cigarette and other tobacco products to a person below the age of 18 years.*
- *Section 6b: Prohibition of sale of tobacco products within a radius of 100 yards of educational institutions.*
- *Section 7: Mandatory depiction of statutory warnings (including pictorial warnings) on tobacco packs.)*
- *Section 7(5): Display of tar and nicotine contents on tobacco packs* [27].

The achievements of this national program are examples of apt implementation. Increase in taxation had led to a reduction in self-reported tobacco sales and consumption at the short-term end-point. The GATS data (2009) indicate that 54.7 and 62.9% are aware of health warnings on cigarette and smokeless tobacco packaging, respectively. Trials of school-based education interventions demonstrated a positive impact on knowledge, advocacy skills and tobacco use. Teaching about the risks of tobacco use for health professional trainees

http://dx.doi.org/10.5772/intechopen.69330

appeared more widespread, but may have reduced slightly post-FCTC. Community-based education interventions and education interventions for adult tobacco users appeared beneficial. Moreover, the secondary outcomes of tobacco control programs observed as cleaner streets and air quality, preservation of forests, increased performance at school/work, reduction in fire hazards, healthy mother and infants and indeed a better quality of life. Tobacco-use outcomes could be improved by school/community-based and adult education interventions and cessation assistance that are facilitated by training for health professionals and schoolteachers [28].

4.4. National fluorosis prevention program

Fluoride is an essential mineral for human health. It widely exists in natural water and in foods such as tea, fish and beer. The twentieth century documented association among reduced level of dental caries with communal fluoridated water consumption. Soon, fluoride has become an effective preventive measure for dental caries. Easy incorporation into toothpaste has improved oral health in some parts of world, particularly in developing countries [26].

However, the other part of world suffers from excessive fluoride in natural environment. Fluorosis, a public health problem, is caused by excess intake of fluoride through drinking water/food products/industrial emission over a long period. Moderate-level chronic exposure (above 1.5 mg/liter of water–the WHO guideline value for fluoride in water) is more common. Acute high-level exposure to fluoride is rare and usually due to accidental contamination of drinking-water or due to fires or explosions. It results in major health disorders like dental fluorosis, skeletal fluorosis and non-skeletal fluorosis. The late stages of skeletal and dental fluorosis are permanent and irreversible in nature and are detrimental to the health of an individual and the community, which in turn has adverse effects on growth, development & economy of the country. There is no treatment for severe cases of skeletal fluorosis, only efforts can be made towards reducing the disability which has occurred. However, the disease is easily preventable if diagnosed early and steps are taken to prevent intake of excess fluorosis through provision of safe drinking water, promote nutrition and avoid foods with high fluoride content.

Fluorosis is worldwide in distribution and endemic at least in 25 countries. It has been reported from fluoride belts: one that stretches from Syria through Jordan, Egypt, Libya, Algeria, Sudan and Kenya, and another that stretches from Turkey through Iraq, Iran, Afghanistan, India, northern Thailand and China. There are similar belts in the Americas and Japan. In India, fluorosis is mainly due to excessive fluoride in water except in parts of Gujarat and Uttar Pradesh where industrial fluorosis is also seen. The desirable limit of fluoride as per Bureau of Indian Standards (BIS) is 1 ppm (parts per million or 1 mg per liter). High levels of Fluoride were reported in 230 districts of 20 States of India (after bifurcation of Andhra Pradesh in 2014). The population at risk as per population in habitations with high fluoride is 11.7 million as on 1.4.2014. Rajasthan, Gujarat and Andhra Pradesh are worst affected states. Punjab, Haryana, Madhya Pradesh and Maharashtra are moderately affected states, while Tamil Nadu, West Bengal, Uttar Pradesh, Bihar and Assam are mildly affected states.

Understanding the clinical manifestations of fluorosis

- *Dental fluorosis*: It is categorized into mild, moderate and severe dental fluorosis depending on the extent of staining and pitting on the teeth. In severe dental fluorosis, unaesthetic & brittle enamel is found. Vitamins A and D deficiency or a low protein-energy diet are also linked to enamel defects. Ingestion of fluoride after 6 years of age will not cause dental fluorosis. The teeth could be chalky white and may have white, yellow, brown or black spots or streaks on the enamel surface. Discoloration is away from the gums and bilaterally symmetrical.
- *Skeletal fluorosis*: The early symptoms of skeletal fluorosis include stiffness and pain in the joints. In severe cases, the bone structure may change and ligaments may calcify, with resulting impairment of muscles and pain. Constriction of vertebral canal and intervertebral foramen exerts pressure on nerves, blood vessels leading to paralysis and pain.
- *Nonskeletal fluorosis/Effects of fluorosis on soft tissues/systems*:
    - Gastrointestinal symptoms: Abdominal pain, excessive saliva, nausea and vomiting are seen after acute high-level exposure to fluoride.
    - Neurological manifestation: Nervousness and depression, tingling sensation in fingers and toes, excessive thirst and tendency to urinate.
    - Muscular manifestations: Muscle weakness and stiffness, pain in the muscle and loss of muscle power, inability to carry out normal routine activities.
    - Allergic manifestation: Skin rashes, perivascular inflammation—pinkish red or bluish red spot, round or oval shape on the skin that fade and clear up within 7–10 days.
    - Effects on fetus: Fluoride can also damage a fetus, if the mother consumes water/food with high concentrations of fluoride during pregnancy/breast feeding. Abortions, still births and children with birth defects are common in endemic areas.
    - Low hemoglobin levels: Fluoride accumulates on the erythrocyte (red blood cells) membrane, which in turn looses calcium content. The membrane which is deficient in calcium content is pliable and is thrown into folds. The shape of erythrocytes is changed. Such RBCs are called echinocytes and found in circulation. The echinocytes undergo phagocytosis (eaten-up by macrophages) and are eliminated from circulation. This would lead to low hemoglobin levels in patients chronically ill due to fluoride toxicity.
    - Kidney manifestations: Low volume, dark yellow to red color of urine is seen.
    - Calcification of ligaments and blood vessel: Forms unique feature of the disease helps in differential diagnosis.

With an aim to prevent and control fluorosis cases, Government of India initiated the National Program for Prevention and Control of Fluorosis (NPPCF) as a new health initiative in 2008–09. During the 11th Plan, 100 districts from 17 States were identified for program implementation. During the 12th 5-Year Plan period, it is proposed to add another 95 districts for prevention and control of fluorosis. In the 12th Plan, the program has been brought under the Non-Communicable Disease Flexi-pool of National Health Mission (NHM).

4.4.1. Goal and objectives

- To collect, assess and use the baseline survey data of fluorosis of Ministry of Drinking Water Supply for starting the project.
- Comprehensive management of fluorosis in the selected areas.
- Capacity building for prevention, diagnosis and management of fluorosis cases.

4.4.2. Strategy

a. *Surveillance* of fluorosis in the community and school children.

b. *Capacity building* at different level of healthcare delivery system for early detection, management and rehabilitation of fluorosis cases.

c. *Diagnostic facilities* in the form of laboratory support and equipment including ion meter to monitor the fluoride content in water and urinary levels at district/hospital/medical college for early detection and confirmation of fluorosis cases.

d. *Health education* for prevention and control of fluorosis: (a) Creating awareness about fluorosis disease, drinking water (safe/unsafe), diet editing and diet counseling through interpersonal communication, group discussions, media, posters and wall paintings. (b) Create awareness and skills among the medical as well as paramedical health workers to detect the disease in the community. (c) Provision of safe drinking water, water harvesting (rain water) and other measures in collaboration with Public Health Engineering Department.

e. *Management* Efforts are aimed to reduce the fluorosis induced disability and to improve quality of life of affected patients. Medical treatment is mainly supplementation of Vitamins C & D, Calcium, antioxidants and treatment of malnutrition. Treatment of deformity includes physiotherapy, corrective plasters and orthoses (appropriate appliances).

4.4.3. Expected outcome

The expected outcome of the National Program for Prevention & Control of Fluorosis in the districts will be:

a. Number of fluorosis cases managed and rehabilitated in the program districts.

b. Capacity for laboratory testing for fluoride in water, urine to be developed.

c. Trained health sector manpower in Government set up for measuring fluoride in urine and water.

d. Improve information base for the community and all concerned in the program districts [29].

Likewise, fluoride is double edge sword, that is, its deficiency and excess both affect the oral health. Hence, science based on effectiveness, safety and benefits should be implemented at different needs at different part of the world.

5. Strategies for oral health promotion

5.1. Generation of strategies based on evidences

WHO aim at building healthy populations involving all communities by combating every possible illness. The organization has recommended strategic framework which focuses and guide on oral health promotion activities/programs.

- *Reduction in oral disease/condition burden and disability, especially in poor and marginalized populations.*
- *Promoting healthy lifestyles and reducing risk factors to oral health that arise from environmental, economic, social and behavioral causes.*
- *Developing oral health systems that equitably improve oral health outcomes, respond to people's legitimate demands and are financially fair.*
- *Framing policies in oral health, based on integration of oral health into national and community health programs, and promoting oral health as an effective dimension for development policy of society* [7].

Program goals are broad statements on the overall purpose of a program. For instance, "to eliminate racial disparities in oral cancer survival rates," "to improve the oral health of nursing home residents" or " to improve the oral health of country's children under 5 years. Program objectives are more specific statements of desired endpoints of program.

Objectives of oral health programs should meet SMART criteria:

Specific—they should describe an observable action, behavior or achievement.

Measurable—they are systems, methods or procedures to track to record the action upon which objective is focused.

Achievable—the objective is realistic, based on current environment and resources.

Relevant—the objective is important to the program and is under the control of program.

Time based—there are clearly defined deadlines for achieving the objective [3].

Designing an oral health promotion program: step by step can be studied as shown in **Figure 2** [1]:

Best practices in oral health promotion and prevention can take various forms, be it education, health promotion, integrating oral health promotion into general health promotion programs, policy changes which promote better oral health, the provision of care services, or programs specifically designed at addressing oral health inequalities. It is interesting to learn how oral

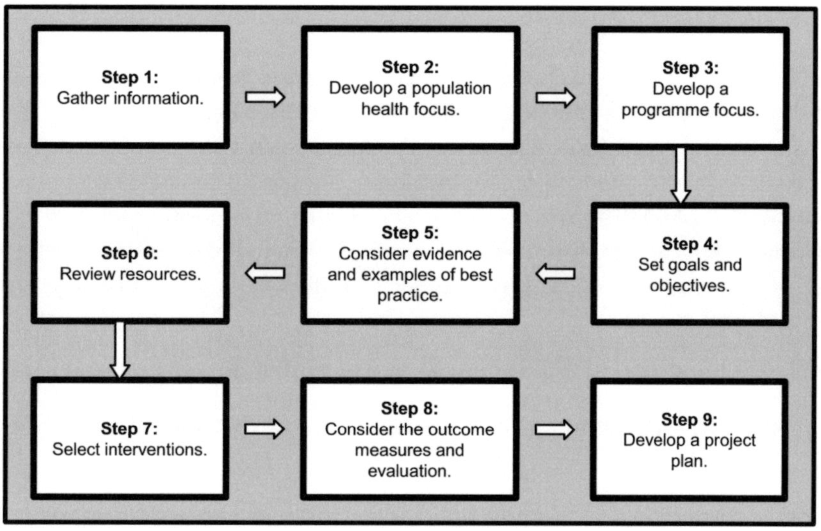

Figure 2. A step-by-step design of an oral health promotion program (based on Ministry of Health, New Zealand, 2006).

health promotion and practices are implemented in through various interventions applying the Ottawa Charter guidelines.

5.1.1. Building healthy public policy

Establishing healthy policies is integral in improving oral health. Based on the needs, evidences and situation analysis, National Government, health ministry, local governments, organizations, communities, schools, primary healthcare settings and local stakeholders forms or reforms the healthy policy. Health promotion advocates hold key responsibility to convey appropriate health needs of the population.

Examples of interventions that build healthy public policy

- Campaigning to extend the coverage of optimal water fluoridation or water de-fluoridation based on needs.
- Supporting early childhood centers and school boards in developing healthy food and nutrition policies.
- Working on policy options that eliminate the advertising of harmful food and beverages to children.
- Working with organizations to promote injury prevention policies, for example, mouthguards in sport or safe play equipment.
- Industrial approach to limit the marketing of carbonated & sugar-containing drinks to children.
- Working to study and develop standards for marketed harmful products to children.
- Developing and implementing smoke free environment policies.

5.1.2. Creating supportive environments

Making the healthy choice easy choice is the aim of health promotion. This can be achieved by creating supportive social, physical, biological and cultural environments. These determinants of health directly and indirectly affect the oral health with or without general health consequences. Hence, the needs of local population should be considered in order to design and implementation of health promotion actions. Health promotion practitioners play a lead role in creating supportive environments along with public health units, government agencies, health organizations, NGOs, professional Dental Association, industry organizations and print and digital media.

Interventions that harness creating healthy supportive environments for oral health

- Provision of fluoridated toothpastes at subsidized cost that low income group can also avail.
- Reforming supermarket's marketing policies for instance replacing sugary products like chocolates.
- Encouragement for usage of smoke-free environment advertisements and sponsorship for oral health promotion.
- Media coverage of healthy food choices which enhance oral health.
- Oral health awareness and promotion through social marketing campaigns.
- Promoting safe water supply at all the public events.

5.1.3. Strengthening community action

Communities are a powerful force for achieving actions for any health promotion program where the key success factors are: *partnership, participation and engagement*. Encompassing all the communities for united efforts to understand their own oral health needs and ascertain to improve the oral health outcomes of their community. These health promotion programs may differ with age, society, culture and environment. Among the five actions themes of Ottawa Charter, community action is unique as concentrate on how particular health actions to be carried out. It eventually may turn out to be effective examples to be followed. Important factor for communities to have equitable access to resources to support the control they must have over their own health and development. Hence, strengthening community action is about providing and facilitating access to sufficient and appropriate resources.

Examples of interventions that strengthen community action for oral health

- Engaging the community to support water fluoridation/de-fluoridation and encourage safe water supply.
- Engaging communities to participate in school oral health programs through leadership activities.

- Empowering communities for healthy eating programs that enhance oral health.
- Specific target-oriented oral health improvement programs based on community cultures.
- Community and school collaboration for establishing playgrounds with safe play equipment, barricades for children safety.

5.1.4. Developing personal skills

Personal skills can help individual to take control of his own health. Empowering people with appropriate knowledge and skills to improve and maintain their oral health is essential. Oral health literacy is the way that provides information, education and skills for oral health improvement. Such things help increases the resources available to people to exercise more control over their own health and environments. Health promotion programs needs to be updated that go collateral with changing environment and culture. Hence, continuum for health education, particularly for oral health, throughout life is necessary. Here, comes the role of oral health professionals who forms the bridge between health promotion advocates and health promotion program communities. At community level or at individual level, they create support system to ingress healthy personal skills to improve and maintain oral health. Oral health professionals fulfill this role of trainer by providing information, resources and training.

Interventions that help developing personal skills

- Oral health promotion though guided tooth brushing using fluoridated toothpaste as self-care habits.
- Smoking cessation actions under the guidance of Oral health professionals.
- Nutritional and dietary education programs which include oral health message.
- Encouraging sports authorities for safe environment at sports events such as making sportsmen to put on mouth guards compulsory when required.

5.1.5. Reorientating health services

Health services carry the burden of all diseases by providing three tier cares. With advancing burden of new diseases and population explosion challenges, reorientation of health services is inevitable. The global burden of oral diseases had led to integrate oral health into general health. Indeed, it is giving a new direction for oral health services and recognizing that oral health is not merely a biomedical process. Health services should be reformed such that they not only treat the diseases but also find suitable solutions for health promotion. Strengthening of health services to analyze needs, to understand the socioeconomic determinants of health of the population is required. Such reformation which reduces oral health inequalities and improves oral health-related quality of life is all about reorienting health services. While prime focus is on primary healthcare services, prevention, allocation, access and cost-beneficial health services are obligatory to achieve this.

Interventions for reorientating health services

- Establishing community-led oral healthcare providers.
- Extensive collaboration with NGOs and social services for oral health promotion, so the curative burden from Government is reduced.
- Linking general health services and children oral health care under primary health centers.
- Training the trainers, that is, training all health professionals about preventive and social components of oral health promotion.
- Facilitating and building knowledge for diagnosing early caries detection programs by primary healthcare professionals.
- Health care led healthy policies supporting access to oral health care.
- Provision of professional fluoride lack and excess treatment facilities delivered by primary healthcare professionals and community [1].

Oral health should be an important agenda on the country's health policy. The above international policy examples envision the challenges and opportunities for better identification, prioritization and integration of oral health services. Collaborative planning and organization may accelerate the process to arrest the global burden of oral diseases and pioneer the oral health promotion. Relevant international developments suggest that some other health promotion frameworks exists that are parallel to Ottawa Charter framework. Although their principles are same, the implementation may differ according to the needs and socio-cultural environment of the region. One can develop or reform a different model based on above evidences for oral health promotion programs at their region.

5.2. Country examples for oral health promotion program

Investment in simple preventive programs is cost-effective for prevention of oral diseases and promotion of good oral health which is already proven in Europe. Twenty eight examples of good practice are presented from across Europe as shown in **Figure 3**. These cover all areas of oral health promotion across the life course and include programs aimed at pregnant mothers, children and adolescents, the elderly and disadvantaged groups. To solve the problem of poor oral health in other parts of world a thorough evaluation of existing successful policies and programs, identification of evidence-based interventions can be learned from these programs.

These programs outline a number of successful initiatives that can help prevent oral diseases, which reduce the social burden and in turn reduce existing inequalities. This is done with various measures, for instance: prevention programs in communities; limiting social, economic, cultural and environmental risk factors for non-communicable diseases, oral hygiene promotion, oral health literacy and an appropriate access to oral health care [30].

http://dx.doi.org/10.5772/intechopen.69330

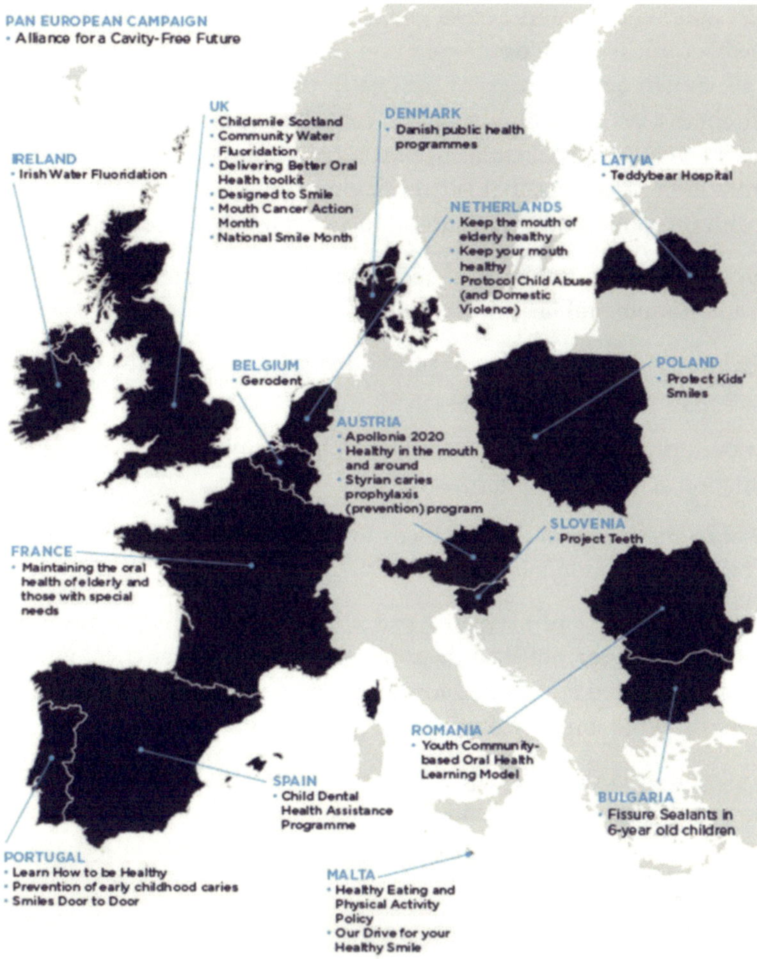

Figure 3. Examples of good practices in oral health promotion programs existing across the Europe.

6. Conclusion

Gradient shift to rural population to urban area, issues of migrants, urbanization, socio, cultural and environmental changes alienate health promotion. Isolated intervention may not be successful at such circumstances. Oral health promotion actions with different approaches can only improve. Health for all is certainly efficient way than the target specific behaviors. It is evident that an effective and sustainable intervention combines health, society and individual through organization, policy and laws to create healthy living conditions which promotes better quality lifestyle.

WHO is considered as an accountable and reliable organization which provide necessary technical and policy support. Their evidence based guidance enable countries to integrate oral health promotion programs into the general health promotion. The organization has different expertise at Collaboration Centers across globe that is resourceful for oral health promotion guidance. However, most of the developed and developing countries utilize own resources and develop their own action program for health promotion. It is based upon local experiences and strengths, active communities to contribute participation facilitate community empowerment by creating sustainable supporting environment. WHO has given a vision to oral health promotion programs, that is, "think globally—act locally." To conclude the chapter, an oral health promotion program should focus on following aspects:

- Recognition of health determinants, capacity building for designing and implementing interventions to promote oral health.
- Community led and based oral health promotion programs, having equal opportunity for marginalized segments of population.
- Planning, monitoring and evaluation strategies to be implemented strictly for national oral health promotion activities/programs.
- Methods and methodological development to analyze the processes and outcomes of national oral health promotion interventions.
- Collaboration with strong of networks and alliances that strengthen local, national and international activities for oral health promotion. Every experience, whether success or failure should be counted and shared to acknowledge the cost-effective and cost-beneficial experience that yield to improve oral health quality of life.

Oral health promotion is one practice that involves strategic planning, integrative activities, evidence-based concepts, evaluation, policy making and other related multifactor. Knowledge generation for oral health promotion through evidence-based concepts is the goal of this chapter.

Abbreviations

WHO	World Health Organization
GBD	Global burden of disease
DALYs	Disability adjusted life-years
YLDs	Years lived with disability
HPS	Health promoting school
NTCP	National tobacco control program
MoHFW	Ministry of Health and Family Welfare
COTPA	Cigarette and Other Tobacco Products Act
GATS	Global Adult Tobacco Survey
NPPCF	National Program for Prevention and Control of Fluorosis
NGOs	Non-government organizations

Author details

Vikram R. Niranjan[1*], Vikas Kathuria[2], Venkatraman J[3] and Arpana Salve[4]

Address all correspondence to: drvikramn@gmail.com

1 Queen Mary University of London, UK and S.D. Dental College, Parbhani, India

2 Consultant Dentist, Hadi Hospital, Jabriya, Kuwait

3 Department of Pathology, Mahatma Gandhi Medical college and Research Institute, Puducherry, India

4 Senior Registrar, Skin & VD Department, Government Medical College & Hospital, Aurangabad, India

References

[1] Ministry of Health. Promoting Oral Health: A Toolkit to Assist the Development, Planning, Implementation and Evaluation of Oral Health Promotion in New Zealand. Wellington: Ministry of Health; 2008

[2] The World Health Organization. The Ottawa Charter for health promotion. Health Promotion. 1986;**1**:i-v. Available from: WHO, Geneva: http://www.who.int/hpr/NPH/docs/ottawa_charter_hp.pdf [Accessed: 15 January 2017]

[3] Rozier G, Pahel B. Patient- and population-reported outcomes in public health dentistry: Oral health related quality of life. In: Oscar A, Chattopadyay A, editors. Dental Clinic of North America: Dental Public Health. 1st ed. India: Sauders; 2008. pp. 333-344. ISBN: 978-81-312-1578-4

[4] Marcenes W, Kassebaum NJ, Bernabé E, Flaxman A, Naghavi M, Lopez A, Murray CJ. Global burden of oral conditions in 1990-2010: A systematic analysis. Journal of Dental Research. 2013;**92**:592-597

[5] The World Health Organization, Oral Health Promotion Through Schools. 1999. Available from: WHO, Geneva: http://who.int/entity/school_youth_health/media/en/89.pdf [Accessed: 24 November 2016]

[6] Northrop D, Lang C. Local Action Creating Health Promoting Schools. The World Health Organization's Information Series on School Health. 2000. Available from: WHO, Geneva: http://www.who.int/school_youth_health/media/en/88.pdf [Accessed: 24 November 2016]

[7] The World Health Organization. Oral Health Promotion: An Essential Element of a Health Promoting School. WHO Information Series on School Health. 2003. Document 11. Available from: WHO, Geneva: http://www.who.int/oral_health/publications/doc11/en/ [Accessed: 24 November 2016]

[8] Young I. Health promotion in schools – A historical perspective. Promotion & Education. 2005;**XII**(3-5):112-117

[9] Gray G, Young I, Barnekow V. Developing a Health-promoting School. International Union for Health Promotion and Education. 2007. Available from: Schools for Health, Eurore: http://ws10.e-vision.nl/she_network/upload/pubs/Developingahealthpromotingschool.pdf [Accessed: 24 November 2016]

[10] Garbin C, Garbin A, Dos Santos K, Lima D. Oral health education in schools: Promoting health agents. International Journal of Dental Hygiene. 2009;**7**(3):212-216

[11] The World Health Organization. Milestones in Health Promotion: Statements from Global Conferences. Available from: WHO, Geneva, 2009: http://www.who.int/healthpromotion/milestones/en/index.html [Accessed: 24 November 2016]

[12] Peterson PE. The World Oral Health Report 2003: Continuous Improvement of Oral Health in the 21st Century – The Approach of the WHO Global Oral Health Programme. The World Health Organization. 2003. Available from: WHO, Geneva: http://www.who.int/oral_health/publications/report03/en/print.html/ [Accessed: 15 January 2017]

[13] Kwan Stella YL, Petersen PE, Pine CM, Borutta A. Health-promoting schools: An opportunity for oral health promotion. Bulletin of World Health Organization. 2005;**83**(9):677-685

[14] Tobler N, Stratton H. Effectiveness of school-based drug education programs: A meta analysis of the research. Journal of Primary Prevention. 1997;**18**(1):71-128

[15] The World Health Organization. The Health Promoting School – An Investment in Education Health and Democracy. Copenhagen: World Health Organization. 1997

[16] Sheiham A, Watt RG. The common risk factor approach: A rational basis for promoting oral health. Community Dentistry and Oral Epidemiology. 2000;**28**(6):399-406

[17] Thomas R, Perera R. School based programming for preventing smoking. Cochrane Database Syst Rev. 2002;(4):CD001293.

[18] Duraisamy P, James E, Lane J, Tan J. Is there a quantity–quality trade-off as pupil–teacher ratios increase? Evidence from Tamil Nadu, India. International Journal of Educational Development. 1998;**18**(5):367-383. Available from: http://www.sciencedirect.com/science?_ob=ArticleURL&_udi=B6VD7-3V72PXC-9&_user=125872&_coverDate=09%2F30%2F1998&_rdoc=1&_fmt=high&_orig=search&_sort=d&_docanchor=&view=c&_searchStrId=1434446368&_rerunOrigin=google&_acct=C000010240&_version=1&_urlVersion=0&_userid=125872&md5=13edd3a0f436133a75223cc179317942#b11 [Accessed: 15 January 2017]

[19] Bruneforth M, Griffin P, Grisay A. Postlethwaite TN, Tran H, Zhang Y. View Inside Primary Schools – A World Education Indicators (WEI) Cross-national Study. 2008. Available from: UNESCO Institute for Statistics: http://www.unescobkk.org/fileadmin/user_upload/efa/Publications/AViewPrimarySchools_comp.pdf [Accessed: 15 January 2017]

[20] Gupta M, Gupta BP, Chauhan A, Bhardwaj A. Ocular morbidity prevalence among school children in Shimla, Himachal, North India, Indian Journal of Ophthalmology. 2009;**57**(2):133-138

[21] Mott JA, Paul AC, Jean RC, Flay B. After-school supervision and adolescent cigarette smoking: Contributions of the setting and intensity of after-school self-care. Journal of Behavioral Medicine. 1999;**22**(1):35-58

[22] Perry C. Parent Involvement with children's health promotion: The Minnesota Home Team. American Journal of Public Health. 1988;**78**(9):11156-11160

[23] St Leger LH, Young I, Blanchard C, Perry M. Promoting Health in Schools: From Evidence to Action. 2010. Available from: International Union for Health Promotion and Education: http://www.iuhpe.org/uploaded/Activities/Scientific_Affairs/CDC/A&E_10June2010.pdf [Accessed: 15 January 2017]

[24] Mid Day Meal Scheme. Department of School Education and Literacy. Available from: Government of India, Department of Elementary Education and Literacy: http://education.nic.in/Sche.asp [Accessed: 15 January 2017]

[25] Ayodele AO. Gender, age and religion as determinants of eating habit of youth in Ikenne local government of Ogun state, Nigeria. African Journal Online. 2010. Available from: http://ajol.info/index.php/ejc/article/view/52673/41277 [Accessed: 15 January 2017]

[26] Public Health England. Delivering Better Oral Health: An Evidence-based Toolkit for Prevention. London: PHE; 2014

[27] Centre for Health Informatics (CHI), National Institute of Health and Family Welfare (NIHFW), Ministry of Health and Family Welfare (MoHFW), Government of India. National Tobacco Control Programme (NTCP) [Accessed 15 January 2017]

[28] McKay AJ, Patel RKK, Majeed A. Strategies for tobacco control in India: A systematic review. Plos One. 2015;**10**(4):e0122610. DOI: 10.1371/journal.pone.0122610

[29] Centre for Health Informatics (CHI), National Institute of Health and Family Welfare (NIHFW), Ministry of Health and Family Welfare (MoHFW), Government of India. National Programme for Prevention and Control of Fluorosis (NPPCF) [Accessed 15 January 2017]

[30] Platform for Better Oral Health in Europe. Best Practices in Oral Health Promotion and Prevention from Across Europe. 2015. Available form: www.oralhealthplatform.eu